Sriharsha. D.S.

WARD'S ANAESTHETIC EQUIPMENT
FOURTH EDITION

WARD'S ANAESTHETIC EQUIPMENT

FOURTH EDITION

John TB Moyle MB, BS, CEng, MInstMC, DPallMed, FRCA
Consultant Anaesthetist, Chartered Engineer
Milton Keynes General Hospital;
Medical Director and Consultant in Palliative Medicine
Willen Hospice, Milton Keynes, UK

and

Andrew Davey LRCP & SI, FRCA
Consultant Anaesthetist
Royal Sussex County Hospital
Brighton, UK

Edited by
Crispian Ward
Consultant Anaesthetist (retired)
The Royal Infirmary Huddersfield, UK

WB Saunders Company Limited
London Philadelphia Toronto Sydney Tokyo

WB Saunders Company Ltd
24–28 Oval Road
London NW1 7DX, UK

The Curtis Center
Independence Square West
Philadelphia, PA 19106–3399, USA

Harcourt Brace & Company
55 Horner Avenue
Toronto, Ontario M8Z 4X6, Canada

Harcourt Brace & Company, Australia
30–52 Smidmore Street
Marrickville, NSW 2204, Australia

Harcourt Brace & Company, Japan
Ichibancho Central Building, 22–1 Ichibancho
Chiyoda-ku, Tokyo 102, Japan

First edition published 1975
Third edition published 1992

A catalogue record for this book is available from the British Library

ISBN 0–7020–2169–5

Typeset by Phoenix Photosetting, Chatham, Kent
Printed and bound at Replika Press Pvt. Ltd. (100% EOU),
Delhi 110 040, India.

CONTENTS

PREFACE

This book has two main purposes. The first is to provide a simple, yet comprehensive, explanation of the function of items of anaesthetic equipment to ensure their safe use in clinical practice by anaesthetists. The second is to provide a source of reference for trainee anaesthetists that covers the relevant syllabus required for the Primary and Final Fellowship Examinations in anaesthesia in the UK and Ireland.

The book will also be of interest to anaesthetic assistants, electronic and biomedical engineers in hospitals, manufacturers representatives and those involved in anaesthesia in other countries where similar equipment is used.

The book has been extensively revised to include new developments and to eliminate obsolete items.

There are new chapters on Equipment for the Inhalation of Oxygen and of 'Entonox', Equipment for Local Analgesia, Advanced Monitoring Systems, Automatic Record Keeping, Surgical Diathermy, Defibrillators and Pacemakers, and Risk Management.

There has been an occasional deliberate repetition of material where the content of some chapters has overlapped. This caters for a reader who may wish to peruse individual chapters rather than read the book from cover to cover.

Finally, the two authors, Dr. John Moyle and Dr. Andrew Davey are greatly indebted to Dr. Crispian Ward who has edited the book with his customary enthusiasm and meticulous attention to detail.

ACKNOWLEDGEMENTS

We are indebted to the many manufacturing companies who have provided us with essential data, illustrations and photographic material. Some of the illustrations have been altered with permission to ensure that they conform to a uniform style. Space does not permit us to acknowledge our gratitude to the individual companies involved but all the companies that have assisted us are listed in Appendix I. To these, we extend our warmest thanks. We are also grateful to the Department of Health and the British Standards Institution for providing several texts, tables, diagrams and permission to reproduce the 'Permit to Work', and to the Association of Anaesthetists for consenting to the reproduction of the Anaesthetic Machine Checklist.

ABBREVIATIONS

ADC	Analogue to digital converter
AICD	Automatic implantable cardioverter-defibrillator
ANSI	American National Standards Institute
APL	Adjustable pressure-limiting (valve)
ATLS	Advance trauma and life support
atm	Atmosphere (unit of pressure)
BOC	British Oxygen Company
BP	British Pharmacopoeia
BPM	Breaths per minute
BS	British Standard
BSP	British Standard Pipe (screw thread)
cmH$_2$O	Centimetres of water (unit of pressure)
°C	Degrees Celsius
CA	Compressed air
cal	Calorie
CFAM	Cerebral function analysing monitor
CMRR	Common mode rejection ratio
COELB	Current-operated earth-leakage circuit breaker
COSHH	Control of Substances Hazardous to Health
CPAP	Continuous positive airway pressure
CPU	Central processing unit
CRT	Cathode ray tube
CSSD	Central Sterile Supply Department
CVP	Central venous pressure
DAC	Digital to analogue converter
DoH	Department of Health (Replaces DHSS Department of Health and Social Security)
DISS	Diameter Indexed Safety System (USA)
EBME	Electronic and Biomedical Engineering (Department)
ECG	Electrocardiogram
EEG	Electroencephalogram
EMC	Electromagnetic compatibility
EMG	Electromyogram
EMI	Electromagnetic interference
EPROM	Eraseable programmable read only memory
EXH	Exhaust
EXP	Expiratory (valve)
FEV	Forced expiratory volume
FEV$_1$	Forced expiratory volume in 1 second
FG	French gauge
FGF	Fresh gas flow
FRC	Functional residual capacity
HbA	Adult haemoglobin
HbF	Fetal haemoglobin
HEI	Health Equipment Information (issued by the DoH)
HFPPV	High frequency positive pressure ventilation
HME	Heat and moisture exchanger
HSC	Health and Safety Executive (UK)
HTM	Hospital Technical Memorandum (issued by HM Stationery Office)
IC	Integrated circuit
ICU/ITU	Intensive care unit/Intensive therapy unit
ID	Internal diameter
IEC	International Electrotechnical Commission
IMV	Intermittent mandatory ventilation
IPPV	Intermittent positive pressure ventilation
IR	Infrared
ISO	International Organization for Standards
K	Degrees Kelvin (always stated without °)
kcal	Kilocalorie
kg/cm^2	Kilograms per square centimetre
kPa	Kilopascal (European standard measurement for pressure)
LCD	Liquid crystal display
LED	Light-emitting diode
LITA	Local instillation of tracheal analgesia
LMA	Laryngeal mask airway
MDM	Monitored Dial Mixer (Quantiflex flowmeter)
MGI	Medical Gas Installations Ltd
MGPS	Medical gas pipeline services
MHz	Megahertz
ml/min	Millilitres per minute
mmHg	Millimetres of mercury (unit of pressure)
MMV	Mandatory minute volume
MV	Minute volume
NAD	North American Dräger

NEEP	Negative end-expiratory pressure	SEF	Spectral edge frequency
NIBP	Non-invasive blood pressure (monitoring)	SI (units)	Système International d'Unites (International System of Units)
NIOSH	National Institute for Occupational Safety and Health (USA)	SIMV	Synchronized intermittent mandatory ventilation
NIST	Non-interchangeable screw threaded (connection)	SVP	Saturated vapour pressure
OD	Outside diameter	TCI	Target controlled infusion
ODC	Oxygen dissociation curve	TIVA	Total intravenous anaesthesia
OMV	Oxford Miniature vaporizer	TILC	Temperature indicated, level compensated (vaporizer)
Pa	Pascal (unit of pressure)	Torr	(Torricelli) mmHg pressure (also used for subatmospheric pressures)
PCA	Patient-controlled analgesia		
PEEP	Positive end-expiratory pressure		
ppm	Parts per million	TSSU	Theatre Sterile Supply Unit
psi	Pounds per square inch (US standard measurement for pressure)	TV	Tidal volume
		TWA	Time-weighted average
PTFE	Polytetrafluorethylene (= Teflon; = Fluon)	USP	United States Pharmacopeia
PVC	Polyvinyl chloride	UV	Ultraviolet
RAM	Random access memory	VC	Vital capacity
RCCB	Residual current circuit breaker	VIC	Vaporizer in circle
R.h.	Relative humidity	VIE	Vacuum insulated evaporator
RF	Radiofrequency	VOC	Vaporizer out of circle
ROM	Read only memory		

— 1 —

PHYSICAL PRINCIPLES

Contents

INTRODUCTION

The art of anaesthesia is essentially practical. For this reason anaesthetists must have an understanding of the physical aspects of the apparatus they use, not only so that they can use it efficiently but also so that they may understand its limitations and use it safely. Many unnecessary accidents and near-misses have occurred as the result of the misuse of equipment because the anaesthetist did not understand the basic principles of its operation.

This chapter is therefore devoted to the basic physics of gases, liquids, vapours and solids, and to the principles of modern control systems, which are increasingly a part of the latest anaesthetic machines. The principles of the electromagnetic spectrum are also discussed at the end of the chapter.

One of the problems besetting the medical profession today is the clinician's inability to discuss his or her requirements with the engineer in terms that they both understand. This problem occurs not only with the development of new equipment, but in discussing faults and difficulties with older equipment.

STATES OF MATTER

In order to understand the functioning of an anaesthetic machine it is necessary to appreciate the difference between the three states of matter: solid, liquid and gas.

A *solid* is compact and relatively dense. It maintains its shape unless subjected to comparatively large forces and is not easily compressed. Its molecules, although in a state of constant agitation, do not change their position relative to one another, hence a solid tends to maintain its shape. Different solids, in contact with each other, do not normally mix.

A *fluid* is a substance that cannot sustain shearing forces or mechanical stress; it easily changes shape when a force is applied to it. Liquids, vapours and gases are all therefore fluids.

A *liquid* is also compact. Its molecules are constantly moving relative to each other and, owing to their being densely packed, there are frequent collisions between them. Because its molecules move freely, a liquid takes the shape of the container in which it is confined and moves from one part of it to another under the influence of gravity. Its shape may be distorted by small forces.

Different liquids, in contact with each other, may or may not mix.

Vapours and *gases* are best characterized as having no inherent boundary or volume; they expand to fill evenly the space within which they are confined. Different vapours or gases in contact with each other normally mix. The terms *vapour* and *gas* are synonymous but vapour is usually used for the gaseous state at a temperature and pressure close to those at which it would condense into a liquid. The scientific distinction between a vapour and a gas is as follows. For any

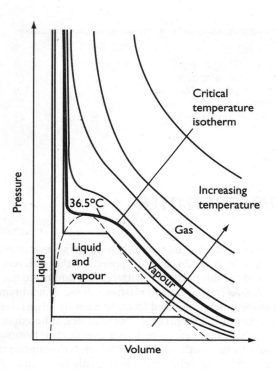

Figure 1.1 Isotherms for nitrous oxide.

substance there is a maximum temperature at which it can be compressed so as to convert it from a gas to a liquid. Above that temperature, known as the *critical temperature*, no amount of pressure will liquefy it. At temperatures lower than the critical temperature the substance may exist as a vapour or as a liquid or, indeed, as a mixture of both depending on its pressure and volume. The relationship between pressure, volume and temperature is usually displayed as a family of *isotherms*. Figure 1.1 shows an isotherm family for nitrous oxide. Each isotherm shows the relationship between pressure and volume at a given temperature. Nitrous oxide may exist as a liquid or a vapour below the critical tempera-

ture of +36.5°C; above this critical temperature it may exist only as a gas. It follows that if a gas is stored below its critical temperature and hence in its liquid/vapour state, assessment of the contents of its container cannot be made from the pressure therein. If a gas is stored above its critical temperature, for example, oxygen which has a critical temperature of −118°C and therefore is in its gaseous state, the quantity of gas will be proportional to the pressure inside its container. The *critical pressure* is that which is required to liquefy a gas at its critical temperature.

BEHAVIOUR OF MOLECULES OF SOLIDS AND LIQUIDS

The molecules of a solid or a liquid attract each other. They may also be attracted by the molecules of another substance. The mutual attraction between the molecules of a substance is termed *cohesion*, and their attraction to those of another substance is called *adhesion*. Suppose that there are three molecules of mercury in a straight row. Each molecule will attract its neighbour, but the first will also attract the third, so that they will at once move to take up a more compact form (Fig. 1.2).

If we now consider a much larger number of molecules of mercury, each one attracting the others, they will tend to take up the shape of a sphere. The force that preserves the periphery of the sphere is called *surface tension*. With an even larger quantity of mercury, the sphere would be so large that it would be distorted by the force of gravity (*G*) and the force of the surface upon which it rests (Fig. 1.3). Note that the edges of the blob are still circular. This may be observed when a small quantity of mercury is spilled and blobs of various sizes are formed. The small ones are nearly spherical whereas the larger ones are flattened.

The molecules of other substances may exert less mutual attraction and so the force of adhesion to another substance may be stronger than the force of cohesion. Thus, if there are several water molecules, for example, on a glass surface, the outer molecules have a greater force of attraction for the glass than for the inner ones, so they 'wet' the surface (Fig. 1.4). However, water will not wet a greasy surface, upon which it takes up a globular form.

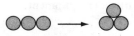

Figure 1.2 The cohesion between three molecules arranged in a straight row causes them to take up a more compact form.

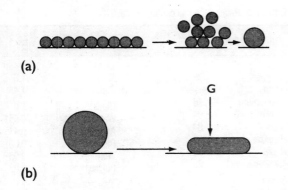

(a)

(b)

Figure 1.3 (a) The cohesion between several molecules causes them to group together in the most compact form, a sphere. (b) The sphere is distorted by the effect of gravity (G).

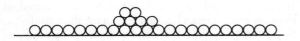

Figure 1.4 The molecules of a substance for which the force of adhesion is greater than the force of cohesion spread out as they wet the surface on which they rest.

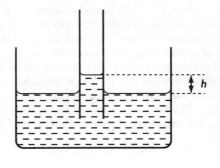

(a)

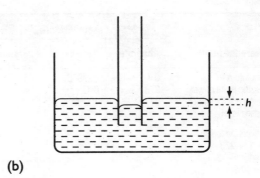

(b)

Figure 1.5 (a) If a narrow tube is dipped into a vessel of water, the wetting effect causes the water to rise up the tube and the edge of the meniscus is turned up. The height h of the water column depends, apart from other factors, on the diameter of the tube. (b) If the same tube is dipped into a vessel of mercury, the level of mercury is depressed and the meniscus is turned down because it does not wet the glass.

HEAT AND TEMPERATURE

Temperature

Temperature means relative hotness or coldness of a substance and is actually a measure of the average kinetic energy possessed by its molecules. Temperature is indicated in degrees on a defined scale. At sea level, at normal atmospheric pressure, pure water freezes at 0°C (degrees Celsius, formerly known as centigrade) and boils at 100°C. Other scales of temperature in common use are Kelvin (absolute) and Fahrenheit.

Kelvin (Absolute) Scale

The SI unit of temperature is the Kelvin (K) and is based on the absolute temperature scale where zero K is the temperature at which molecular motion ceases. It

If a vertical dry glass tube of about 1 cm in diameter is dipped into a vessel of water, the upper surface within the tube forms a *meniscus* with an upturned edge because the water wets the surface of the tube (Fig. 1.5a). Water is drawn a little way up the tube by molecular attraction, against the force of gravity. However, if the water is replaced by mercury, which does not wet the glass, the shape of the meniscus is reversed and the edges are depressed (Fig. 1.5b) since the edge of the meniscus is pulled inwards by cohesion and it resembles the blob of mercury described above (Fig. 1.3).

Returning to the case of the tube filled with water, if it has a very narrow bore it is known as a *capillary* tube and the water may be drawn up a considerable amount by the wetting effect on the inside of the tube. The force of attraction of the wall of the tube on the column determines the height to which the column of water will be raised. This phenomenon is known as capillary action or *capillarity*. It may also occur, for example, when two closely fitting smooth surfaces of any shape are separated by a thin film of water. Considerable force may be needed to prise them apart.

Use is made of capillarity when a wick is used in a vaporizer. Because it dips into the liquid agent, the liquid rises up the wick and so presents a larger surface area from which vaporization may occur.

is equivalent to −273°C on the Celsius scale, which is also allowed as an SI scale of temperature. It will be seen from Charles' law (see Properties of Gases) that the volume of an ideal gas (whose molecules have zero volume) is proportional to its temperature. Zero Kelvin is known as absolute zero, as though if a gas could be cooled to 0 K it would disappear. Of course this does not happen as the gas liquefies before this low a temperature is reached. Table 1.1 compares absolute, Celsius and Fahrenheit scales.

Table 1.1 Comparison of the absolute, Celsius and Fahrenheit temperature scales

Reference point	Temperature		
	Absolute	Celsius	Fahrenheit
'Absolute zero'	0 K	−273°C	−459°F
Freezing point of water	273 K	0°C	32°F
Boiling point of water (at sea level)	373 K	100°C	212°F

Conversion formulae:
$K = °C + 273$
$°C = \frac{5}{9}(°F − 32)$
$°F = \frac{9}{5}°C + 32$

Heat

In order to raise the temperature of a substance, energy, in the form of heat, must be added to it. The SI unit of heat is the *joule* but the most commonly used unit is the *calorie*. One calorie raises the temperature of 1 g of water by 1°C from 14.5 to 15.5°C. The calorie is a very small amount of heat and therefore heat energy is usually expressed in kilocalories (kcal), which is often written as Calories.

$$1 \text{ Cal} = 1 \text{ kcal} = 1000 \text{ calories} = 4200 \text{ joules}$$

Heat may be transferred from one object or substance or from one part of an object or substance to another by conduction, convection or radiation.

Conduction

In *conduction*, heat simply travels along a substance from molecule to molecule. Metals, such as copper, are good conductors of heat, whereas, for example, glass and expanded polystyrene are poor conductors. Very poor conductors of heat are termed thermal insulators (Table 1.2).

Table 1.2 Relative thermal conductivity at 0°C

Good conductors		Poor conductors	
Silver	428	*Liquid state*	
Copper	403	Nitrous oxide	1.5
Gold	319	Carbon dioxide	1.45
Aluminium	236		
Nickel	94	Glass	1.0
Iron	84	Water	0.561
Bronze	53	Asbestos	0.11
Lead	36	Paper	0.06
Stainless steel	25	Wool	0.05
		Polystyrene	0.035
		Gaseous state	
		Oxygen	0.0245
		Nitrous oxide	0.015

Convection

If part of a fluid, be it a liquid or a gas, is heated, it expands and becomes less dense than the fluid around it. Being free to move, it rises, and as it travels upwards, its place is taken by the cooler, denser fluid from around it, which in turn is heated and rises. There is, therefore, a constant rising stream above the source of heat and the heat is carried by *convection*.

Radiation

The amount of heat radiated from a surface depends not only on its temperature but on its nature. A matt black surface radiates far more than a smooth, shiny one. Radiated heat 'rays' can be focused and directed, as is seen in the electric radiant heater with a reflector. Radiation is defined as energy that is transferred directly from a source, and propagated as wave energy in straight lines from a source.

Specific Heat

The quantity of heat required to raise the temperature of a given mass of a substance by a certain amount varies from one substance to another. This is termed *specific heat capacity*, which is defined as the amount of heat required to raise the temperature of 1 kg of the specified substance by 1 K.

Latent Heat

Considerably more heat is required to vaporize a liquid than to raise its temperature from room temperature to its boiling point. The heat required to vaporize a liquid is called the *latent heat of vaporization*. For water, this is 539 cal/g at 100°C and normal atmospheric pressure. The heat required to melt a solid is known as the *latent heat of fusion*. For ice this is 80 cal/g at 0°C and normal atmospheric pressure.

Vaporization

Molecules of a liquid are in constant motion, but they also have a mutual attraction for each other.

If the liquid has a surface exposed to air or other gases, or to a vacuum, some molecules will escape from the surface when their energy exceeds that of their mutual attraction for other molecules at the surface. This is the process of *evaporation*. Its rate is increased if the temperature of the liquid is raised, since the molecules move faster and possess more energy. If the atmosphere is enclosed, some of the molecules that have escaped while moving freely in the gaseous state will impinge on the surface of the liquid and re-enter it. The vapour formed by the molecules exerts a pressure which is known as *vapour pressure*. Within a confined space there may occur an equilibrium in which the number of molecules re-entering the liquid equals the number leaving it. At this stage the vapour pressure is at a maximum for the temperature and is called *saturated vapour pressure* (SVP). If the liquid is heated, a point is reached at which the SVP becomes equal to ambient atmospheric pressure. Vaporization now occurs not only at the surface of the liquid but also in the bubbles that develop within its substance. The liquid is *boiling* and the temperature is its *boiling point*. From this it is evident that the boiling point of a liquid depends on the ambient pressure. At high altitudes there is a significant depression of the boiling point.

Expansion of Gases

The molecules of a gas are far more widely separated than those of a solid. This results in two phenomena that do not occur in the case of solids or liquids:

- A gas expands to fill evenly the space within which it is confined.
- Gases expand to a greater extent when heated than do solids or liquids.

PROPERTIES OF GASES

As is the case with all substances, the smallest particle of a gas that can exist separately is a molecule. Gas molecules are in constant motion, moving about in all directions and occasionally bombarding the walls of the space in which they are confined. It is this bombardment of the walls that exerts the pressure due to the gas.

A vessel may be occupied by more than one gas, in which case the total pressure within it is the sum of the pressures exerted independently by each of the gases.

Each gas is said to exert a partial pressure. If a gas is heated, the movement of its molecules becomes more energetic and this leads to a rise in pressure. If the volume in which it is confined is constant, its pressure varies directly with temperature. These facts are expressed in Dalton's, Boyle's and Charles' laws as follows.

Dalton's law relating to vapours. The pressure exerted by a vapour or a gas in a closed space, at a given temperature, depends only on that temperature, and is independent of the pressure of other vapours or gases (provided they have no chemical action upon it). When several vapours or gases, having no chemical action upon each other, are present in the same space, the pressure exerted by the mixture is the sum of the pressures that would be exerted by each of its constituents if it was separately confined in the same space.

Boyle's law. Boyle's law states that, at a constant temperature, the volume of a mass of gas is inversely proportional to the pressure.

Charles' law. Charles' law states that the coefficient of expansion of any gas at a constant pressure is $1/273$.

From the last two laws we may derive the equation:

$$\frac{P_1 V_1}{T_1} = \frac{P_2 V_2}{T_2}$$

where P_1, V_1 and T_1 are the pressure, volume and temperature of one case and P_2, V_2 and T_2 are the corresponding quantities of a second case. T must be expressed on the absolute scale (i.e. in Kelvin). The above formula may be used to calculate the results of a change of pressure, temperature or volume of a gas.

The Poynting Effect

The Poynting effect is also known as the *overpressure effect*.

The critical temperature and critical pressure of one gas may be affected by its admixture with another. If a cylinder is partially filled with liquid nitrous oxide, inverted, and then further filled from a high-pressure source of oxygen, an unexpected phenomenon occurs. This may be viewed through the glass observation window of a high-pressure rig. The bubbles of oxygen diminish in size as the gas is partially dissolved in the liquid nitrous oxide through which it passes. Simultaneously, the volume of the liquid nitrous oxide diminishes as it evaporates and mixes with the oxygen. Eventually the cylinder, filled to a pressure of nearly 137 000 kPa (2000 psi), contains mixed oxygen and nitrous oxide both in the gaseous state. A 50:50 mixture of these two gases is marketed under the name Entonox. Further details of the use of this mixture and the correct handling of the cylinders are given on p. 27 and p. 185. Precautions concerning cooling of cylinders of the mixture are necessary as the critical temperature of the nitrous oxide changes from 36.5°C to a *pseudocritical* temperature of −6°C.

Viscosity

The *viscosity* of a fluid is a measure of its resistance to flow. Consider a fluid passing along a tube: the fluid in the centre of the tube flows more rapidly than that at the periphery, which tends to adhere to the walls of the tube. Imagine that there are layers of fluid slipping over each other. It is the friction between these layers that causes viscosity. Viscosity is measured in *poise* (1 poise = 0.1 pascal second), named after the French physiologist Poiseuille, but a more useful measure for both liquids and gases is the coefficient of viscosity as compared with that of water.

TEMPERATURE CHANGES IN ANAESTHETIC APPARATUS

The performance of some items of anaesthetic equipment is affected by changes in temperature. A rise in temperature:

- increases the vaporization rate of volatile agents;
- causes a fall in density of fluids due to expansion;
- reduces viscosity of liquids;
- increases the viscosity of gases owing to the increased molecular activity.

THE FLOW OF FLUIDS THROUGH TUBES AND ORIFICES

By definition, a tube has a length considerably greater than its diameter, whereas an orifice has a diameter greater than its length. Three factors affect the rate of flow of a fluid through a tube or an orifice, namely its density, its viscosity and the pressure difference across the tube or orifice. The resistance to flow also depends on the diameter and length of the tube, or the diameter of the orifice.

Both the viscosity and density of a fluid are affected by changes in temperature. In the case of an orifice, the density has the most effect and in the case of a tube, the viscosity.

The Flow of Fluids through a Tube

The relationship between the factors relating to a fluid (which may be a liquid or a gas) flowing with laminar flow (see below) through a tube are:

Flow rate $\propto 1/L$ where L = length of tube

Flow rate $\propto P$ where P = the pressure difference between the two ends of the tube

Flow rate $\propto 1/V$ where V = the viscosity of the fluid

Flow rate $\propto r^4$ where r = the radius of the tube (Poiseuille's law)

Thus

$$\text{Flow rate} \propto \frac{P \times r^4}{L \times V}$$

Laminar and Turbulent Flow

The above formulae refer to fluids when the entire stream flows in a straight line. This is known as *laminar* flow. However, under certain circumstances, although the general flow is in a straight line, eddy currents occur. This is known as *turbulence*. These eddy currents cause resistance to flow. For any system there is a critical velocity, above which the flow becomes turbulent and below which it remains laminar.

Turbulence may also be caused by the flow being deflected by rough areas, passing through a tube of irregular diameter, or passing around sharp bends (Fig. 1.6). As examples, the design of the inlet to a flowmeter tube is important, since turbulence would render the reading inaccurate, and in breathing systems, especially those of the circle type, it increases the resistance and therefore increases the work done in spontaneous breathing. Where there is turbulence, a greater pressure is required to maintain the same rate of flow.

The wider the tube, the lower the flow velocity for the same flow rate (volume per unit time) and therefore the less the likelihood of turbulence.

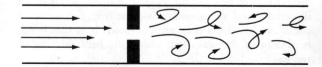

Figure 1.6 Laminar flow becoming turbulent as its smooth pathway is obstructed by an obstacle.

The Flow of Fluids through an Orifice

When a fluid passes through an orifice there is usually turbulence. The flow rate is determined by the pressure difference across the orifice, the density of the fluid and the area of the orifice. Thus:

Flow rate $\propto \sqrt{P}$ where P = the pressure difference across the orifice

Flow rate $\propto \dfrac{1}{\sqrt{D}}$ where D = the density of the fluid

Flow rate $\propto r^2$ where r = the radius of the orifice

Thus

$$\text{Flow rate} \propto \frac{\sqrt{P}(r^2)}{\sqrt{D}}$$

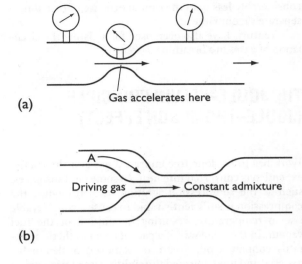

(a)   Gas accelerates here

(b)   A   Driving gas   Constant admixture

Figure 1.7 (a) The Bernoulli effect. (b) The venturi.

The Effect of Changing the Bore of a Tube

Where the bore of a tube is diminished, the flow velocity is increased, since the flow rate (volume per unit time) must remain the same. The change in diameter acts to some extent as an orifice, and because of this, and the fact that turbulence may occur, the density of the fluid becomes significant. The kinetic energy required to accelerate the fluid through the narrower part of the tube can be calculated and may be expressed as resistance or the pressure difference required to overcome it.

It will be seen, therefore, that for any system through which fluids flow there are three elements of resistance to overcome: (a) those due to the dimensions of the tube, (b) those of an orifice, and (c) those associated with initiating the flow and changing its velocity. A combination of all three is always present, but one or another tends to dominate under different circumstances.

The fact remains that the passages in anaesthetic equipment should be as wide, short, smooth, straight and uniform as possible.

The Bernoulli Effect and the Venturi

Let us consider a tube that has a constriction along part of its course. When a gas passes through the tube it will accelerate when it encounters the constriction.

If pressure gauges are attached at various parts of the tube it is found that as the gas accelerates, the pressure falls (Fig. 1.7a). This is known as the Bernoulli effect. When the gas emerges from the constriction into the wider tube the linear velocity of flow decreases and

the pressure increases again. The pressure may rise to a level almost as high as that before the constriction, the extent of this rise being dependent on the design of the tube and the constriction.

Advantage of this phenomenon was taken by Venturi, who found that if the shape of this constriction was suitably designed, and there was a side branch to the tube in a suitable position, fluid from the branch would be entrained by the main stream (Fig. 1.7b). In order to achieve this, not only must the constriction be of a suitable shape, but also the distal limb of the tube needs to be of gradually increasing diameter.

The rate of flow of fluid per unit time is a function of the cross-sectional area of the tube and the flow velocity. Energy is expended in accelerating the flow of fluid to increase its velocity as it passes into the constriction. When it leaves the constriction it will tend to continue to flow at the same velocity, but since the cross-sectional area of the tube is gradually increasing, either it will be slowed down or further fluid may be entrained through the side branch mentioned above or the fluid close to the walls of the tube of expanding diameter will stagnate.

It is one of the features of a venturi that provided the velocity of the driving gas is adequate, and there is no change in the configuration of the orifice from which it emerges, or of the side branch, the volume of gas entrained will bear a constant proportion to the driving gas. It may, therefore, be used for the mixing of nitrous oxide and oxygen in an anaesthetic machine or in mixing valves such as some oxygen/air blenders.

Apart from their use in mixing of gases, venturis may also be used to provide a medical vacuum. Very often the extra cost of using oxygen to drive the venturi is considerably less than the capital expense of installing a separate vacuum line.

Venturis have also been used for assisting the circulation of gases in a breathing system.

THE JOULE–KELVIN PRINCIPLE (JOULE–THOMPSON EFFECT)

Work has to be done to compress a gas and the energy expended is converted into heat. In some circumstances, such as the compression–ignition (diesel) engine, the compression is sufficiently rapid to cause a considerable rise in temperature, resulting in ignition of the fuel vapour. In the same way, if a part of an anaesthetic apparatus contained oil, grease or some other flammable material and was subjected to a sudden rise of pressure in the presence of oxygen, as when a cylinder is turned on suddenly, an explosion could occur. For this reason all apparatus using high-pressure oxygen must be free of oil, grease or other flammable material. Pressure gauges are fitted with a constriction in the inlet to reduce the shock wave that occurs when a cylinder is turned on.

Conversely, when a gas expands, it does work and the temperature drops. Under normal circumstances in anaesthetic practice, the expansion of a gas leaving the cylinder is not sufficiently rapid to cause a great fall in temperature. The fall in temperature is, for example, much less than that due to the latent heat of vaporization, which is the main cause of cooling of cylinders of nitrous oxide when in use.

ELECTRONICS AND CONTROL SYSTEMS

Electronics in any more than the broadest of terms is outside the scope of this book. However, some basic points will be elucidated so that the terms used in this book and in general when discussing modern medical equipment may be understood.

Analogue Versus Digital

Modern electronic techniques have invaded almost every area of technology in medicine. The reason for this is that logic and computing power of great complexity is now feasible, economically and with high reliability. Electronic techniques may be subdivided into two broad groupings, namely analogue and digital, both of which are employed in most equipment.

Analogue circuits are those that handle continuously variable quantities (i.e. without discrete steps) such as pressure, flow, temperature, voltage or current. Digital circuits may handle the same variables but do so in discrete steps, of which there may be only two states (yes/no, high/low, go/no-go), or in many steps that may be very small, so small that the impression is given of a smooth transition. Most variables are expressed in decimal form, that is with a base of 10, i.e. using the digits 1, 2, 3, 4, 5, 6, 7, 8, 9, 10. This would require digital electronics to have 10 stable states in each of its circuit elements, which would be extremely difficult to implement. As digital electronics is based upon two stable states, it requires the conversion of the variable into a binary or base-2 number code (Fig. 1.8).

Decimal	Binary							
	MSB 2^7	2^6	2^5	2^4	2^3	2^2	2^1	LSB 2^0
0	0	0	0	0	0	0	0	0
1	0	0	0	0	0	0	0	1
2	0	0	0	0	0	0	1	0
3	0	0	0	0	0	0	1	1
4	0	0	0	0	0	1	0	0
5	0	0	0	0	0	1	0	1
6	0	0	0	0	0	1	1	0
7	0	0	0	0	0	1	1	1
8	0	0	0	0	1	0	0	0
9	0	0	0	0	1	0	0	1
10	0	0	0	0	1	0	1	0
200	1	1	0	0	1	0	0	0
255	1	1	1	1	1	1	1	1

MSB = Most Significant Bit
LSB = Least Significant Bit

Figure 1.8 Binary representation of decimal numbering.

An analogue signal is converted into a digital format using a circuit-block called an analogue-to-digital converter (ADC). An ADC integrated circuit has a single input connection for the analogue signal and multiple pins for the digital output. ADC integrated circuits may have 8, 12, 16 or even more output pins, each representing an output bit; the higher number of bits allows higher precision of conversion, i.e. each step represents a smaller change in the analogue signal: 256 steps with 8 bits, 4096 with 12 bits and 32768 with 16 output bits.

A digital-to-analogue converter (DAC) has the reverse function of converting a signal in a digital format into an analogue form.

Almost all modern electronic instrumentation and control systems use a combination of analogue and digital circuitry. An input pressure, flow or temperature (a measurand) is converted by a transducer to a voltage or current whose magnitude is an analogue function of the measurand. However, in all but the most simple cases, computation or manipulation of this signal is more conveniently carried out by digital techniques, usually by use of a microprocessor. The analogue signal from the transducer is converted to a digital format by an ADC. The output of the microprocessor, which is also in a digital format, may directly control solenoids, solenoid valves, motors, etc., or may be re-converted back to an analogue format by a DAC. The reasons for this seemingly complex conversion from analogue to digital and back again are as follows.

- Complex mathematical and logical functions between input and output are easier to implement with digital circuitry.
- The calibration and 'zero' of digital circuits do not drift as analogue circuits tend to.
- The calibration of digital circuitry is easier and more accurate.
- Major or minor changes in any mathematical functions can be enacted simply by software changes.
- Digital circuitry is cheaper and easier to design and manufacture.
- Digital circuitry tends to be more reliable than its analogue counterpart.

Microprocessor Systems

Embedded microprocessors are microprocessors which, although the integrated circuits comprising them are identical to those of a small computing system, are an integral part of the equipment into which they have been built, and the user will not necessarily appreciate their presence in the equipment. Such microprocessors are all composed of similar components (Fig. 1.9).

The central component of any microprocessor system is the central processing unit (CPU), which is a single integrated circuit (IC) with 40 or even 64 connection pins. The CPU is the heart of the system where all the mathematical and logic functions are carried out. However, the CPU is useless without its support ICs. Input and output (I/O) packages control the already digitized signals for the CPU. Input packages allow several different signals to be applied in turn to the CPU. Output packages similarly allow the output of the CPU to be applied between, say, solenoid valves, motors and display systems. This switching may be so rapid that the user is unaware that the CPU is carrying out many functions sequentially. The CPU cannot carry out any functions at all without a program or software which is held in non-volatile memory.

Non-volatile memory is permanent memory unaffected by the equipment being switched off, in which the program is stored in binary digital form, usually in a read only memory (ROM), so called because it cannot be altered by the functioning of the microprocessor system.

Embedded microprocessors also need *volatile* memory, which can be altered by the CPU. It is said to be volatile because this form of memory, random access memory (RAM), is cleared by the disconnection of the power supply. It is used as a 'scratch-pad' by the CPU for

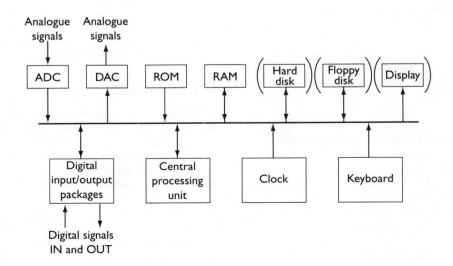

Figure 1.9 Schematic diagram of the components of any microprocessor-based system.

(a)

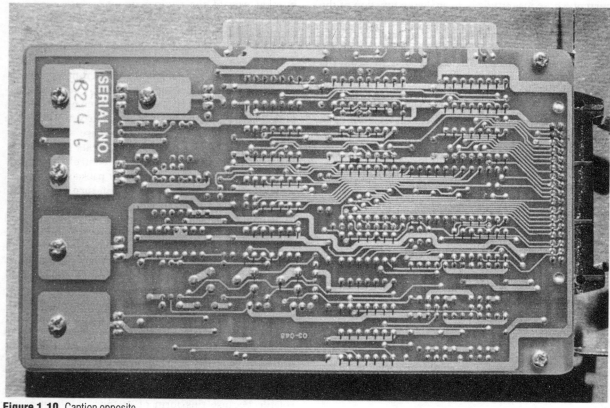

Figure 1.10 Caption opposite.

making its calculations, 'remembering' trends, and assembling information for any display device.

As microprocessor systems use the binary numbering system, it is necessary to use multiple connections between each of the ICs, usually 8, 16 or 32. These interconnections are usually referred to as buses, a contraction from the term bus-bar used in the electrical industry. There are three buses in a microprocessor-based system: a data bus which carries the actual data being manipulated; an address bus which carries the addresses of the 'pigeon holes' containing data stored in the memories; and a control bus which, as the name implies, carries all the control and timing signals. Synchronism is maintained by a crystal controlled clock or oscillator, which is usually at a fixed frequency of usually greater than 5 MHz.

Where data in large quantities have to be retained, then a *hard disk* drive may be included. Disk drives are non-volatile but slow compared with silicon memory. Hard disks are not removable from computing systems and may hold up to 500 megabytes of information. If it is necessary to move data by hand then this is done with small 'floppy' disks, so called because they used to be protected by a flexible cardboard casing. Currently used

'floppies' are smaller and protected by a firm plastic casing.

Because of the complexity of the interconnections involved in modern electronics, these interconnections are always made by use of 'printed' circuitry (Fig. 1.10). Once the printed circuit has been designed it has the advantage of ease of economic manufacture without wiring errors and with high reliability.

Control Systems

The term *control systems* may be used when the control of anything is any more complicated than, for example, the direct manual manipulation of a valve to control gas flow. A simple example of a control system would comprise a *control loop* consisting of an *actuator* which operates on, say, a valve; a *transducer* senses the flow and the signal from the transducer forms a *feedback* to the actuator. This seemingly complex system is arranged so that any change in pressure which would cause an alteration in flow may be automatically corrected very rapidly. A separated input, which may be either manual or from some other part of a larger system, may be arranged to alter the target flow level.

(b)

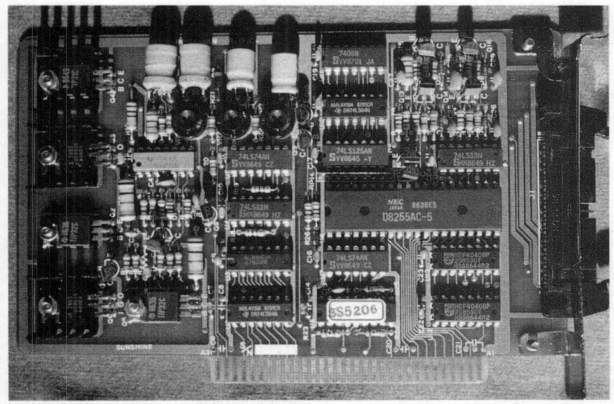

Figure 1.10 Printed circuit board. (a) The track side; (b) the component side. Note there are conductive tracks on both sides of the board. The components may be conventionally attached to the board by passing their leads through holes in the board and then soldering the connection to make it permanent. 'Surface mount' components are now also available that have shorter connections which are soldered to the same surface of the board as the component is mounted.

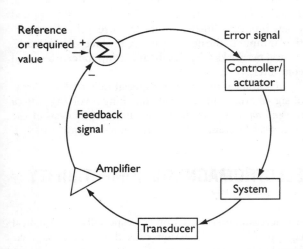

Figure 1.11 The principle of a servo control loop.

Table 1.3 Common transducers

- Temperature
- Pressure
- Flow
- Force
- Position
- Acceleration
- Sound (and ultrasound)
- Light (ultra violet – visible – infrared)
- Ionizing radiation
- Chemical composition

Table 1.4 Physical properties used in transducers

- Resistance
- Capacitance
- Inductance
- Thermoelectricity
- Piezo-electricity
- Photovoltaic
- Electrochemical
- Nuclear magnetic resonance
- Ionization

Transducers

A *transducer* is a device that converts one form of energy into another (Table 1.3). Most transducers convert to a electrical signal, which then may be used to display or record some measurement modality or used as part of a control system.

Many different physical, and in some cases chemical, properties are used in transducers (Table 1.4); individual transducers will be discussed in the relevant chapters.

Displays

In previous decades, electronic displays were limited to physiological monitoring equipment; it is now common practice to use various forms of electronic display in anaesthetic delivery machines to indicate gas flow, gas and vapour concentrations, ventilator parameters, and the safety status of the machine. Displays may be analogue in the form of meters or *optoelectronic*. Optoelectronic displays of simple alpha-numerical data may be done with light emitting diode (LED) displays or liquid crystal displays (LCD); more complex displays including graphical representations of dynamic pressure and flow require some form of picture display, for example a cathode ray tube (CRT) as in a television. Although it is possible to use a graphical LCD as in a portable computer, the CRT is generally used in anaesthetic machines for this type of display as it is easier to read in high ambient light and from angles other than the perpendicular. The disadvantage of the CRT type of display is that it requires very high voltages (5–15 kV but at very low current) whereas the LCD operates from very low voltages (5–10 V) Other types of graphical display, for example the electronic 'plasma' display, have not yet come into common use in anaesthetic equipment.

New Terms

The are a few new terms that have recently come into common use with regard to control and measurement systems. They are often used in sales literature and by sales representatives. These terms include *fuzzy logic*, *neural networks* and *artificial intelligence*.

'Fuzzy' Logic

As already mentioned, in most logical situations, there are just two conditions: on/off, go/no-go, one/zero, yes/no. There are, however, several situations where things are not so clear-cut: for example, at what point is an arterial blood pressure considered as being 'hypertensive'? (Fig. 1.12). Fuzzy logic allows logical manipula-

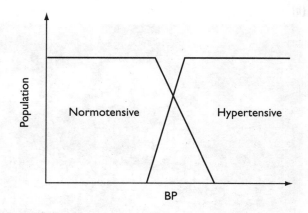

Figure 1.12 Example of fuzzy logic sets.

tions to be made from data where there is this blurring of change-over point.

Neural Computing

The origins of *neural computing* date back to the 1940s but have been overshadowed by advances in conventional computing, especially with the advent of large-scale integrated circuits. Neural computing is now rapidly expanding but must not be considered a competitor but rather complementary to conventional digital computing. The main difference between conventional and neural computing is that conventional computers have to be *explicitly* programmed, whereas neural computers *adapt* themselves during a period of *training* based upon examples with solutions presented to them. Neural computing is so called because the basic unit of the system is similar in function to a neurone (Fig. 1.13a). During the training period the 'weight' applied to any input is adjusted to vary the 'strength' of any particular input to the neurone where the 'decision' is made. Neural networks (Fig. 1.13b) are set up to form a neural computer.

Neural computing has a special role to play in areas of signal processing and data handling involving *pattern recognition*, for example in the automatic analysis of the electrocardiogram and electroencephalogram.

ELECTROMAGNETIC COMPATIBILITY

An increasingly serious problem, especially with medical equipment, is malfunction caused by *electromagnetic interference* (EMI). Electronic equipment may, intentionally or otherwise, emit electromagnetic radiation. If the intensity of this radiation is high enough it may

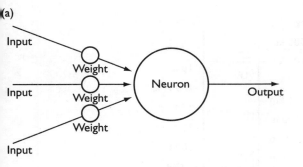

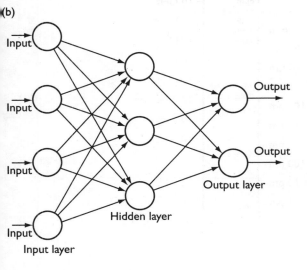

Figure 1.13 Neural networks. (a) The structure and function of a single 'neurone'; (b) a typical three-level neural network.

interfere with nearby electronic circuitry, which in the case of infusion pumps and ventilators may be life-threatening. This problem is becoming more serious as modern equipment has become more *susceptible* than its more antique counterparts and with the ever increasing amount of electromagnetic 'smog'. Figure 1.14 shows how this problem has increased in recent years and how the European EMC Directive, which came into force in 1995, legislates to improve design of equipment both to reduce unwanted emissions and susceptibility.

The increasing reliance upon electronics and especially information technology related equipment, communication and navigation has led to this enormous pollution or *smog*. The trend from vacuum valves through discrete semiconductors to large-scale integrated circuits has increased the susceptibility. This has also recently been made worse by the use of menu-programming rather than thumbwheel switches to select, for example, infusion rate and also by the replacement of metal cases and enclosures by moulded plastic, which is cheaper and easier to manufacture. Some EMI is unavoidable, as for example with communications equipment.

Any transmitting device, be it walkie-talkie, cordless phone, radio-controlled model or cellular telephone, emits an electromagnetic field that has a strength known as the *field strength*, which is measured in volts per metre (V/m). Most electronic equipment in use in health care facilities should be able to function normally if the field strength is <1 V/m. Susceptibility also varies with the frequency of the transmitting source. Future design recommendations say that the equipment should be able to withstand 10 V/m.

A serious danger has recently come to light in the form of *cellular telephones*. Normally radiotelephones

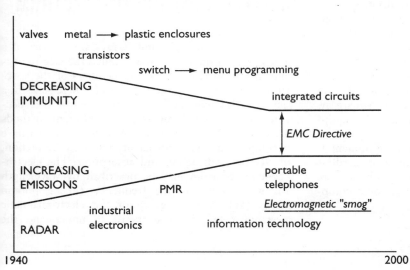

Figure 1.14 The EMC Gap. Since the early 1940s there has been an increasing pollution with electromagnetic energy, both useful emissions (communication and radar) and 'interference' or 'waste'. During the same period, the immunity of electronic equipment to interference has decreased. The EEC EMC Directive (1989) is part of a world-wide initiative to stabilize the situation.
PMR, private mobile radio.
(Reproduced from *EMC for Product Engineers*, 2nd edn, with permission from Butterworth-Heinemann, Oxford.)

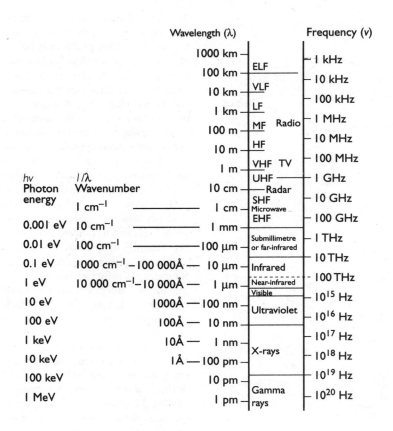

Figure 1.15 The electromagnetic spectrum.

only rarely come in close enough proximity to medical equipment to present a risk. However, pocket-sized cellular telephones at the bedside produce enough electromagnetic energy to change the settings of infusion pumps and ventilators. Most users do not realize that cellular telephones emit pulses intermittently, even when they are not being used, so long as they are switched on. The risk decreases by an inverse-square law as the distance between the telephone and the equipment increases.

Until the susceptibility of medical equipment is improved it should be made a rule that cordless 'phones, walkie-talkies and cellular telephones are kept at least 5–10 m from medical electronic equipment.

THE ELECTROMAGNETIC SPECTRUM

Radio waves, heat, light and X-rays are all part of a family of electromagnetic waves called the electromagnetic spectrum (Fig. 1.15). All members of the spectrum travel with the same velocity of 3×10^8 m/s in a vacuum. Although the various members of the spectrum have different properties and different methods of generation, absorption and detection, they all have in common the phenomena of reflection, refraction, interference, diffraction and absorption. The electromagnetic spectrum may be described by wavelength (λ), wavenumber ($1/\lambda$), frequency (v) or photon energy (hv). A basic grasp of the electromagnetic spectrum helps the anaesthetist to understand the principles behind the various forms of gas analysis, pulse oximetry and other monitoring techniques as well as those of surgical diathermy, radiology and nuclear medicine with which he or she is likely to come in contact during the course of the working day.

FURTHER READING

Department of Health (1994) *Portable, Cordless and Cellular Telephones: Interference with Medical Devices*, Safety Action Bulletin (94)49 November 1994. London: DoH.

European Commission (1989) *European EMC Directive 89/336/EEC*.

Horowitz P, Hill W (1989) *The Art of Electronics*, 2nd edn. Cambridge: Cambridge University Press.

Morris NM (1991) *Control Engineering*, 4th edn. London: McGraw-Hill.

Mushin WW, Jones PL (1987) *Physics for Anaesthetists*, 4th edn. Oxford: Blackwell Scientific.

Padmore GRA, Nunn JF (1974) SI units in relation to anaesthesia. *British Journal of Anaesthesia* 46: 236–243.

Williams T (1992) *EMC for Product Designers*. Oxford: Newnes.

— 2 —

THE SUPPLY OF ANAESTHETIC GASES

Contents

INTRODUCTION

The gases used in anaesthesia may be supplied in cylinders small enough to be manhandled or in bulk in liquid form which is vaporized and transmitted to the anaesthetic machine via pipelines.

CYLINDERS

Modern cylinders are manufactured from molybdenum steel and, because of the greater strength of this alloy, they have thinner walls than their larger carbon steel predecessors and are therefore lighter. Aluminium alloy cylinders are not, as yet, widely used in the medical field in the UK.

Oxygen, nitrogen, air and helium are stored in cylinders as compressed gas (see the inside front cover). Nitrous oxide and carbon dioxide, being strictly speaking vapours and not gases, liquefy at the pressures to which the cylinders are filled. Indeed, the greater part of the contents of cylinders of these 'gases' is in the liquid form when full. The cylinder is not completely filled with liquid since, if it were, a comparatively small rise in temperature would lead to a very large rise in pressure, which would result in rupture. It is filled to a *filling ratio* which is the weight of the substance with which it is actually filled divided by the weight of water that it could hold. In the UK, which has a temperate climate, nitrous oxide and carbon dioxide cylinders are filled to a ratio of 0.75; in tropical climates this is reduced to 0.67. Since they contain liquid, it is important that cylinders of nitrous oxide and carbon dioxide are mounted in the vertical position, with the outlets uppermost, when in use. The temperature of the cylinder and its contents drops during vaporization, and where high flow rates of nitrous oxide are taken from a small cylinder, the fall of temperature, and consequently pressure, may be marked. Water vapour from the surrounding air condenses on the exterior of the cylinder as it cools and if the temperature falls still further this may freeze. In a 'dental gas session' the pressure in a 3600–litre cylinder may fall from 50 000 to 35 000 kPa (750–500 psi) before the liquid nitrous oxide is exhausted.

In the case of oxygen and other gases that do not normally liquefy, the contents of the cylinder may be estimated with a pressure gauge, since the amount of gas is proportional to the pressure. Fluctuations of pressure caused by changes of ambient temperature are not usually of a significant order in clinical practice. However, in the case of nitrous oxide and carbon dioxide, it is not until all the liquid content has evaporated that the pressure within the cylinder falls appreciably, provided that there has not been significant cooling. Therefore, in this case the contents gauge falls rapidly only when the contents are nearly exhausted. Some contents gauges for

Table 2.1 Physical properties of compressed vapours and gases

	Oxygen	Nitrous oxide	Entonox	Carbon dioxide
Symbol	O_2	N_2O	$O_2 + N_2O$	CO_2
Physical state in cylinder	Gas	Liquid	Gas	Liquid
Pressure when full (15°C)				
psi	1980	639.5	1980	723
kg/cm²	139.2	44.9	139.2	50.8
atm	134.7	43.5	134.7	49.2
$10^3 \times$ kPa	136.5	4.4	136.5	5
Type of cylinder valve*	PI BN HW	PI HW	PI	PI
Critical temperature (°C)	−118.4	36.5	(Gases separate at −6°C)	31
Critical pressure (atm)	50.14	71.7	—	72.85
Boiling point (°C at 1 atm)	−183	−89	—	−78.5
Flammability	Supports combustion	Supports combustion	Supports combustion	No
Approximate weight (for calculation of cylinder contents)				
g/litre	—	1.87	—	1.87
oz/gallon	—	3.3	—	3.3

* PI, pin index; BN, bull-nose; HW, handwheel.

these gases are therefore calibrated with a wide segment marked 'Full at varying temperatures'. The pressure of gases in full cylinders is shown in Table 2.1.

The contents of nitrous oxide, carbon dioxide and cyclopropane cylinders are more accurately determined, if required, by weighing the cylinders. As shown in Fig. 2.1a, the weight of the empty cylinder (Tare) is stamped on the side of the valve block. The weight of the gas in terms of its density in ounces per gallon or grams per litre is shown on the label on the neck of the cylinder, and by weighing the cylinder and subtracting its empty weight, the weight of the contents of the cylinder can be estimated at any time. The densities of various gases are shown in Table 2.1.

The cylinder for each gas is painted in a distinctive colour. They are also marked with the chemical symbol for the gas they contain. Throughout the equipment the colours shown in Table 2.2 are used to identify the gaseous pathways.

Medical gas cylinders are hydraulically tested every 5 years and this test is recorded by a mark which is stamped on the neck of the cylinder. Other marks on the neck and the valve block (Fig. 2.1) relate to the name of the owner, the serial number of the cylinder and the pressures to which the cylinder has been tested and may safely be filled.

Pin Index System (International Standard)

This system has been devised in order to prevent the accidental fitting of a cylinder of the wrong gas to a yoke, thus making interchangeability of cylinders of different gases impossible. One or more pins project from the yoke, and these locate in holes bored in the valve block of the cylinder (Fig. 2.2). The configuration of the pins

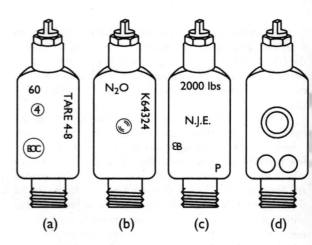

Figure 2.1 The four faces of a pin index cylinder valve block. Note on (a) the weight of the empty cylinder, 'tare' in pounds and ounces (or kg); on (b) the symbol for nitrous oxide; on (c) the pressure of the hydraulic test; on (d) the outlet and pin index holes.

Table 2.2 Colour codes for medical gases and vacuum

Gas	Symbol	ISO and UK	USA	Germany
Oxygen	O_2	White on black	Green	Blue
Nitrous oxide	N_2O	Blue	Blue	Grey
Carbon dioxide	CO_2	Grey	Grey	—
Air (medical)	AIR	White and black on black	Yellow	Yellow
Entonox 50/50 N_2O/O_2	$N_2O + O_2$	Blue and white on blue	—	—
Vacuum	—	Yellow	—	—

varies for each gas, as illustrated in Fig. 2.3. If the wrong cylinder is accidentally offered up to a yoke, it is impossible to fit it. When piped medical gas systems were first employed, the supply hose to the anaesthetic machine often terminated in a block similar to the valve block of a cylinder and drilled for the appropriate pin index. Full details of the pin index system are given in British Standard 1319 of 1955.

The then Department of Health and Social Security advised in 1973 that pipeline hoses should be connected permanently to anaesthetic machines using a union such as a cap and liner.

Medical gases are also supplied in cylinders other than those with pin index outlets, and those still available in the UK are shown in Fig. 2.4. Note that the 'handwheel' type cylinders (Fig. 2.4b) of nitrous oxide and oxygen,

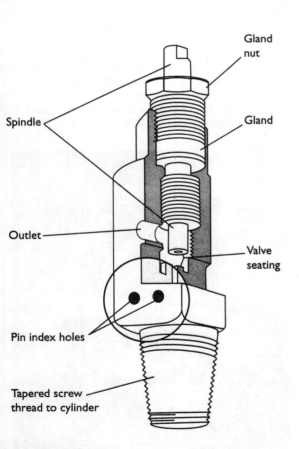

Figure 2.2 A section through a pin index cylinder valve block, showing the position of the pin index holes.

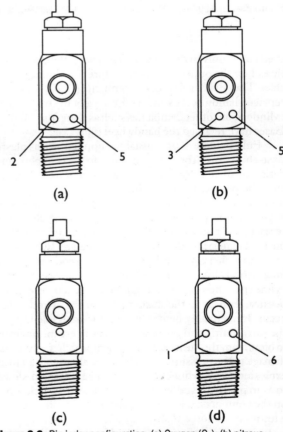

Figure 2.3 Pin index configuration. (a) Oxygen (O_2); (b) nitrous oxide (N_2O); (c) Entonox (50% N_2O + 50% O_2); (d) carbon dioxide (CO_2).

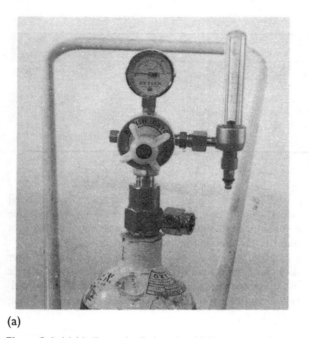

(a)

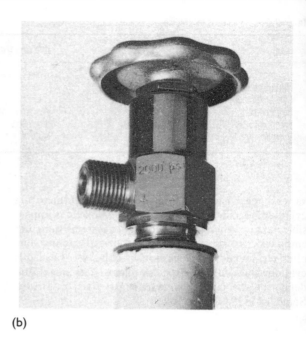

(b)

Figure 2.4 (a) A bull-nosed cylinder valve. (b) A hand-wheel cylinder valve. These are for larger cylinders.

used commonly in dental practice, have different sizes of thread on the outlet and are therefore non-interchangeable. The British Oxygen Company (BOC) has now replaced handwheel cylinders for oxygen by 'bull-nosed' cylinders, but other companies such as Kingston Medical Gases have retained the handwheel type.

Full cylinders are usually supplied with plastic dust-covers over the outlet in order to prevent contamination by dirt or grit; these should be removed immediately before fitting the cylinder. When a cylinder is fitted, care should be taken to see that the sealing washer is present and in good order. If it is not so, it should be replaced by a new one, and this must be of non-combustible material. ('Bodok' seals supplied by BOC have a metal periphery, which keeps them in good order for a long period (Fig. 2.5).) The screw or clamp securing the cylinder in the yoke should not be tightened excessively because damage to the washer or even the cylinder may occur. Immediately before fitting, it is advisable to open the valve gently and to allow some gas to escape, in order to blow from the outlet any dirt or grit which might cause damage to the pressure regulator or could even lead to an explosion. The cylinder valve should be opened slowly so as to prevent a sudden surge of pressure (shock wave) on the contents gauge and regulator. It should be closed with no more force than is sufficient, or damage to the seating of the valve may result. If, after a cylinder has been turned on, there appears to be a leak, this may be tested for with water or a soapy solution. Occasionally

there is a leak of gas around the spindle of the valve; this can be prevented by gently screwing down the gland nut (see Fig. 2.2). If high-pressure oxygen is allowed to come into contact with combustible materials, especially oil or grease, fire or an explosion is liable to occur.

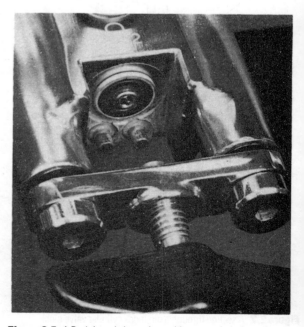

Figure 2.5 A Bodok seal shown in position on a pin index yoke.

In the USA, cylinders are fitted with a Wood's metal fusible plug in the valve block that melts at low temperature. This is to prevent the risk of explosion if the cylinders are exposed to very high temperatures, such as in a fire. (In the UK the sealing material between the valve and the neck of the cylinder is often made of a fusible material that in the event of involvement in a fire would melt and allow the contents of the cylinder to escape around the threads of this joint.)

Cylinders should be stored in a clean place in order to prevent the admission of dirt and possible infection to the operating theatre. They should be kept in a rack in such a manner that they are used in rotation, to prevent any being stored for a long period, thereby reducing the possibility of their being empty when brought into use. Cylinders of Entonox (50% nitrous oxide plus 50% oxygen) should never be stored under conditions in which the temperature might fall below 0°C, since if the temperature falls below the pseudocritical (condensation) temperature for this mixture, the nitrous oxide and oxygen could laminate (separate). If this does happen, the instructions for remixing the contents, printed on the neck of the cylinder, should be followed. This involves gentle rewarming and repeated inversion of the cylinder.

Empty cylinders should be stored separately from full ones and marked accordingly. The valves of empty cylinders should be closed to avoid the ingress of water vapour, water or dirt. Faulty cylinders should be appropriately marked and returned to the supplier. Cylinders should not be stored under conditions where very high temperatures may occur.

OXYGEN CONCENTRATORS

The desirability of the local 'manufacture' of oxygen, obviating the need for the provision of cylinders or liquid oxygen, has led to the development of methods of separating oxygen from air. Oxygen concentrators may be required for the following reasons:

- economy
  - (a) very large bulk users;
  - (b) domestic users;

- convenience
  - (a) aircraft;
  - (b) ships;

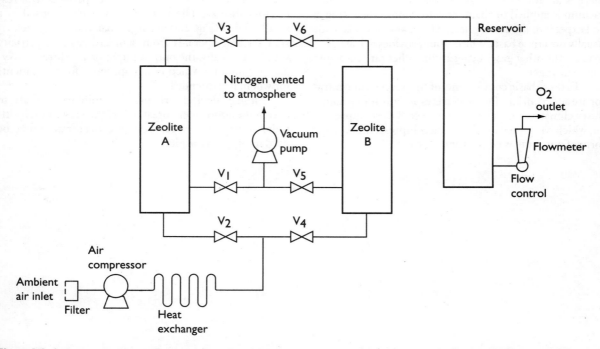

Figure 2.6 An oxygen concentrator. To start, valves V_1, V_4 and V_6 are closed. Compressed air passes via V_2 into cylinder A, where the nitrogen is absorbed by the zeolite, and concentrated oxygen passes out via V_3. When the capacity of cylinder A is used up, valves V_1, V_4 and V_6 are opened and valves V_2, V_3 and V_5 are closed. Cylinder B then takes over the function, while nitrogen from cylinder A is discharged to the atmosphere via the vacuum pump.

- logistics
  - (a) armed forces;
  - (b) geographical;
    - (i) developing countries;
    - (ii) mission hospitals;
    - (iii) expeditions.

In theory, oxygen concentrators could use as a power source any source of mechanical energy, since the only energy-consuming component is a compressor. All currently manufactured oxygen concentrators are electrically powered.

The principle of the oxygen concentrator depends on the property of an *artificial zeolite* (dust-free aluminium silicate, sometimes referred to as a molecular sieve) to adsorb molecules of nitrogen onto the very large surface area presented, and to allow oxygen to pass through.

The component parts of the oxygen concentrator are shown in Fig. 2.6. The two chambers, A and B, are identical and contain the zeolite. Initially, chamber A is charged with compressed air; the nitrogen is retained in the zeolite, while the remainder of the gas, comprising more than 92% oxygen, passes on to a reservoir and from there to the patient. When the zeolite in chamber A is calculated to have been fully charged with nitrogen, there is an automatic change-over to chamber B and a vacuum is applied to chamber A to remove the nitrogen and expel it to the atmosphere. The change-over is made usually on a time basis. The output provides at least 92% oxygen, the other gases being argon, other rare gases and a little nitrogen.

To these basic components of the oxygen concentrator are added an air filter, which is especially important in dusty climates, a heat exchanger to cool the compressed air, which has gained heat by being compressed, and some form of output flow control and meter.

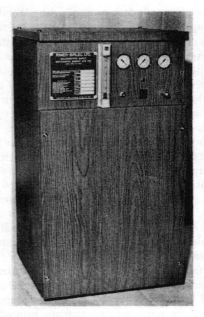

Figure 2.7 A small domiciliary oxygen concentrator.

Small oxygen concentrators are in regular use for the treatment, in their own homes, of patients with respiratory disease. The whole equipment is housed in a small cabinet (Fig. 2.7) no larger than the average television set and operates from standard mains electricity supply. Typically, the output might be 2–3 litres of oxygen per minute, which is the optimum for the patients for whom it is intended.

Similar devices are used in military aircraft to enrich the atmosphere breathed by the crew at high altitudes. Very much larger oxygen concentrators may be used to supply a hospital.

− 3 −

MEDICAL GAS SERVICES

Contents

INTRODUCTION

The most economical way to supply a large institution with a medical gas supply is to deliver it in bulk to a single convenient site on the premises and subsequently decant it through a network of pipes to the areas where it is required. The advantages of piped gases are not only that there may be a reduction in the cost of the gases and rental of cylinders (which often may be the more expensive), but also that there is a saving of the cost of labour for transporting cylinders and also a reduction in medical accidents caused by small cylinders becoming exhausted. By virtue of the installation of a medical gas pipeline system, the need for provision of large quantities of small 'duty' cylinders of gas such as oxygen and nitrous oxide on anaesthetic machines and similar items is dispensed with. (However, BS 4272 Part 3: 1987 (UK) requires that some equipment such as anaesthetic machines must have a reserve supply of oxygen and so even though some small cylinders are therefore necessary, the number in 'reserve' may be greatly diminished.)

Much publicity has been given in recent years to the few accidents that have occurred in connection with piped medical gas supplies, but it is not easy to make a rational comparison between the number of accidents before and after the introduction of pipelines, owing to the great increase in the amount and complexity of work undertaken.

The information given in this chapter refers mainly to the practice in the UK, though similar systems have been used for many years in other countries. In some of these other systems the nominal pressure for piped medical gas is 310 kPa (45 psi) rather than the British Standard of 420 kPa (60 psi). In some systems a higher pressure is used for oxygen than for other services.

Medical gas pipeline services (MGPS) may be considered in five sections:

1. The bulk store or production plant.
2. The fixed distribution pipework.
3. The terminal outlets.
4. The flexible hoses, flowmeters and vacuum controllers, which are all detachable.
5. The connections between the flexible hoses and the anaesthetic machines.

Items 1 and 2 above may be considered as 'behind the wall' and it is usually felt that, apart from broad strategy, this is the province of the Engineering, Supplies and Pharmacy departments. The anaesthetist has to take it on trust that the correct gases will be supplied and cannot be held responsible for what goes on 'behind the wall'. With items 4 and 5, the anaesthetist takes a share of the responsibility to ensure the maintenance of good standards, of checks and of tests and to prevent abuse. The terminal outlet is the interface between the two.

Of the rare accidents that have occurred, most have been between the wall and the patient. These could be deemed possibly to be the most preventable, though several deaths have occurred in the UK and elsewhere due to cross-connections (called 'confusion') which have led to gases other than pure oxygen being delivered from the oxygen outlet. It should be stressed that nearly all accidents have been caused by alterations or faulty repairs made by incompetent and sometimes unauthorized people rather than because the installation was that of one manufacturer or another or of a more modern or an older model (prior to the introduction of a British and International Standard). It has also been suggested that if oxygen only were supplied by pipeline, there would be no possibility of confusion.

BULK STORAGE AND SUPPLY OF GASES

Liquid Oxygen

In the case of large consumers, oxygen is delivered and stored on site in the liquid form. It is transported in specially insulated tankers and is delivered into a vacuum insulated evaporator (VIE) (Fig. 3.1). This consists of an inner shell of stainless steel, separated from an outer shell of carbon steel by a space in which is maintained the greatest degree of vacuum possible and which also contains perlite, an insulating powder, so that heat gain to the inner chamber from the outside is minimized in the event of loss of vacuum. The temperature within the inner chamber is around $-183°C$, which is above the critical temperature of liquid oxygen and since the container cannot be a perfect insulator arrangements are made to maintain this very low temperature (see below, Mode of operation). There are four connections to the inner cylinder:

- The filling port, through which fresh supplies of liquid oxygen are introduced.
- A gaseous withdrawal line at the top of the cylinder, from which, during periods of low demand, gaseous oxygen may pass via a restrictor plate to a superheater and from here to the control system and distribution pipework. The purpose of the superheater (a length of copper tubing about 2.5 cm in diameter on which are mounted metallic fins to conduct ambient heat) is to raise the temperature of the gaseous oxygen to that of the ambient air, for otherwise dangerously cold oxygen might be delivered to the terminal outlets in those parts of the hospital close to the VIE.
- A liquid withdrawal line, which during periods of high demand may withdraw liquid to enter the main flow downstream from the restrictor and upstream from the superheater.

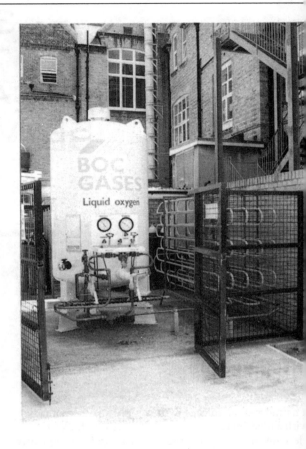

Figure 3.1 A VIE plant for liquid oxygen.

- A second liquid withdrawal line, which may pass through an evaporator and then either into the distribution network or back into the gaseous compartment of the container.

Mode of Operation of a Liquid Oxygen Plant
(Fig. 3.2)

Since no insulation can be perfect, the inner container is continually receiving heat from the exterior; the effects of this are offset by the evaporation of liquid oxygen thus helping to keep the liquid at the appropriate temperature. If there is no demand for oxygen for a period of time, the pressure within the chamber may rise above normal (around 1055 kPa), and at a predetermined pressure a safety valve opens to allow the escape of some gas. The loss of oxygen due to this venting is, as a rule, fairly small. Conversely, if the demand for oxygen is increased there may be a fall of pressure within the vessel. In this case a control valve opens in the lower liquid withdrawal line and liquid passes through an evaporator and then either to the pipeline or to the gaseous compartment of

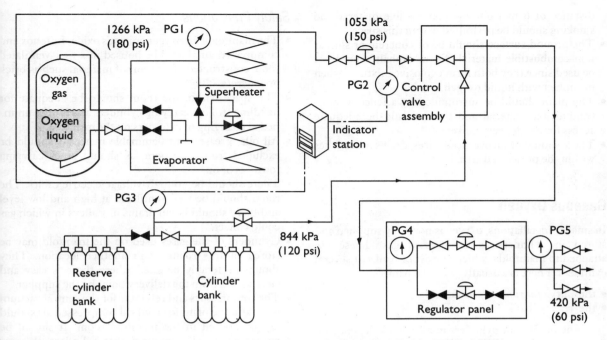

Figure 3.2 A simplified schematic diagram of a liquid oxygen plant and standby (reserve) cylinders (see text for details).

the VIE until the pressure within it is restored to normal. In the event of an exceptionally high demand for oxygen, liquid may pass through the upper liquid withdrawal line directly to the superheater and via the control panel to the distribution system.

A cause of considerable waste is that during the delivery of fresh supplies of liquid, the hose between the tanker and the VIE needs to be cooled to below the critical temperature of oxygen before delivery can be effected. Cooling is achieved by allowing liquid to escape from the tanker through the hose to the atmosphere. The oxygen delivered is metered at the tanker and, on occasions, it has been found that as much as one-quarter of the total delivery has been required for this pre-cooling.

Estimation of Contents
Older versions of the VIE rested on three legs, two of which were on hinged supports. The third rested on a simple steelyard weighing device with an appropriate counterweight. The liquid content of the VIE was expressed in weight and indicated on a dial.

Currently, the estimation of liquid contents is assessed by measuring the pressure differential between the top and bottom of the VIE. The pressure at the bottom of the VIE is greater than at the top because of the added effect of gravity on the mass of liquid oxygen. With evaporation, this mass reduces causing the pressure at the bottom to do likewise. A differential pressure

gauge (Barton gauge) compares the pressures at the top and bottom of the VIE and the scale on the dial converts the difference into contents. The gauge is calibrated for each model of VIE as their shapes and sizes differ.

The VIE is sited outside a building but within an enclosure that also houses two banks of reserve cylinders in a manifold (see below under Gaseous Oxygen). The reserve cylinders automatically take over the load if the output from the VIE falls below a predetermined level.

Relative Capacities of Cylinders and the VIE
The pressure within a full cylinder of oxygen is 13 700 kPa (1980 psi). Thus, when used on a pipeline, a cylinder can be expected to give approximately 130 times its capacity of oxygen at atmospheric pressure. Compared with this, one volume of liquid oxygen gives 842 times its volume of gas at 15°C and normal atmospheric pressure. Since the VIE has a very much greater capacity than a cylinder, it will be obvious that it can deliver a far greater volume of oxygen than a whole manifold of cylinders. It should also be large enough to provide 10 days' consumption on site. The reserve cylinder manifold should be large enough for 1 day's supply.

Safety Precautions
- Liquid oxygen plants should not be housed within a building. They should be sited in the open, a minimum

distance of 6 m from any combustible material; no smoking should be permitted within this space.

- The ground surface should be of concrete or similar non-combustible material. Tar or asphalt should not be used since they both form explosive mixtures when in contact with liquid oxygen.
- The plant should be surrounded by a fence of non-combustible material and there should be adequate access for the delivery tanker.
- There should be no overhead wires, drains or trenches within the prescribed area.

Gaseous Oxygen

In smaller installations, oxygen is normally supplied and stored in cylinders as compressed gas. These are attached to manifolds, which consist of banks of several cylinders. There are usually two such banks:

- the *'duty' (or running)* bank; and
- the *'reserve'* bank.

The number of cylinders in each bank depends on the expected demand. The cylinders in each bank are all turned on and interconnected. However, the flow of oxygen from one cylinder to another is prevented by non-return valves. When the duty bank is almost exhausted the supply is automatically switched to the reserve bank. This now becomes the duty bank and an indication is given that this has occurred. The exhausted cylinders must now be replaced by full ones, and if this is not done before the second bank reaches a certain level of exhaustion, a compelling warning is given (see below). Linked to this manifold is a smaller one for use as an emergency back-up. It may be used to continue the supply during periods of maintenance or repair, when the main manifold is out of action. Under these circumstances, the pipeline is isolated by manually closing the main manifold valve and opening the emergency manifold valve. There is also a pressure relief valve, which, like that on the main manifold, is vented to the outside rather than to an enclosed area where it might be dangerous. The valves on the cylinders of the emergency manifold are kept open during periods of standby, in order to show by means of the contents gauge on the pressure regulator that they are full, and by the regulated pressure gauge that the regulator is correctly set. Figure 3.3 shows a typical modern, automatic manifold.

In many instances relatively small establishments such as dental clinics have piped gas installations with very few outlets. In the UK those employed by general dental practitioners are provided and owned by individual practitioners. However, these installations are required to meet the appropriate standards in the UK (855 5682: 1984).

Safety Precautions

- The manifolds for oxygen, nitrous oxide, Entonox and compressed air should be housed in a well-ventilated room constructed of a fireproof material such as brick or concrete.
- The space within the room should be adequate for handling trolleys carrying cylinders and for the unimpeded changing of cylinders on the manifold.
- All oils, greases and flammable materials should be excluded from the room, as should pipes carrying town gas or oil.
- There should be no high-voltage electric cables. The room should be well ventilated at high and low level and there should be no drains or gulleys in which gas could collect.
- Cylinders of the gases used on the manifold may be stored in this room or in another location. They should preferably be sited where there is easy and close access from the delivery point by the supplier.
- The compressors and reservoir for the central vacuum plant and the plant for medical compressed air should not be housed in the manifold room. It should be impressed on all personnel that cylinders of compressed gas, particularly oxygen, can be dangerous if mishandled. Provisions should be made for securing the cylinders to the wall.

Nitrous Oxide

As stated previously, nitrous oxide liquefies at room temperature when stored under pressure in a cylinder. It is therefore supplied to a piped medical gas system from a manifold of cylinders similar to those for oxygen described above.

When considering the size and number of cylinders to be installed in each bank, thought must be given to the maximum demand that will be required. This is because nitrous oxide cools not only as it expands but also because of the latent heat required to vaporize the liquid. If a heavy demand is taken from a bank of small capacity, the gas may cool to such a low temperature that water vapour in the ambient atmosphere condenses, and may even freeze, on the surface of parts of the pipework and in particular the pressure regulators. In the days when nitrous oxide cylinders contained some water vapour, this used to freeze within the regulator, causing obstruction. For this reason a regulator heater, thermostatically controlled at 47°C, may be fitted to warm the gas and prevent condensation. A typical nitrous oxide manifold is similar to the oxygen manifold (Figure 3.3). No practical method for the local manufacture of nitrous oxide yet exists, though progress in this field is being made.

(a)

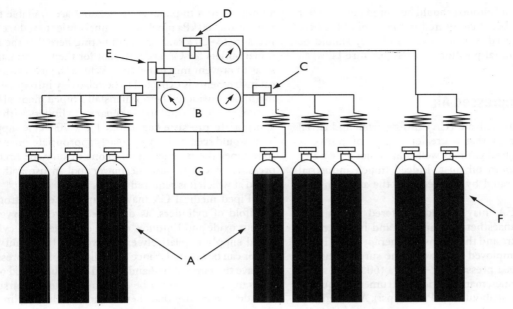

(b)

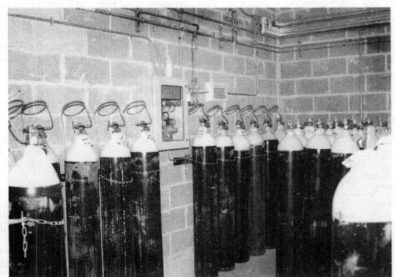

Figure 3.3 (a) A major oxygen manifold. A, cylinder banks; B, control panel that includes the regulators, pressure gauges and automatic switches; C, isolating valve for a main cylinder bank; D, isolating valve for emergency cylinder bank; E, isolating valve for main cylinder manifold; F, emergency cylinder bank; G, alarm indicator panel.
(b) A major oxygen manifold. The coils in the pipework provide greater flexibility so as to prevent damage to the pipes during cylinder changes.

Entonox (50% Nitrous Oxide + 50% Oxygen)

This mixture is used for the administration of inhalational analgesia, principally in the obstetric department. The manifolds employed are essentially the same as those for nitrous oxide and oxygen, but additional safeguards are required in the handling of the cylinders. This is because the mixture has a pseudocritical temperature of approximately −6°C and if the cylinder were allowed to cool below this point, the nitrous oxide and oxygen might separate out by a process known as *lamination*.

The large cylinders for Entonox manifolds have pin index outlets and, unlike smaller cylinders for this purpose, there is an internal tube from the valve block, leading down to within 10 cm of the bottom of the cylinder. The contents are supplied through this tube, the position of which would prevent the discharge of pure nitrous oxide if lamination had occurred. Excessive cooling of the cylinders is prevented by ensuring that there are a sufficient number of cylinders on the manifold and that all of them are turned on at the same time. No single cylinder should supply gas at a rate greater than 300 litres/min.

Cylinders of Entonox should be stored for 24 h after delivery before being connected to the manifold. There should be a special store for them and they should be kept in a horizontal position at a temperature between 10°C and 38°C.

Medical Compressed Air

Medical compressed air (CA) differs from industrial compressed air in that a greater degree of purity is required. Industrial CA may well contain not only water vapour but also an oil mist. Indeed, much industrial equipment operated by CA requires the addition of a lubricant.

Medical CA may be administered to patients through both anaesthetic equipment and lung ventilators in the theatre and the Intensive Therapy Unit (ITU) and it is also employed to power some surgical instruments. Whereas a pressure of 420 kPa (60 psi) is sufficient for the former, many surgical instruments require a higher pressure of about 700 kPa (105 psi). Although the CA driving surgical instruments is not intentionally administered to the patient, it would, if not clean, contaminate the operating field.

At first sight it might be thought that a 700 kPa compressed air system would on its own be suitable to supply a hospital (this pressure being required for surgical instruments); however, it must be borne in mind that this might present difficulties in the Intensive Care Ward, where blenders are used for mixing oxygen with medical CA to achieve the appropriate mixtures for administration to patients. Regulators are available that plug into a 700 kPa pipeline terminal outlet to reduce the pressure to 420 kPa. It is worth noting here that the terminal outlets for CA are different for the two pressures so as to prevent misconnection. Where the use of surgical instruments is expected to be relatively infrequent, it might be considered better to install a piped medical CA system at 420 kPa and to use separate cylinders with the appropriate pressure regulators for a 700 kPa supply. This would seem to be particularly appropriate since it is sometimes the practice of surgeons to vary the precise pressure of CA to suit the power tool in use and the speed at which it is required to run.

Piped medical CA may be supplied either from a manifold of cylinders, as described above for oxygen, nitrous oxide and Entonox, or by a compressor. A cylindered supply is relatively expensive, but the quality of the air can be assured. Since the cylinders of compressed air have the same right-hand thread on a bull-nosed outlet as oxygen, care must be taken in the storage of such cylinders to ensure that they are not accidentally interchanged. It is recommended that the storage bins be separated from each other, for example, by a wall or partition, and that they be clearly marked.

In a larger hospital it may well be economical to install a compressor. In this case the air has to be both dried and filtered at the outlet of the compressor in order to achieve adequate quality. A scheme for such a compressed air plant is shown in Fig. 3.4. A single plant may be used both to provide medical CA and to run an oxygen concentrator.

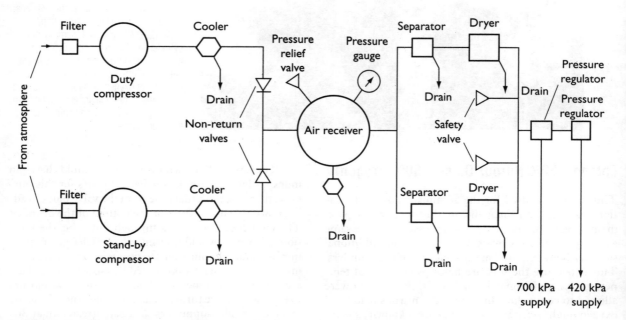

Figure 3.4 Simplified diagram of a medical compressed air plant.

In some instances it has been considered appropriate to install a small local compressor for a particular department in order to save extensive pipework. If this is done, it is essential to ensure that there is adequate oil separation and filtration to suit the requirements of that department. This is often lacking in small compressors.

Indicators and Alarms

The gauges and indicators that are an integral part of a major manifold are shown in Fig. 3.3b. A typical arrangement has one green indicator marked 'running' or 'duty' and one red indicator marked 'empty' for each bank of cylinders. Thus when the first bank of cylinders becomes exhausted, the green 'running' indicator on that side is extinguished and the red 'empty' indicator on that side is illuminated. At the same time the green indicator marked 'running' for the second bank will illuminate. The red indicator on the first bank stays lit until the cylinders have been replaced by full ones and have been turned on.

Since the manifolds are usually remote from the users and the members of staff responsible for changing the cylinders, repeater indicators should also be installed – for instance at the telephone switchboard or in an operating theatre suite.

The above indicators may be expected to operate when the installation is running normally. Warning signals, which may consist of a red or orange flashing light, and an audible alarm are given when there is some impending failure, for example if one bank is empty and the pressure in the cylinders in the other bank falls to a predetermined level, i.e. if there has been a failure to heed the indication that one bank of cylinders needs replenishing. Another warning may be given if the pressure in the output of the manifold falls below a predetermined level. The audible alarm may be muted temporarily (15 min intervals) but never immobilized.

The indicators for a liquid oxygen plant may show 'normal running', 'running from cylinders', 'first bank of cylinders empty' and 'low line pressure'.

PIPED MEDICAL VACUUM

In the UK, guidance on the design and installation of piped medical vacuum services is set out in Hospital Technical Memorandum (HTM) No. 2022 as revised in 1994.

Figure 3.5 shows the layout of a typical vacuum plant. The precise details of this may vary according to the type of pump in use.

The distribution pipework may take the form of a 'ring main', the two ends of which each pass towards the pump through an isolating valve and then a drainage trap in which any aspirated liquid or condensed vapour, for example from body cavity drainage, may separate out and be removed. The pipes then pass through bacterial filters and from there to the vacuum reservoir. At the bottom of the reservoir is a drainage pipe, with a manual drain valve, to evacuate any liquid that may collect.

The connection between the reservoir and the vacuum pumps is made through flexible hoses in order to reduce vibration and the noise that this might transmit through the pipework. There are two pumps, each of which is adequate for the needs of the system. Thus one pump may be 'on duty', whilst the other is on standby or being serviced.

There are various types of vacuum pump, but particular mention should be made of those that are oil-lick lubricated. It has been suggested that if the vacuum system is employed for the purpose of scavenging waste anaesthetic gases, the vapour of halothane and other anaesthetic agents may be absorbed by the lubricating oil, and by reducing its efficiency may cause failure of the pump. Furthermore, the Department of Health in the UK does not recommend the use of medical suction systems for scavenging, because the high inflow of anaesthetic gases will reduce surgical suction below desired levels and because experience has shown that such high vacuum levels can injure the patient if safety devices fail.

The output of the pump passes through a silencer to be exhausted at a suitable point, such as above roof level where the gases may be vented to the atmosphere without risk of polluting the air breathed by staff or patients.

Performance Levels and Specifications for a Medical Vacuum Service

For the UK the specifications for a piped vacuum service are laid down in BS 4957 of 1973. A few of these are quoted below, but for more complete information the full specifications should be consulted.

- A vacuum of at least 53 kPa (400 mmHg) below the standard atmospheric pressure of 101.3 kPa (760 mmHg) should be maintained at the outlets, each of which should be able to take a flow of free air of at least 40 litres/min.
- There should be at least two outlets per operating theatre, one per anaesthetic room and one per recovery bed.

(a)

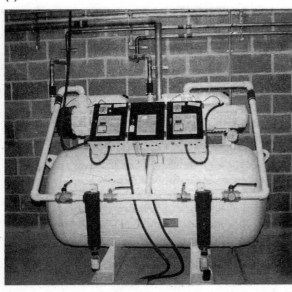

Figure 3.5 (a) A medical vacuum plant showing the 'duty' and 'standby' electric pumps, their control panels and duty reservoir. (b) A simplified diagram of a piped medical vacuum plant.

(b)

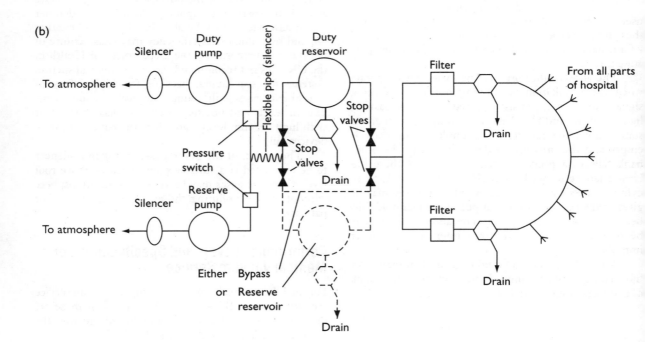

ELECTRICAL SUPPLY TO MGPS

The pumps for compressed air and vacuum should be powered by the 'non-interruptible' supply, which is backed up by the emergency generator. If possible, the manifold controls and warning lights should also have their own emergency supply. Some manifolds are so constructed that if there is total power failure the indicators and warning lights will fail, but all the cylinders, of both banks, are switched on so as to continue the supply. Other manifold controls have a manual override that may be used to switch from one bank to the other.

DISTRIBUTION PIPEWORK

The 'gases' that are commonly supplied by pipeline are oxygen, nitrous oxide, Entonox (a nitrous oxide/oxygen mixture), compressed air and vacuum. Other gases such as helium and hydrogen are supplied in piped services to pathology laboratories and the like, but are not frequently used in direct connection with patients. They are not, therefore, considered in this book.

For detailed information concerning the regulations and standards required for fixed distribution pipework, those imposed by the appropriate Government or Health Ministries should be consulted. In the UK these are quoted in HTM 2022 and its supplement, which refer to the 'permit to work' system laying down the procedures to be adopted when service maintenance, repair or alterations are to be undertaken.

In this chapter only a brief description can be given of the fixed pipework; because this part of the installation is 'behind the wall', it is more properly the concern of the hospital engineer. The anaesthetist should, however, be aware of the nature of the installation and should always be informed and consulted before any alterations to it are made.

The tubes used are copper, of a special degreased quality. Before they are delivered to the site, i.e. prior to installation, the ends are sealed so that there can be no ingress of dirt or other foreign material. The copper is also of a special alloy that prevents degradation of the gases. These rules may be relaxed in the case of the vacuum installation. The fittings are of degreased brass and joints are made by brazing rather than with soft solder or compression fittings. A system of brazing without the use of a flux has been developed and this results in a greatly reduced incidence of corrosion of both the surface and interior of the pipe and fittings. The diameter of pipe is determined by the demand that it will carry. Commonly, it may start from the manifold with a diameter of 42 mm, but after branching to supply one or more areas, pipes as narrow as 15mm may be employed.

Large installations may be divided into sections, supplying various departments. Each of these sections may be isolated by valves. Each department or ward, or section thereof, may be further isolated by a valve that is readily accessible to the staff, which may be used to turn off the gas supply in case of fire, fracture or other catastrophe.

Area valve and service units (Fig. 3.6) may be installed in such positions as to protect several departments or wards. These consist of a locked box containing an isolating valve, upstream and downstream of which are branches with the appropriate NIST (non-interchangeable screw thread) unions that are normally

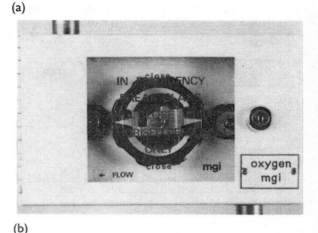

(a)

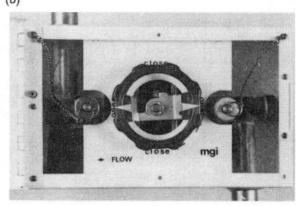

(b)

Figure 3.6 An area valve box: (a) with the door in the normal closed position; (b) with the door open, showing the NIST connections.

closed with a blanked-off NIST nut. The NIST union also contains a self-sealing valve. When the blanking nut is removed and the appropriate NIST connection is made, the self-sealing valve is automatically reopened. These branches may be used to purge pipelines or to introduce a local supply during alterations or breakdowns. The box also contains a 'spade', which may be used to ensure absolute closure of the pipeline, irrespective of the action of the valve.

Regional flowmeters may be incorporated in piped medical gas systems to detect the section in which an excessive leak or wastage of gas is occurring. Moisture traps may also be installed.

The pipework itself should be identified by labels placed upon it at regular intervals, in accordance with the identification code described in Fig. 3.7. Indeed, it is good practice for all pipework, whatever substances are carried, to be correctly labelled at regular intervals. The pipework may be hidden behind the wall or buried within the plaster, or alternatively it may be

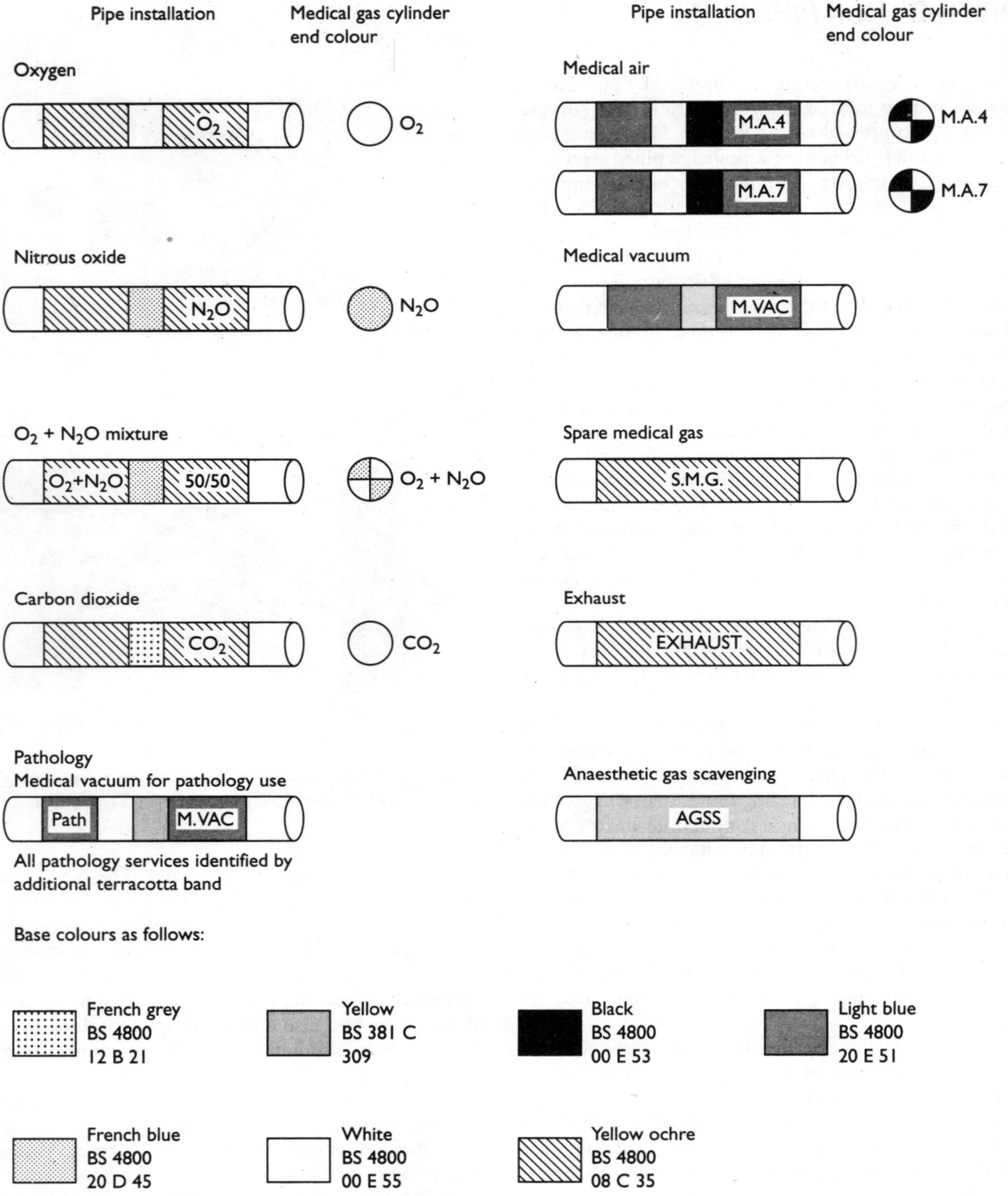

Figure 3.7 Colour code for the identification of medical gases, vacuum and active gas scavenging pipeline installations in the UK. Flexible hoses must be colour-coded throughout their length, or by means of the coloured bands shown (in the form of a tubular sleeve), which must be securely fitted at both ends (BS 5682:1984). 'BS' refers to the appropriate British Standard (e.g. BS 4800:1972) defining the colours used. Each colour shade has a specific number – e.g. French blue is 20 D 45.

Note that medical air is supplied at two different pressures: MA4 refers to medical air at 420 kPa pressure (60 psi), which supplies respiratory equipment; MA7 is medical air supplied at 700 kPa (105 psi) primarily to power air-operated surgical equipment.

mounted on the surface. The latter arrangement is not only aesthetically less attractive, but also less satisfactory from the standpoint of general hygiene and cleanliness.

The pipework for medical gases and vacuum, and their fittings should be separated from other pipework so as to avoid confusion and the isolating valves should be clearly labelled and positioned so that they may be closed by the retreating staff in the event of a fire.

TERMINAL OUTLETS

The distribution pipework terminates in outlets that are in the form of self-closing sockets (Fig 3.8).

In 1978 a British Standard was published (BS 5682, upgraded in 1984) that laid down a specification for the design of terminal units. It specifies that the terminal unit should consist of two sections:

- The first, *a termination assembly*, should be permanently attached to the appropriate pipeline.
- The second, the '*Schrader*' socket assembly, can be removed by a service engineer but must be designed so that it cannot be accidentally connected to a different gas service.

A termination assembly for a pressurized gas (but not a vacuum) must have an isolating valve so that work can be carried out on any terminal unit without shutting down all the terminal units for that gas in that area. It should be designed to operate automatically as soon as the socket assembly is removed. Furthermore, the identity of the gas for that terminal unit should be permanently displayed on the socket.

The 'Schrader socket' will accept a probe with a collar indexing system that is unique to each gas service.

FLEXIBLE PIPELINES

The flexible pipeline connects the terminal outlet to the anaesthetic machine. It has three components:

- a Schrader probe that fits the terminal outlet;
- a flexible hosepipe;
- a NIST connection that fits the anaesthetic machine.

The Pipeline Probe for the Terminal Outlet

The design of the Schrader probe is such that it is the same size for all gases. To prevent connection to the wrong gas service, the probe for each gas supply has a protruding indexing collar (see Fig. 3.9). This collar has a unique diameter that fits only the matching recess fitted to the socket assembly for that gas. The British Standard also stipulates the following:

- It must not be possible to twist the probe while it is connected to the unit. To this end, the collar is provided with a notch that fits over a rigid pin in the socket assembly.
- It must be possible to insert or remove the probe simply and quickly using one hand only. The socket assembly has a spring-loaded outer ring, which when depressed releases the locking mechanism holding the probe, and causes the probe to be ejected.
- The unit must seal off the flow of gas when the probe is withdrawn.

The Flexible Hose

This is the section of the system in which damage and wear are most likely to occur. Originally the hose for each gas was constructed of the same black reinforced rubber or neoprene tubing, identified only by a short length of

(a)   (b)   (c)   (d)

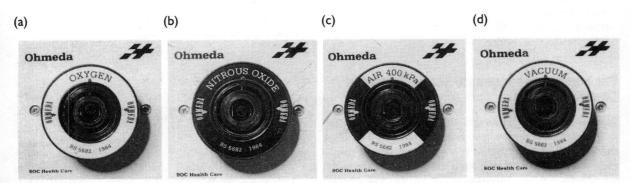

Figure 3.8 The GEM 10 terminal outlets for (a) oxygen, (b) nitrous oxide, (c) compressed air and (d) medical vacuum.

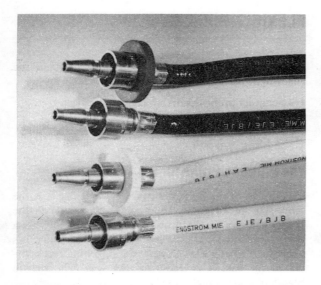

Figure 3.9 Pipeline probes for the terminal outlets. From top to bottom: nitrous oxide, compressed air, oxygen and medical vacuum. Note that the metal collars have different diameters so that each one will only fit its matching socket.

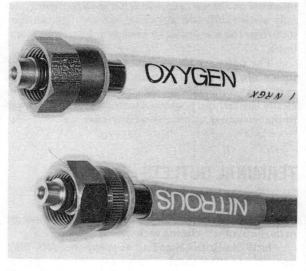

Figure 3.10 Nut and probe (nipple) connection to an anaesthetic machine. Note the different sizes of shoulders of the male probes (nipples) for the different gases.

coloured sheath at each end. Several accidents, some resulting in fatalities, have been caused by the connection, or reconnection, of the probe for one gas at the upstream end of such a hose, but with the socket or union for another at the downstream end.

The incidence of such accidents should be reduced by the current practice of most manufacturers, which is:

- To produce hoses for the different gas services, complete with the appropriate connections, in different factories or different areas of one factory. Furthermore, it is now a recommended practice that a damaged hose should not be repaired on site but should be returned in its entirety to the manufacturer in exchange for a factory-made service replacement.
- To use characteristically coloured tubing for each gas. The development of such self-identifying tubing was unfortunately delayed by the difficulties involved in manufacturing it with the necessary antistatic (electrically conductive) properties.

The Non-interchangeable Screw-Threaded Connection

To ensure that the gas services are attached correctly to the anaesthetic machine, each hose is fitted with a unique connector. This takes the form of a nut and a probe (nipple) (Fig. 3.10). The probe has a unique profile for each gas supply and fits only the union on the anaesthetic machine for that gas and hence is *non-interchangeable*.

The nut has the same diameter and thread (in the UK) for all the gas services but can be attached to the anaesthetic machine only when the probe is correctly engaged. The term 'non-interchangeable screw-threaded connection' is ambiguous as it can give the impression that the screw threads are different and cause the unique fit, which is untrue.

The connections between the hose and fittings must be secure and tamper-proof. Both the Schrader and NIST probes have serrated spigots, which are pushed into the ends of the hosepipe. To prevent their working loose, a stainless steel sleeve (ferrule) is placed on the outside of the hosepipe and spigot and compressed (crimped) by a 30-ton press. The ferrule is sufficiently robust to defy all but the most determined attempts at removal as well as compressing the hosepipe onto the spigot with such force that if an attempt were made to pull the two apart, the hose would stretch and break before the components separated.

TESTS AND CHECKS FOR MGPS

- Anaesthetists should be held responsible for checking only that part of the MGPS system between the terminal outlet and the patient. They should be able to take for granted the quality and unfailing supply of gases.

- Quality control is usually considered to be the province of the hospital pharmacist, who should order, or make, tests to confirm the identity of the gas, its purity and composition, and freedom from contaminants, including solid particulate matter. Compressed air should also be examined for water vapour and oil mist. The pharmacist is usually responsible for maintaining adequate supplies of cylinders.
- The engineering department is responsible for organizing both planned preventive maintenance and emergency repairs.
- Designated theatre staff are usually responsible for changing cylinders and holding a store of portable oxygen cylinders with flowmeters and suction equipment for use in emergencies or during shutdown for maintenance and alterations.

- The anaesthetist is responsible for the correct insertion of the pipeline probes and any necessary adjustments. A fuller description of 'cockpit drill' is to be found in Appendix IV.
- The supplement to HTM 2022, which should be consulted for further details, describes a 'permit to work' system. Essentially this is a code of practice for repairs and preventive maintenance on the MGPS system in which the engineer discusses with the appropriate people the nature of the work to be done and ensures that independent services for medical gases such as oxygen and vacuum may be made available as required. The 'permit to work' document (Fig. 3.11) with no less than six parts to be completed (depending on the degree of hazard) may at first seem to be yet another proliferation of the already burdensome paperwork in hospitals. It does, however, increase safety and improve the relationships between departments.

HOSPITAL ....   PERMIT: 0789

PERMIT TO WORK FOR PIPED MEDICAL GASES

System to be isolated   OXYGEN: N₂O: VACUUM: ENTONOX: MEDICAL AIR: ....
Delete as necessary.

PART 1   The piped medical gas system indicated above, supplying the following area,

....

may be taken out of service without hazard to patients
From ....   AM/PM on ....   date
until ....   AM/PM on ....   date
Signed ....   Medical/Nursing Officer ....   date .... time am/pm

---

PART 2   The piped medical gas system indicated above is isolated as follows at:-

The following work ONLY shall be carried out:-

Other associated Permits to Work in use are (a) Number .... issued to .... date ....
                                              (b) Number .... issued to .... date ....

Signed Authorized Person ....   date .... time .... am/pm

---

PART 3   **I accept responsibility** for carrying out the work detailed in PART 2.

No attempt will be made by me or any person under my control to work on any other part of the installation. Should the work transpire to exceed that indicated in Part 2, I will advise the Authorized Person **IMMEDIATELY**.

Signed Competent Person ....   date .... time .... am/pm

---

PART 4   I declare that:-   * this permit to work is cancelled;
                                  * the work described in Part 2 has been completed;
                                  * all modifications have been incorporated on Drawing No. ....
* delete if inapplicable   * the tests initialled overleaf have been carried out;
                                  * all valve keys have been returned;
                                  * the system is safe for use by patients

Signed Authorized Person ....   date .... time .... am/pm

---

Figure 3.11 A 'permit to work' form. (Continued overleaf.)

PART 5   I have been advised by the Authorized Person named in PART 4 that the system named above is now available for use.

Signed .... Medical/Nursing Officer .... date .... time .... am/pm

I acknowledge receipt of the following valve keys:-

Signed Competent Person .... date .... time .... am/pm

I acknowledge return of the following valve keys:-

Signed Authorized Person .... date .... time .... am/pm

I declare that in conjunction with the work detailed in PART 2, the following tests and/or procedures were carried out:-

Test	Initials	Date
Valve Tightness		
Pipeline Pressure Tests		
Anti-confusion Tests		
Flow Rate Tests		
Delivery Pressure		
Alarm Test		
Cleaning Procedure		
Purging Procedure		
Purity Test		
Manifold Changeover		
Relief Valve Operation		

Signed Authorized Person .... date .... time .... am/pm

Figure 3.11   A 'permit to work' form (continued).

FURTHER READING

BOC (1990) *Gas Safe – Gas Safe – in the Hospital. A Guide to the Safe Use of Medical Gas Cylinders*. Guildford, Surrey: BOC Ltd.

Brancroft ME, du Moulin GC, Hedley-Whyte J (1980) The hazards of hospital bulk oxygen delivery systems. *Anesthesiology* 52: 504–510.

British Standards Institution (1984) *Terminal Units, Hose Assemblies and their Connectors for Use with Medical Gas Pipeline Systems*, BS 5682. Milton Keynes, Bucks, UK: British Standards Institution.

Grant WJ (1978) *Medical Gases: Their Properties and use*. Aylesbury: HM&M.

Howell RSC (1980) Piped medical gas and vacuum systems. *Anaesthesia* 35: 676–698.

HTM 2022 (1994) *Medical Gas Pipeline Services*. London: HMSO.

HTM 2022 (1994 Suppl.) *Permit to Work Systems*. London: HMSO.

International Standards Organization (1989) *Low Pressure Flexible Connecting Assemblies (Hose Assemblies) for Use with Medical Gas Systems*, ISO 5359, 1st edn. Geneva: ISO.

International Standards Organization (1990). *Terminal Units for Use in Medical Gas Pipeline Systems*, ISO 9170, 1st edn. Geneva: ISO.

Jones PE (1974) Some observations on nitrous oxide cylinders during emptying. *British Journal of Anaesthesia* 46: 534–538.

— 4 —

MEASUREMENT OF GAS FLOW AND PRESSURE

Contents

INTRODUCTION

Before discussing the design of modern anaesthetic equipment, this chapter will introduce the basic building blocks of any system where accurate measurement and control of gas flows is concerned. Gases *flow* between two points of unequal *pressure*, from a higher pressure to a lower one.

FORCE AND PRESSURE

It is important to understand the terms force and pressure.

Force causes an object to move in a certain direction. The amount of force does not vary with the area over which it is exerted. The unit of force is the *newton*. One newton causes a mass of 1 kg to accelerate by 1 metre per second per second (1 m/s²). Other units are the kilogram-force (kgf) and the pound-force (1bf), a thrust of 1 kg and 1 lb, respectively.

Fluid pressure is exerted in all directions and is a measure of force *per unit area*, i.e.

$$\text{Pressure} = \frac{\text{Force}}{\text{Area}}$$

Hydrodynamic pressure (in a fluid) is exerted in all directions. Consider the hypodermic syringe. The user exerts a force on the plunger in one particular direction. The pressure of the fluid in the syringe is exerted in all directions, and if there were a leak in the barrel of the syringe, the liquid would squirt out sideways (Fig. 4.1). If a wide-bore syringe is used, the same force exerted by the thumb acts over a large area and so the pressure in the syringe is lower than it would be if the same force were exerted on the plunger of a narrower bore syringe.

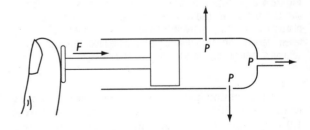

Figure 4.1 When the user exerts a force *F* on the plunger of an intravenous syringe, it is applied in one direction only, but the resulting fluid pressure *P* is exerted in all directions.

Pressure and Partial Pressure

The air in which we live exerts a pressure. At the surface of the earth, this *atmospheric* pressure is due to the influence of gravity on the mass of air supported, as may be demonstrated as follows.

A long transparent tube, closed at one end, is filled with mercury and then inverted so that its open end rests in a reservoir of mercury, as shown in Fig. 4.2. The column of mercury falls until its meniscus is about 760 mm above the level in the reservoir. Above the meniscus is a vacuum (or near vacuum). The atmospheric pressure acting on the reservoir supports a column of mercury 760 mm high and is said to be 760 mmHg (or 760 Torr).

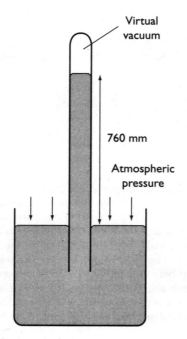

Figure 4.2 A simple barometer. The long tube is closed at the top and, although it was filled with mercury before being inverted and placed in the mercury reservoir, the mercury level in the tube has fallen, leaving a virtual vacuum at the top of the tube. The height of the column of mercury indicates the atmospheric pressure.

If the column had a cross-sectional area of 1 cm², it would weigh 1033 g, so the pressure can be said to be 1.033 kg/cm². The average atmospheric (barometric) pressure at sea level is therefore 1033 kg/cm² = 15 psi = 1.01×10^5 newtons/m² (pascals) = 1 bar = 1000 millibars.

Partial Pressure

As already stated, the pressure (or partial pressure) of a gas is the result of energy expended by its molecules impinging on its confines, and if two or more gases are mixed the total pressure is the sum of all the partial pressures measured as if they were acting independently of each other.

If the pressure of a mixture of two gases is 760 mmHg, the partial pressures of each of the two gases added together equals 760 mmHg. If, for simplicity, we consider that air contains 20% oxygen and 80% nitrogen, then the partial pressures (disregarding other gases and water vapour) and the barometric pressure equals 760 mmHg (152 mmHg + 608 mmHg).

As the altitude above sea level increases, the barometric pressure decreases because for each unit of area a shorter column of air is being supported. The relationship between altitude and average barometric pressure is shown in Fig. 4.3.

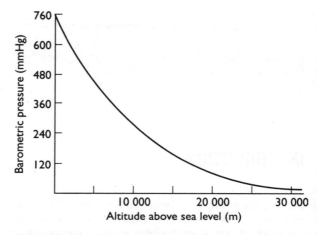

Figure 4.3 The relationship between barometric pressure and altitude above sea level.

When treating patients at high altitudes, a larger percentage of oxygen in the inspired gas mixture is required to maintain the same partial pressure, and it is the partial pressure rather than the percentage of oxygen that is important (refer to the oxygen dissociation curve). The relationship between altitude and the partial pressure of the components of the atmosphere is shown in Fig. 4.4.

Direct Methods of Measuring Pressure

Simple Manometer

Figure 4.5 shows the principle of a simple manometer, which is a U-tube partially filled with liquid, in this case water. A gas at pressure P has been applied to end A of the tube and end B is open. The pressure P causes the water to be pushed across to the opposite limb of the tube. At a the water level has been depressed by 5 cm from its former position and at b it has been raised by 5 cm. The pressure P is therefore 10 cm of water. If the U-tube were filled with mercury, the pressure would be expressed in millimetres of mercury (Torr).

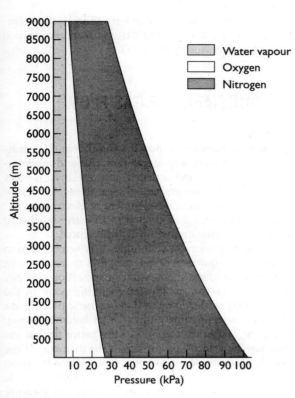

Figure 4.4 Variation with altitude of components of inspired air. Saturation with water vapour by upper airways is assumed.

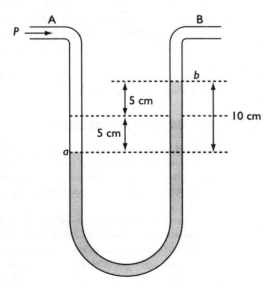

Figure 4.5 A simple manometer. A pressure *P* is applied at A. This causes a depression of the fluid level at *a* and a corresponding rise of the fluid level at *b*. In this case the tube is filled with water and the pressure is 10 cm of water. (See also p. 269.)

Pressure Gauges

There are basically two common types of mechanical pressure gauge: the *Bourdon* gauge and the *aneroid* gauge.

As shown in Fig. 4.6, the Bourdon gauge consists of a curved and flattened tube, elliptical in section. When pressure is applied to it, the tube expands and the curvature is partially straightened out. This movement is translated via levers, gear-train or a rack and pinion mechanism to movement of the dial pointer. The inlet to the gauge is fitted with a constriction to prevent sudden surges of pressure damaging the mechanism. The Bourdon pressure gauge is:

- robust;
- inexpensive;
- able to indicate and withstand high pressures;
- low precision;
- used to indicate cylinder and pipeline pressures.

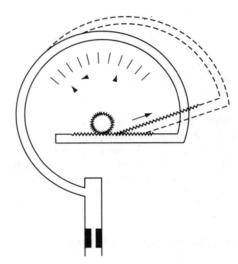

Figure 4.6 The principle of the Bourdon tube pressure gauge. Note the constriction at the inlet.

Figure 4.7 shows a typical low-pressure aneroid gauge. This consists of a small flexible capsule which may be made of metal alloy, synthetic rubber or a plastic material. This capsule expands and contracts with an increase or decrease in pressure. Any change in the size of the capsule is indicated by a pointer on a scale calibrated in pressure. The aneroid pressure gauge is:

- delicate;
- sensitive;
- comparatively expensive;
- able to indicate low pressures;
- used for airway pressure and blood pressure measurement.

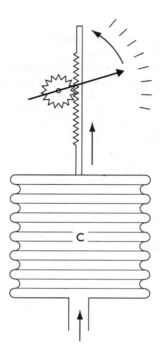

Figure 4.7 A low-pressure aneroid gauge. C, low-pressure chamber.

Pressure Transducers

Electronic devices may measure pressure, or changes in pressure, by means of a transducer, which converts the pressure into electrical units. Often, the transducer consists of a semiconductor, the shape of which is deformed by the application of pressure, thus altering its electrical conductivity.

Calibration of Pressure Gauges

Pressure gauges for high pressures are usually calibrated in psi, kg/cm², atmospheres (1 atm = 15 psi = 1.03 kg/cm²), kPa or bar. They are normally calibrated in *gauge pressure*, i.e. the pressure *above atmospheric pressure*. In this case 'g' may be written after the pressure.

In some circumstances gauges are calibrated in *absolute* pressure (P_{abs}). In such a case a pressure gauge open to the air would indicate a pressure of 15 psi or 1 atm. Examples are the barometer and gauges used in connection with hyperbaric oxygen therapy. Where it is not stated which of these units is used, as in this book, it is usually understood that gauge pressures are being described. It is important to make this distinction in apparatus such as hyperbaric oxygen equipment, where a gauge pressure of, say, 2 atm may be used, which equals an absolute pressure of 3 atm. This is discussed in Chapter 30. For lower pressures, gauges are often calibrated in millimetres of mercury (mmHg) or centi-

metres of water (cmH_2O). The term 'Torr' is now commonly used in place of millimetres of mercury (normal atmospheric pressure = 760 Torr).

MEASUREMENT OF GAS FLOW

The measurement of gas flow is a complex and fascinating subject. Knowledge of gas flow rate and measurement of inhaled and exhaled gas volumes is very important to the safe practice of anaesthesia. In view of the current and future development of electronic measurement and control of gas flow in anaesthesia, a broad survey of flow measurement will be presented.

Flow measurement techniques may be classified in several ways. Flowmeters may respond to gas velocity, volumetric flow, gas momentum or mass flow. *Velocity meters* measure the gas flow at a specific point in the cross-section of the flow and in anaesthetic practice are calibrated to approximate to the total volume flowing. *Volumetric flowmeters* respond to the entire flow of gas whatever the velocity profile across the diameter of the tube. An example of a volumetric flowmeter is the positive-displacement meter used for measuring domestic gas consumption, also used in medicine to measure exhaled minute volume. *Differential pressure flowmeters* respond to the momentum of the moving gas. *Mass flowmeters* measure directly the total mass of gas passing during a period of time.

There are many thousands of designs of flow-metering devices but those relevant to gas flow in anaesthesia may be classified as follows: differential pressure, variable area, inferential, positive-displacement, anemometric, ultrasonic and fluidic. The choice of flow measurement technique depends, in the main, upon the characteristics required, as shown in Table 4.1.

Differential Pressure Flowmeters

The differential pressure flowmeter is very versatile and probably the most common flowmeter used for industrial flow measurement. It finds application in anaesthesia both for machine gas flow and respiratory gas flow measurement.

A constant resistance is applied to the total gas flow and the pressure drop across the resistance is measured with a pressure gauge, manometer or, for very rapid response to changes in flow rate, an electronic pressure transducer. The resistance may be tubular, when the flow rate is proportional to the differential pressure; an orifice, in which case the pressure drop is proportional to the square of the flow rate; or a venturi (Fig. 4.8).

Table 4.1 Characteristics of flow and volume measurement in anaesthesia

Gas flow *into* breathing system
Continuous flow
Dry gas
Resistance to flow irrelevant
Slow response to change in flow rate
Single or mixed gases
Gas flow and volume *within* breathing system*
Intermittent flow
Wide range of flow rates
Rapid response
Very low resistance to flow
Mixed gas composition
High humidity
Integration of flow, breath by breath

* NB *Exhaled* volumes should *always* be measured rather than inspiratory volumes, as then the anaesthetist always has an indication that *at least this volume* has been exhaled despite any leaks in the system.

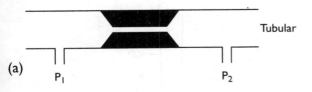

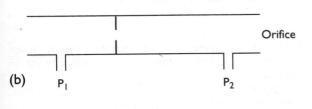

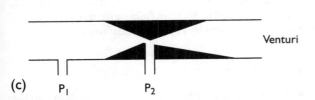

Figure 4.8 Differential pressure flowmeters. P_1, P_2, differential pressures.

The Fleisch pneumotachograph is a constant orifice differential pressure flowmeter designed to have a very low resistance to flow and a fast response rate

necessary for the measurement of respiratory gas flows (Fig. 4.9). A linear flow resistance is provided by a bundle of small-bore parallel tubes in the gas pathway. Its accuracy, sensitivity and response rate are dependent on the quality of the differential pressure transducer. The Fleisch screen is electrically heated to prevent water condensation affecting the calibration.

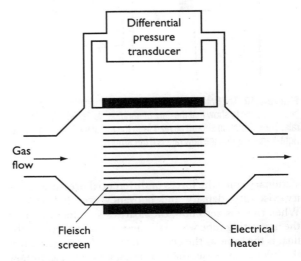

Figure 4.9 Fleisch pneumotachograph.

In the venturi flowmeter, the gas is passed through a narrowed portion of tubing. The gas accelerates in that portion and the pressure is less than in the broader part of the tube. The pressure difference is approximately proportional to the square of the flow rate and thus may be used to indicate flow.

Variable-Area Constant Differential Pressure Flowmeters

In the variable-area constant differential pressure flowmeter the size of the orifice varies with flow rate. The variation in size of the orifice maintains a constant pressure differential, and gives the indication of the flow rate. The most common constant pressure variable-area flowmeter in anaesthetic practice is the Rotameter. Strictly speaking, Rotameter is the trade name used by one manufacturer, Elliot Automation, but it has become synonymous with this type of flowmeter. The Rotameter is the final development in a line of earlier constant-pressure flowmeters (Coxeter, Heidbrink, McKesson, Connel) that have been used in anaesthesia.

The Rotameter (Fig. 4.10) consists of a vertical tapered metering tube and a float which is free to move up and down in it. For a given flow rate, the float remains

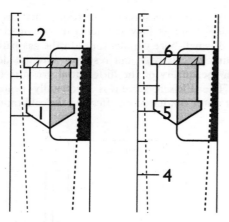

Figure 4.10 The Rotameter. In each case a portion of the tube has been cut away to show that the gap, or annulus, varies with the flow rate. The calibration should be read from the top of the float (e.g. in the right-hand diagram the flow rate is 6 litres/min).

stationary since the forces of differential pressure, gravity, viscosity, density and buoyancy are all balanced. When there is zero flow, the float rests at the bottom of the measuring tube where the maximum diameter of the float is the same as the bore of the tube. When gas enters the inlet at the base, the float rises, allowing gas to flow through the annular space between the float and the wall of the tube. The float moves up or down in proportion to the increase or decrease in the gas flow rate such that the pressure drop across the float remains constant, higher flows requiring a larger annular area than lower flows. At low flow rates, flow is a function of viscosity because the comparatively longer and narrower annulus behaves like a tube. With higher flow rates, the annulus is shorter and wider and behaves like an orifice and is therefore density dependent. The float has oblique notches cut in the rim so that it rotates freely in the middle of the gas stream and should normally not touch the walls of the tube. There is therefore no tendency for it to stick unless the Rotameter is out of the vertical plane. The taper of the bore of the Rotameter tube may be constructed so that it varies in order to elongate part of the scale, as shown in Fig. 4.11. This has the advantage that, even with a short tube, low flows may be measured accurately, while high flows are also indicated.

Calibration of Rotameters

Rotameters may be calibrated with great accuracy. Flowmeter tubes are calibrated individually, with their floats, at a specific pressure and temperature. Should there be any back-pressure, for example when a minute volume divider ventilator is used, the density of the gas is increased and therefore the calibrations become

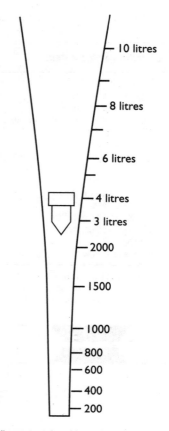

Figure 4.11 A flowmeter tube with varying taper to give an elongated scale at lower flow rates but allowing calibration for high flow rates also.

inaccurate. Changes in temperature, except when extreme, cause inaccuracies that are insignificant in clinical practice.

Flowmeters should be read from the top of the float. They are not calibrated from zero to the top of the scale, but from the lowest accurate point, and this is the lowest mark on the scale. Readings by extrapolation below this mark should not be attempted. A typical tube may be calibrated from 100 to 8000 ml/min, with the lower part of the scale elongated by a more gradual taper.

Causes of Inaccuracy in Rotameters

- *Tube not vertical.* The orifice between the float and the tube is an annulus of complex shape (Fig. 4.12). If the tube is not vertical, the shape of the annulus becomes asymmetrical and at certain flow rates there is a significant variation in the proportion of the orificial and tubular elements of the resistance, and therefore inaccuracies occur. If the flowmeter is grossly out of the vertical position, then the float may come into contact

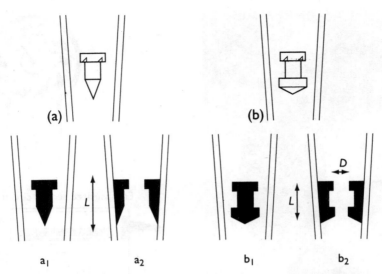

Figure 4.12 The annulus of flowmeter floats; (a) and (b) are two different types of float, a_1 and b_1 show the space around them; a_2 and b_2 show how the effective tubular and orificial elements of these annuli differ. Note that this is a two-dimensional representation of a three-dimensional situation. L, length of tube or orifice; D, diameter of bore of tube or orifice.

with the wall of the tube and the resulting friction will cause even greater inaccuracy.

- *Static electricity.* The float may also stick to the side of the tube as a result of static electricity, particularly in very dry atmospheres. Moist air can discharge static from the outside of the tube. The effects of static may be reduced by spraying the outside of the tube with an antistatic agent. Improvements may also be made by coating the inside of the tube with a transparently thin layer of a conductor such as gold.
- *Dirt.* Dirt on the tube or float may also cause sticking, especially in the case of nitrous oxide. Even if they do not cause sticking, particles of dirt either on the float or on the inner wall of the tube can change the effective diameter of the annulus and therefore cause an inaccurate reading.
- In some older machines, the wire stop at the upper limit of the Rotameter was shaped in such a way that the float could become impaled upon it. When the gas supply is turned off or fails, the float may remain at the top of the tube and give the impression that there is still a high rate of flow.
- Some flowmeters of the Rotameter type are so constructed that the top of the tube is hidden behind the bezel, so that accidental high flow rates of carbon dioxide may not be observed.

Causes of Failure of Rotameters

On a number of occasions patients have suffered oxygen deprivation because of leakage from a cracked or broken flowmeter tube in a flowmeter block arranged so that the oxygen is at the upstream end. If, for example, the carbon dioxide tube is broken, the force of the nitrous oxide flow will tend to cause a much higher proportion of oxygen than nitrous oxide to leak out of the fractured tube. This is prevented by making sure that the oxygen is the last gas to enter the mixed gas flow (*see* Fig. 6.18, p. 85). In fact, ISO 5358 requires that '. . . the oxygen shall be delivered downstream of all other gases . . .'.

Inferential Flowmeters

The most common example of the inferential type of flowmeter in anaesthetic practice is the Wright's respirometer (Fig. 4.13) which is, in fact, an integrating flowmeter since it indicates volume rather than flow rate.

The Wright's respirometer is a turbine flowmeter, the principle of which is shown in Fig. 4.14. Exhaled gas is induced to flow around the stator, which has a series of tangential slits that cause a circular motion of the gas flow that produces rotation of the vane. In the mechanical version, the rate of rotation of the vane is reduced by a gear-train so that a single revolution of the appropriate hand on the dial indicates 1 litre of gas having passed through the device. One of the problems of measuring exhaled gases is that they contain water vapour, which condenses on the internal parts of the respirometer. The mechanical version of the Wright's respirometer has a mercury seal interposed between the turbine and the

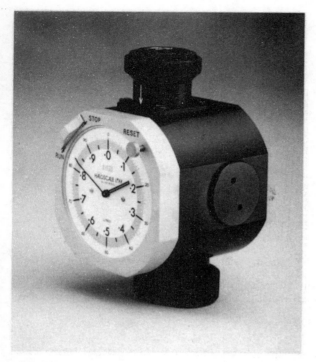

Figure 4.13 Inferential type flowmeter, colloquially referred to as the Wright's respirometer.

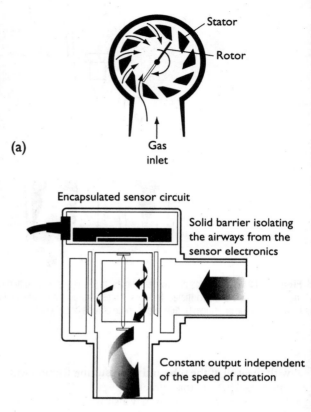

(a)

(b)

Figure 4.14 (a) Plan view of the Wright's respirometer; (b) side view of the electronic version of Wright's respirometer.

gear-train, to prevent water vapour condensing and the gears becoming corroded. It is also constructed so that only gases entering by the radial port cause movement of the vane, so that if it were mounted in a to-and-fro part of the breathing system, as when attached to a catheter mount, only gases passing in one direction would be measured.

Modern versions of the Wright's respirometer (Fig. 4.14b) overcome the water vapour and other problems by doing away with the gear-train and mechanical display and replacing them by detection of the rotation of the vane by means of a light source and photodetector or a Hall effect detector. The Hall effect detector is a semiconductor device that responds to very small changes in a magnetic field. These pulses are then converted electronically into indications of tidal and minute volume. Another advantage of these electronic versions is that alarms for minimum volumes and respiratory rate may be incorporated.

The Wright's respirometer is most accurate at 'normal' gas flow rates; its accuracy decreases at very low and also at very high flow rates.

Positive-displacement Flowmeters

Positive-displacement flowmeters are mechanical meters that measure total volumetric flow over the entire diameter of the pipe through which the gas is flowing. Two types of positive-displacement flowmeters are used in anaesthesia, namely the intermeshing figure-of-eight rotors type and, less commonly, the diaphragm meter.

The Dräger volumeter (Fig. 4.15) consists of a pair of intermeshing rotors connected via a gear-train to an analogue scale, as is the case with the Wright's respirometer. Again, its accuracy and susceptibility to water vapour are improved by using an electronic transducer rather than the gear-train.

The diaphragm or bellows flowmeter is a simple, inexpensive and reliable meter of moderate accuracy, widely used as a domestic gas meter. It will not be described in detail here as it finds application mainly in physiological research for measuring minute volume.

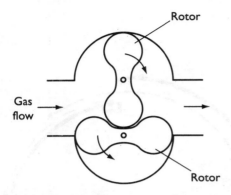

Figure 4.15 Principle of the Dräger volumeter.

Anemometry

Anemometers measure gas velocity at a given point, and do not necessarily give the actual total flow rate along the tube. For this reason they are sometimes referred to as insertion meters, especially when the point of velocity measurement is very small compared with the total cross-section of the tube.

The *hot-wire anemometer* is the only type of anemometer used in anaesthetic practice and has only recently been introduced. This is because it is dangerous to use it in the presence of flammable anaesthetic agents. An electrically heated element in the form of a very fine resistance wire, a thin metallic film or a thermistor is placed within the stream of gas. The passing gas tends to cool the element, and the higher the flow rate the greater the cooling; the change in temperature causes a change in electrical resistance. If a constant current is used to heat the element, then the voltage across the element will vary inversely with flow rate. The finer the element, the faster the response time. A hot-wire anemometer transducer is very small, lightweight and easy to sterilize or make disposable. It has a very low resistance to gas flow. However, the wire may be very delicate and there is a need for fairly frequent calibration.

Fluidic Flowmeters

Fluidic flowmeters rely on some dynamic instability in the gas which generates an oscillation whose frequency is proportional to the flow rate.

Ohmeda uses a flowmeter in its current machines that uses a series of fixed vanes to induce a swirl that is detected by causing the rotation of a single vane, as shown in Fig. 4.16. The rotation of the vane is sensed optically.

The vortex-shedding flowmeter has a very low resistance to gas flow and no moving parts. A laminar flow of gas is passed along a smooth-bore tube that has a bluff

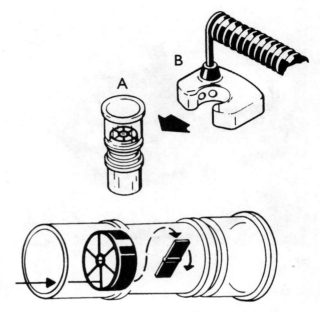

Figure 4.16 Sensor components for the Ohmeda respiratory volume monitor. This sensor assembly is composed of two parts: A, cartridge; and B, optical sensor clip.

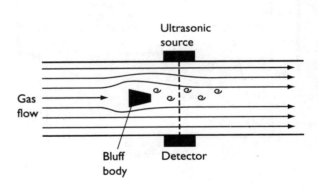

Figure 4.17 Vortex shedding flow transducer.

body causing a very small obstruction. Vortices are generated when the gas hits the bluff body (Fig. 4.17). The frequency of shedding is linearly proportional to the flow rate. In anaesthetic practice, the vortices are detected by their interruption of a narrow ultrasonic beam.

Ultrasonic Flowmeters

The term ultrasonic indicates that 'sound' above the reception capability of the human ear is the physical principle of operation. Frequencies used are usually over 1 MHz. There are two ways of measuring flow

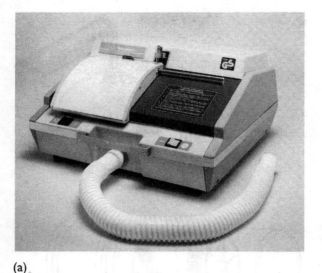

(a)

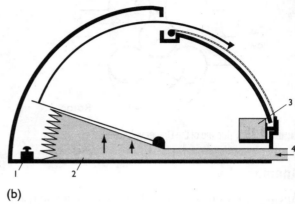

(b)

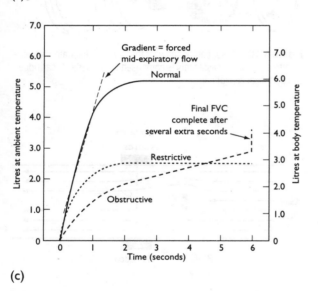

(c)

Figure 4.18 (a) The Vitalograph Bellows spirometer. (b) Exhaled breath direct from the patient's mouth passes through the inlet (4) causing the bellows (2) to inflate and the stylus to mark the paper proportional to the exhaled volume. As the bellows lift off the switch (1), the paper carriage is moved horizontally by the motor (3) at a constant rate so that exhaled volume is recorded against time. Typical tracings are shown in (c).

ultrasonically. The Doppler principle is not applicable to respiratory gas flow measurement as the technique requires particulate impurities to be present in the gas to reflect the 'sound'; Doppler flowmetering is very successful in measuring liquid flow as most liquids contain minute bubbles and blood contains cells. Ultrasound can be used to measure gas flow by using the 'time-of-flight' or 'transit time' principle. Sound takes a finite time to travel through a gaseous medium. If short pulses of ultrasound are injected into a gas flow and then detected at a fixed distance from the source, the time taken will be altered proportionately with the rate of gas flow. This type of flowmeter has a low resistance to flow, very fast response, and is easily sterilized. However, it is very expensive.

Spirometers

Spirometer is a term used to describe devices that are used to measure exhaled tidal volumes and flow rates. The most common single-breath spirometer in clinical use is manufactured by Vitalograph and is shown in Fig. 4.18. Exhaled gas from the patient causes a lightweight bellows to be filled, causing a stylus to move across a chart at the same time as the chart is moved at a constant speed at right angles to the stylus movement. Thus a chart of exhaled volume against time is plotted from which volumes and flow rates may be deduced.

There are now available several inexpensive, pocket-sized 'spirometers' that use microprocessor techniques to measure FEV (forced expiratory volume), FEV_1

(forced expiratory volume in 1 s) and VC (vital capacity), using differential pressure flow transducers. These devices are especially useful for quick preoperative assessment.

Calibrated bellows may also be used to measure exhaled gas volume. A very lightweight bellows is inflated against gravity by the gas exhaled from the patient. These are usually part of the ventilator and may be inaccurate because of leaks in the breathing attachment or around the endotracheal cuff, and also because of the comparatively enormous compliant volume in the expiratory limb of some ventilators.

FURTHER READING

Clutton-Brock TH, Hutton P (1994) Gas pressure, volume and flow measurement. In: *Monitoring in Anaesthesia and Intensive Care*. London: WB Saunders.

Hayward AJT (1979) *Flowmeters*. London: Macmillan.

— 5 —

VAPORIZERS

Contents

INTRODUCTION

Many inhalational anaesthetic agents are liquids under normal storage conditions and need to be in a vapour form before they can be administered to a patient. In order that they may be administered safely, an understanding of the phenomenon of vaporization is required.

LAWS OF VAPORIZATION

Molecules of a liquid have a mutual attraction for each other (a phenomenon called *cohesion*) which is sufficiently great for them to remain in close proximity. However, they also possess varying levels of kinetic energy and are in constant motion, colliding with each other. If the liquid has a surface exposed to air or other gases, or to a vacuum, some molecules with a high kinetic energy will escape from this surface. This is the process of *evaporation* or *vaporization*. The molecules from the liquid which exist in the gaseous phase are known collectively as a *vapour*. This vapour exerts a pressure on its surroundings which is known as *vapour pressure*. If the space above the liquid is enclosed, some of the molecules that have escaped while moving freely in the gaseous state will collide with the surface of the liquid and

re-enter it. Eventually, there will occur an equilibrium in which the number of molecules re-entering the liquid equals the number leaving it. At this stage the vapour pressure is at a maximum for the temperature of the liquid and is called *saturated vapour pressure* (SVP).

Factors Affecting Vaporization of a Liquid

These include:

Temperature

Vaporization is *increased* if the temperature of the liquid is raised, since more molecules will have been given sufficient kinetic energy to escape. Figure 5.1 shows the vapour pressure curves of volatile anaesthetic agents (as well as water) and shows how they vary with temperature. If the liquid is heated, a point is reached at which the SVP becomes equal to ambient atmospheric pressure. Vaporization now occurs not only at the surface of the liquid but also in the bubbles that develop within its substance. The liquid is *boiling* and this temperature is its *boiling point*.

The boiling point of a liquid may therefore vary with *atmospheric pressure*. At high altitudes (where the air is 'thinner' and has a lower ambient pressure) there is a significant depression of the boiling point. This may render the use of agents with low boiling points such as ether difficult. Figure 5.2 shows the depression of the

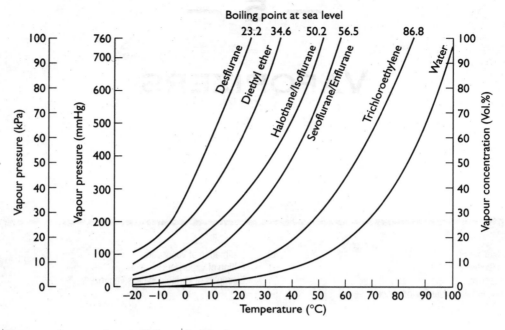

Figure 5.1 Vapour pressure curves for anaesthetic agents and water vapour.

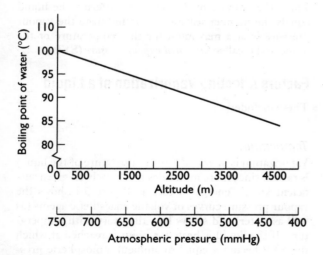

Figure 5.2 Variation of boiling point of water with atmospheric pressure or altitude.

boiling point for water with change in atmospheric pressure.

Volatility

The ease at which a liquid vaporizes depends not only on its temperature but also on its volatility. A more volatile liquid has weaker cohesive forces between its molecules so that they require less energy (i.e. a lower temperature) to vaporize (see Fig. 5.1).

The Surface Area of the Liquid

The greater the surface area of the liquid, the more space there is for molecules to leave the liquid. Vaporization is therefore proportional to the surface area of the liquid.

Removal of Vapour from the Vicinity of Liquid

If the container holding the liquid is not closed, molecules will still leave the liquid and some will escape into the atmosphere. Some, however, will collide with adjacent vapour molecules and be bounced back into the liquid. If a gas is passed across the surface of the liquid, vapour will be removed more quickly allowing fresh vapour to form. Vaporization is therefore proportional to gas flow (convection) across the surface of the liquid (*provided the temperature of the latter remains constant*).

N.B. A liquid at a given temperature has a mixture of molecules with varying energies. Molecules entering the vapour phase tend to be the ones with the highest energy (the hottest). The remaining liquid molecules have a lower average kinetic energy (and therefore a lower temperature). Fewer molecules remain with sufficient energy to form a vapour and so vaporization decreases.

VAPORIZING SYSTEMS

The various liquids that possess anaesthetic properties are too potent to be used as pure vapours and so are diluted in a carrier gas such as air and/or oxygen, or nitrous oxide and oxygen. The device that allows vaporization of the liquid anaesthetic agent and its subsequent admixture with a carrier gas for administration to a patient is called a *vaporizer*.

Historically, the early vaporizers were constructed of a wire frame that was placed over a patient's nose and mouth (Schimmelbusch mask). The frame was covered in gauze to provide a sufficient surface area which was then impregnated with anaesthetic liquid. When the patient inhaled, air passed through the gauze and removed vapour that was forming. The concentration could be altered by increasing or reducing the rate at which the liquid agent was added to the gauze to replace that which had been vaporized. These devices produced unknown quantities of anaesthetic vapour because of:

- Variable working temperatures: the vaporizer (the gauze and liquid) cooled rapidly, as vaporization took place.
- Variable surface area: the vaporizing surface diminished as ice from exhaled water vapour formed as crystals in the gauze.
- Variable removal of vapour as the flow rate of the carrier gas (air) varied both with inspiration and depth of anaesthesia.

TYPES OF VAPORIZER

Modern vaporizers are now designed to include features that overcome these problems and so provide a more stable and predictable concentration of anaesthetic vapour. In addition to this, a suitable method of calibrated dilution of the vapour is required as even the least potent of volatile anaesthetic agents is too powerful to be administered as a saturated vapour.

This may be achieved by either:

- Splitting the carrier gas flow so that only a portion passes through the vaporizer. This picks up saturated vapour and then leaves to mix with the remainder of the gas that has gone through a bypass. The final concentration may be altered by varying the splitting ratio between bypass gas and vaporizer gas using an adjustable valve. This type is often referred to as a *variable bypass vaporizer* (Fig. 5.3).
- Alternatively, some vaporizers heat the anaesthetic agent to a temperature above its boiling point (in order

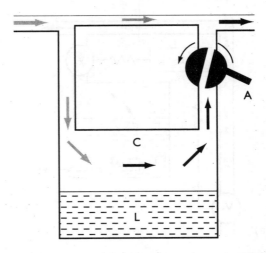

Figure 5.3 A schematic diagram of a variable bypass vaporizer. A, flow splitting valve that can be rotated to alter the relative diameters of the vaporizer and bypass channels and so vary the flows through them; L, liquid; C, vaporizer chamber.

that it may behave as a gas) and which can then be metered into the fresh gas flow (Fig. 5.4a). Similarly, a vaporizer may contain a fine metal sieve that is submerged in the anaesthetic agent and through which a small independent gas supply (normally oxygen) can be made to pass. The minute bubbles produced have a very large surface area and produce a saturated vapour at ambient pressure which can then be passed through a flowmeter into the fresh gas flow (Fig. 5.4b). These types of vaporizer are often referred to as *measured flow vaporizers*.

It should also be taken into account that the various inhalational anaesthetic agents currently available have widely differing potencies and physical properties and hence require vaporizers constructed specifically for each agent. Very potent agents (halothane, enflurane, sevoflurane, isoflurane and desflurane) require vaporizers that can accurately control the concentration of vapour leaving the vaporizer. However, agents such as diethyl ether, with a lower potency, may be used safely with simpler apparatus (if necessary) in which the vapour concentration is not accurately known, since there is less risk of over-dosage.

Variable Bypass Vaporizers

Design Features
Surface area of contact between carrier gas and the liquid
Vaporizers that are required to be very accurate should always present a saturated vapour to the carrier gas across a wide range of flows. To ensure sufficient vaporization at the highest planned flow, a sufficiently large

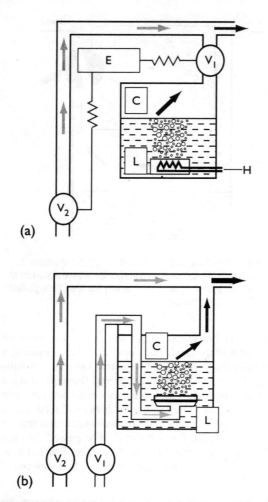

(a)

(b)

Figure 5.4 Schematic diagrams of measured flow vaporizers. (a) H, electric heater; L, liquid anaesthetic agent; C, vaporizer chamber; V_1, V_2, flow control valves; E, electronically controlled proportioning of flows through the valves. (b) L, liquid anaesthetic agent; C, vaporizer chamber; V_1 V_2, flow control valves.

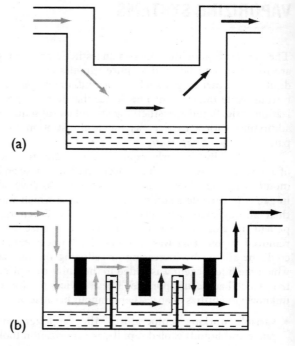

(a)

(b)

Figure 5.5 Vapour pick-up in vaporizers. (a) Carrier gas passing over a small surface area of liquid anaesthetic agent. (b) The surface area for vaporization is increased by porous wicks dipped into the liquid. The carrier gas is also made to pass close to the surface of the liquid by the baffles and thus increasing vapour pick-up.

surface area of liquid should be present. This size is also governed by the *volatility* of the agent used. A highly volatile liquid will require a smaller surface area. The surface area for vaporization of a liquid can be increased by causing it to spread (by capillarity) over a large sheet of porous material, which may be folded in such a way that the carrier gas passes across its entire surface (Fig. 5.5).

Temperature As vaporization progresses, the liquid as well as the vaporizer itself cools, and the quantity of vapour produced decreases. In an attempt to retain the performance of the device, the temperature drop is minimized or prevented by the incorporation of a heat source (heat sink). This normally takes the form of a water bath or substantial metal jacket or even a heating element surrounding the vaporizing liquid. These devices may also control the temperature of the carrier gas entering the vaporizer. Metal jackets and water baths, however, can only transfer a finite quantity of heat and so only minimize the inevitable fall in temperature.

In order to maintain the expected output of the vaporizer when this occurs, a greater proportion of carrier gas is required to pass through the vaporizing chamber in order to collect sufficient vapour molecules. This is achieved by using devices that sense temperature changes (*temperature-compensating devices*, see Fig. 5.6) and which then alter the flow rate through the vaporizer. Two types are commonly used:

- The first (Fig. 5.6a and b) consists of two dissimilar metals or alloys placed back to back (i.e. a bi-metallic strip). The two metals have different rates of expansion and contraction with temperature change so that when this occurs the device bends. It can therefore be used to vary the degree of occlusion in the aperture of a gas channel (usually the bypass) and thus alter the flow rate of carrier gases through it.

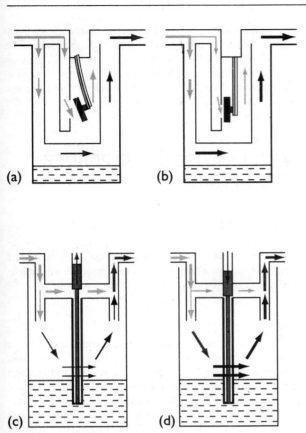

Potency of anaesthetic agent All currently used anaesthetic agents are too potent to be used as saturated vapours at ambient temperatures. They require suitable dilution. Therefore, only a proportion of the gas intended for the patient is diverted into a vaporizer to collect vapour. This amount may be varied to produce the desired concentration by using an adjustable flow-splitting valve. This is a rotary valve incorporated within the vaporizer inlet. It proportions the flow of gas between the vaporizing chamber and the vaporizer bypass system, thus controlling the final vapour composition (i.e. the more gas going through the vaporizer chamber, the greater the amount of vapour leaving the vaporizer). The flow-splitting valve is calibrated in percentage of the vapour in the final gas/vapour composition. However, this valve is accurate only if the vaporizer is temperature-compensated (see below). As both the temperature-compensating mechanism and the flow-splitting valve work by altering resistance through the vaporizer chamber, the devices are dependent upon each other. Therefore, each vaporizer for a designated anaesthetic agent should be individually calibrated at the factory (see below) for that agent and at a specific temperature and flow rate of carrier gas.

As the potency of anaesthetic agents varies widely, the flow splitting ratios must be individually tailored for each agent and vaporizer design. Agents with high potency will require a wide splitting ratio so that a smaller amount of gas passes through the vaporizer. This produces a lower final concentration when mixed with bypass gas.

Figure 5.6 Temperature-compensating devices. (a) The bimetallic strip in a vaporizer bypass operating at ambient temperature. (b) The same device operating at a cooler temperature; the bimetallic strip has moved closer to the inflow increasing the resistance in the bypass and increasing the amount of gas passing through the vaporizing chamber and therefore increasing vapour pick-up. (c) A bimetallic rod that works on a similar principle. The outer jacket is in contact with the vaporizing liquid and is made of an expansile metal (brass). (d) When this contracts (with cooling) it drags the choke on the inner rod into the bypass, increasing the resistance to flow through it.

Volatility The flow splitting ratio must also be adjusted to match the volatility of the agent. For example, at any given temperature, a very volatile agent may produce a higher saturated vapour pressure than a less volatile agent even though they may have similar potencies. The former, however, requires a flow splitting valve with a wider ratio so as to increase the dilution in order to provide a similar concentration. Table 5.1 shows the relative potency and volatility of some liquid anaesthetic agents that influence vaporizer design.

- A second arrangement (Fig. 5.6c and d) has the metals as two concentric rods. The outer one, which is more expansile, is anchored at one end. Subsequent expansion/contraction of the latter causes the asymmetric tip of the inner rod to move within a gas channel and alter its aperture. This movement changes in one plane and hence produces a linear change in gas flow resistance (making calibration easier). The resistance produced by a bi-metallic strip is non-linear.

Heating elements fitted to a vaporizer may be thermostatically controlled and are therefore automatically temperature compensated and do not require the addition of the devices above.

Types of Variable Bypass Vaporizers

Draw-over vaporizers The early vaporizers relied on the patient's respiratory effort to draw gas over the vaporizing surface (hence their name). Unfortunately, draw-over systems are subjected to very variable flow rates, i.e. from 0 to 60 litres/min (the peak inspiratory flow in a hyperventilating adult). At these higher flows the carrier gas usually produces a more rapid dilution of the available vapour resulting in a reduced concentration leaving the vaporizer. Furthermore, the gas pathways must offer very little resistance to flow so as not to compromise the

Table 5.1 Relative potency and volatility of some liquid anaesthetic agents

Agent	Volatility			Potency
	Boiling point (°C) at 100 kPa	SVP at 20°C (kPa)	SVP at 20°C (mmHg)	MAC (vol. %) in 100% O_2
Desflurane	23	88.5	669	6
Diethyl ether	35	57.9	440	19
Isoflurane	48	31.5	240	1.15
Halothane	51	31.9	243	0.76
Enflurane	56	23.1	175	1.68
Sevoflurane	58	21.3	156–170	2

MAC, minimum alveolar concentration
SVP, saturated vapour pressure

patient's inspiratory effort. This restricts the design of the vaporizer components, especially the flow splitting valve (see above) which must have sufficiently wide a bore. It is very difficult to design a flow splitting valve that will work accurately over a wide range of flow rates, i.e. 1–60 litres/min. In a draw–over vaporizer, the valve must present a low flow resistance so that at flows of 60 litres/min (the peak flow in a patient breathing spontaneously) no respiratory embarrassment is caused. However, if the flow across this valve drops to about 4 litres/min, the resistance through the valve will be so low that carrier gas will preferentially pass across the bypass channel rather than through the vaporizing chamber where it has to mix with and then push the 'heavy' vapour out into the attached breathing system. At this flow and below, there is therefore bound to be a marked fall in vaporizer performance.

Plenum vaporizers A vaporizer could be made more accurate if the carrier gas were pressurized to make it as dense as the vapour so that at lower flows it would more readily mix with the latter rather than tend to pass above it in the vaporizing chamber. Furthermore, if a smaller, continuous flow of gas, i.e. 0–15 litres/min were used, there would be a less rapid removal of vapour ensuring that a saturated vapour was present at all times. This would allow the vaporizer to be calibrated very accurately. This type is usually referred to as a *Plenum vaporizer* (plenum being the term that describes a pressurized chamber). The typical flow resistance (2 kPa (22 cm H_2O) at 5 litres/min) found in Plenum vaporizers renders them unsuitable for use as draw-over vaporizers. The high intermittent flow rates in a breathing system generated by a spontaneously breathing patient or a mechanical ventilator are accommodated by siting a reservoir (bag or bellows) downstream, which stores gas and vapour during exhalation.

Flowmeters on an anaesthetic machine are calibrated for use at or around atmospheric pressure. The final design of a Plenum vaporizer therefore develops from a compromise between the high carrier gas pressures required for accurate vapour delivery and the low pressures required to maintain the accuracy of the flowmeters.

FACTORS AFFECTING VAPORIZER PERFORMANCE

Extremes of Temperature
It is obvious that a temperature-compensating mechanism can operate only within a reasonable temperature range. At too low a temperature, vaporization will be low, and it may be uncontrollably high when it is too hot.

Barometric Pressure
Ideally, a vaporizer should also be calibrated at a specific barometric pressure. Strictly speaking, as a saturated vapour is altered only by temperature, one might expect the calibration of a vaporizer to be independent of barometric pressure. However, changes in barometric pressure affect the carrier gas composition passing through the vaporizer, which in turn affect the concentration of vapour in the mixture leaving it. For example, when the barometric pressure is reduced (at altitude) the number of molecules of carrier gas flowing through the vaporizer is reduced. However, the number of vapour molecules collected by the gas in the vaporizing chamber remains unchanged, although these now represent a higher percentage of the total number of molecules leaving the vaporizer. This effect, however, is so small under normal operating conditions that it is inconsequential. However, extremes of pressure may have a significant effect. For example, at very high altitude (low barometric pressure), a very volatile liquid such as ether may boil at ambient temperature. This may render the use of such agents difficult. Figure 5.2 (p. 50) shows the variation of boiling point with atmospheric pressure.

Pumping Effect
When a resistance is applied to the outlet of the anaesthetic machine such as that which occurs when manually assisted or controlled ventilation is used, or with ventilators that are powered by the fresh gas flow (e.g. minute volume divider ventilators), there is an increase in the anaesthetic gas pressure which is transmitted back to the vaporizer. This back-pressure is intermittent or variable. When it occurs, it causes carrier gas within the vaporizer

to be compressed. When the back-pressure is released, the expanding carrier gas, which is saturated with vapour, surges out through both the inlet and outlet of the vaporizer. The gas that leaves the inlet enters the bypass and adds to the vaporizer output to increase the final vapour output. Figure ·5.7 demonstrates the sequence of events.

This effect is now minimized by the fitting of internal compensating mechanisms. It may be achieved either by:

• Increasing the resistance to flow through the vaporizer and bypass so that the carrier gas develops a constant higher pressure within the vaporizer so as to reduce

the pumping effect. (However, the pressure increase due to vaporizer design should be as small as possible as these pressures are transmitted back to the flow-meters, which are calibrated for use at atmospheric pressure.)

• Building an elongated flow passage into either the inlet or outlet of the vaporizer to minimize the effect of surges in pressure (Fig. 5.8). Some vaporizer designs employ both mechanisms. (Neither can be fitted to draw-over vaporizers as they would produce too great a resistance to flow; see below.)

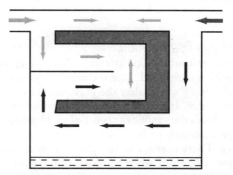

Figure 5.8 Elongation of the inflow channel in a vaporizer preventing saturated vapour reaching the bypass.

Furthermore where Plenum vaporizers are fitted, some anaesthetic machines now incorporate a non-return valve on the end of the back bar so that the back-pressure surges on the vaporizer are reduced. However, pressure still builds up to some extent in the back bar when the non-return valve closes because of higher downstream pressure.

Gas Direction

With some vaporizers, a higher concentration of vapour is given if, by misconnection, the gas is made to pass in the reverse direction.

Liquid Levels

The liquid level within the vaporizing chamber may affect performance. If the vaporizer is overfilled, insufficient exposed surface area of wick may cause a drop in output concentration of vapour. On the other hand, overfilling may result in dangerously high concentrations, owing to spilling of liquid agent into the bypass.

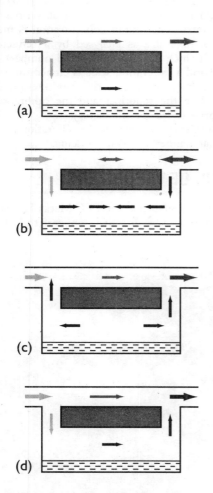

Figure 5.7 (a) Flow through vaporizer with no back pressure. (b) Back-pressure and/or reverse flow causing build-up of carrier gas in the vaporizer chamber. (c) Release of back-pressure causing gas and saturated vapour to escape through the vaporizer inlet and outlet and into the bypass. (d) Anaesthetic vapour in the bypass gas added to that from the vaporizer outlet so increasing the final vapour concentration.

Anaesthetic Agents

The anaesthetic agent halothane contains a stabilizing agent, thymol. This is a waxy substance which, if allowed to accumulate in the vaporizer, clogs the wick, reducing the potential surface area for vaporization. This then reduces the vaporizer performance. Thymol may also 'gum up' the vaporizer making the control knob difficult to adjust, as well as compromising the internal mechanism. The manufacturers therefore advise that the liquid agent be drained off and replenished at intervals of 2 weeks. This advice should be tempered by consideration of economy and the frequency with which the vaporizer is employed.

Carrier Gas Composition

Vaporizer output may be affected when the carrier gas composition is changed. This is due to changes in viscosity and density which alter the performance of the flow splitting valve. Increasing the concentration of nitrous oxide reduces the vapour concentration. However, this is not great enough to be of any importance in clinical practice. There is also a further but temporary decrease in vaporizer output when nitrous oxide concentrations are increased: nitrous oxide dissolves in volatile agents, so that the effective total gas flow through the vaporizer is temporarily reduced.

Stability

Many vaporizers, if tilted, may allow the liquid agent to contaminate the bypass. A fatal outcome has occurred when a vaporizer was accidentally overturned. Liquid halothane was thought to have run into the bypass and into the patient's lungs. Even if the spilled agent found in the breathing system did not reach the patient as a liquid, the vapour concentration could be so high as to have fatal results.

Summary of Vaporizer Performance

Vaporizer performance can thus be affected by:

- temperature (unless the vaporizer includes some compensatory device that minimizes the effect of temperature, such as a heat sink and/or temperature compensator);
- flow rate (all vaporizers are affected to some degree by flow (see performance data supplied with the various vaporizers described). Plenum vaporizers perform better than draw-over vaporizers;
- barometric pressure (minimal effect in clinical practice);

- variable vaporizer working pressures (back-pressure surges);
- liquid levels within the vaporizer;
- movement and tilting of vaporizers (see under specific vaporizers below);
- carrier gas composition;
- stabilizers in the inhalational agent (e.g. thymol).

CALIBRATION OF VAPORIZERS

Vaporizers designed to give an accurate output are individually calibrated prior to leaving the factory. Typically, they are filled with the designated anaesthetic agent and left in a room at a standard temperature (23°C) for 4 h. A blank dial (linked to a computer) is attached and rotated at various carrier gas flow rates. The output concentration is measured using a sample that is analysed by a refractometer. The dial (which has a unique serial number) is then removed and a calibration scale is etched onto it from the information stored on the computer. It is then reattached to the vaporizer and the calibration confirmed prior to leaving the factory.

Vaporizers may also have the calibration confirmed in a similar manner following servicing.

FILLING OF VAPORIZERS

In early systems (such as the TEC Marks 1, 2 and some 3's (Fig. 5.9), a screw-threaded stopper in the filling port

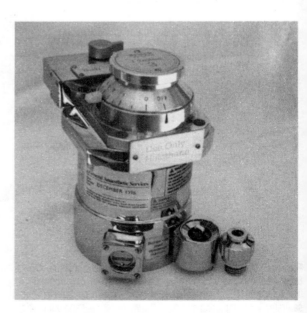

Figure 5.9 The TEC 3 vaporizer showing the open filling port and screw-threaded stopper.

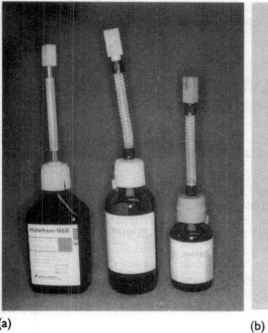

(a)

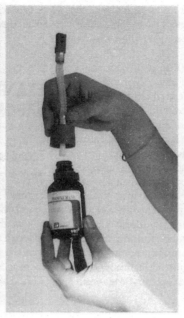

(b)

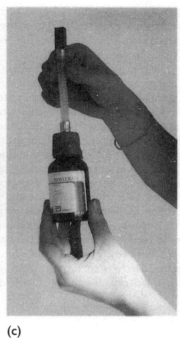

(c)

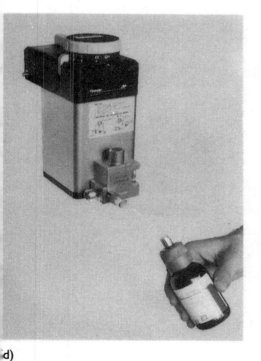

(d)

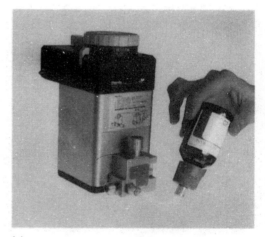

(e)

Figure 5.10 (a) Fraser Sweatman pin safety system for (left to right) halothane, enflurane and isoflurane. Note that the tops have unique grooves (shape and position) that fit only the specific filling ports on matching vaporizers. The screw caps for the bottles have unique grooves that fit only the collars on matching bottles. (b and c) A pin safety system being attached to a bottle for isoflurane; (d and e) the connection and filling of a vaporizer.

was simply unscrewed, liquid agent was added and the stopper reconnected. However, these systems were criticized because the vaporizer could easily be filled with the wrong agent.

Agent-specific filling devices (Fraser Sweatman pin safety system) were introduced by Cyprane (now Ohmeda) in the early 1980s. In these the distal end was keyed to fit a vaporizer calibrated and labelled for a specific agent and the proximal end keyed to fit only the neck of the bottle for that agent (Fig. 5.10). Although this device goes some way to reducing the potential for filling vaporizers with the wrong agent, it is by no means foolproof. Some countries take supplies of agent in large bottles and then subsequently decant into smaller bottles. Early supplies of isoflurane into the UK could be fitted (prior to 1984) to enflurane-keyed fillers. The two most recent agents, sevoflurane and desflurane, are presented in sealed bottles to which only the agent-specific filling device may be fitted. The bottle (desflurane) and the filler (sevoflurane) also have valves that are opened only when inserted fully into their respective filler ports so as to prevent spillage (see Fig. 5.11).

EXAMPLES OF VARIABLE BYPASS VAPORIZERS

Temperature-Compensated Vaporizers

TEC 3 (Ohmeda)

Figure 5.12 shows a Fluotec version of the TEC 3 (with a keyed filler) and its mode of operation.

In this vaporizer, gases destined for the patient pass through the vaporizer by two channels. In the OFF position the channel to the vaporizing chamber is occluded so that all the inflow (1) passes through one channel. This leads through a bypass (2) and the temperature-

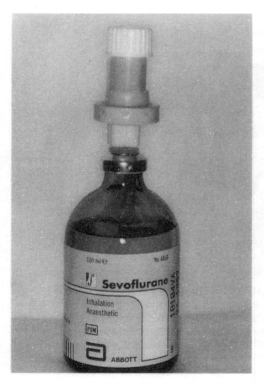

(a)

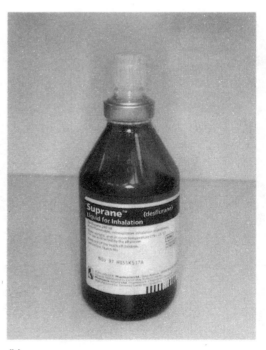

(b)

Figure 5.11 (a) A sealed bottle of sevoflurane with its uniquely shaped filler connected. Note that the stopper on the bottle is secured by a crimped metal seal. (b) Similarly, a sealed bottle of desflurane; the filler is attached at manufacture. As the contents are pressurized at ambient temperature, the glass bottle is encased in a plastic coat to prevent it exploding if damaged.

compensating device (7) and leaves through the outflow (4) without coming into contact with anaesthetic vapour.

In the ON position, both channels are open. The vaporizer channel has an elongated passage (8) that funnels carrier gas to the bottom of the vaporization chamber. Inside the latter, two concentric wicks separated by a nickel-plated copper helix (5) are placed so that their bases are immersed in the reservoir of anaesthetic liquid. The latter is drawn up into the wicks, which become saturated with agent and present a very large area from which it evaporates. The gases passing through the chamber become saturated with vapour by the time they have passed between the wicks and have travelled upwards in the gaps made by the helical spacer to the rotary valve in the control knob (3).

The proportion of gases passing the two channels is determined by (a) the resistance to flow in the temperature-compensating device (7) and (b) the calibrated control knob (3) which varies the resistance through both the bypass (9) and the vapour chamber exit (10). The percentage of vapour at the outlet depends on the amount of vapour-laden gases that is mixed with the fresh gases passing through the bypass. As the temperature within the vaporization chamber falls (reducing the vapour concentration produced), the thermostatically operated valve closes. This causes a greater proportion of the total gas flow to pass through the chamber; by this means the vapour concentration in the output is kept constant.

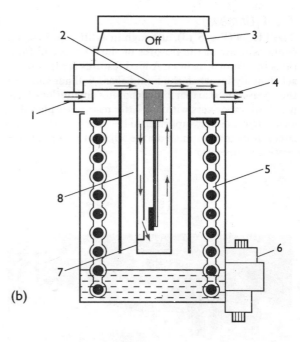

(b)

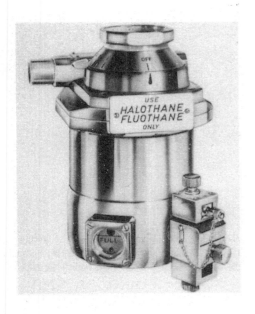

(a)

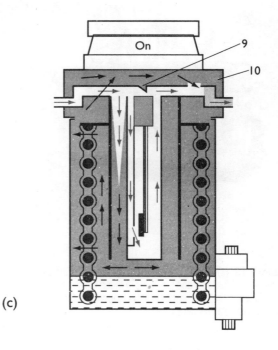

(c)

Figure 5.12 (a) The TEC 3 vaporizer. (b) The gas flow through the vaporizer when switched off. 1, inlet; 2, bypass in the OFF position; 3, control knob that houses the flow splitting (rotary) valve; 4, vaporizer outlet; 5, concentric wicks separated by the helical spacer; 6, agent-specific filling port; 7, temperature-compensating device. 8, elongated inflow channel to the vaporizing chamber. (c) The vaporizer in the ON position. 9, variable resistance acting on the bypass channel causing more gas to pass through the temperature compensating device; 10, vapour chamber exit.

TEC 4 (Ohmeda)

The TEC 4 (Fig. 5.13), although in a different housing, contains many of the features of the TEC 3 and functions in a similar manner. Added features are that if it is accidentally inverted, the liquid agent will not spill into the bypass and also that it incorporates an interlock facility. If two vaporizers with this latter feature are placed on a back bar, the first vaporizer to be switched on extends lateral rods that impinge on the adjacent vaporizer preventing its operation.

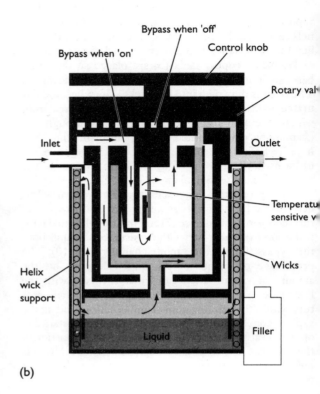

(b)

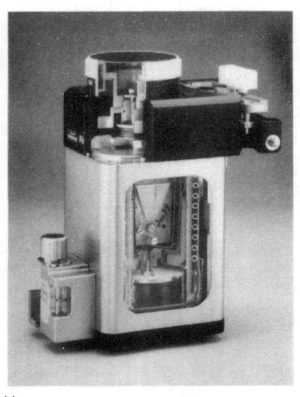

(a)

Figure 5.13 (a) The TEC 4 vaporizer. (b) Working principles. Although this vaporizer is in a different housing from the Mark 3, it contains many of the features of the latter and functions in much the same way. Added features are that if it is accidentally inverted, the liquid agent will not spill into the bypass and that, in one model, if two vaporizers are mounted side by side on the appropriate back bar a push-rod mechanism prevents their both being turned on at the same time.

TEC 5 (Ohmeda)

The TEC 5 (Fig. 5.14) has several design improvements over previous models. The wick assembly is constituted of a hollow cloth tube held open by a steel wire spiral and which is wound into a helix within the vaporizer. This arrangement greatly increases the surface area for vaporization over previous TEC models. Two additional features are the improved key filling action (c) and an easier mechanism than the TEC 4 for switching on the rotary valve and lock (now a single-handed action).

Table 5.2 highlights the differences between the TECs 3, 4 and 5.

Table 5.2 Comparison of TEC vaporizers (using halothane).

Element	Vaporizer		
	Cyprane TEC 3	Cyprane TEC 4	Ohmeda TEC 5
Nominal working range			
Flow (litres/min)	0.25–15	0.25–15	0.25–15
Ambient temperature (°C)	18–35	18–35	18–35
Capacity			
With dry wicks (cm³)	135	135	300
With wet wicks (cm³)	100	100	225
Graduations % Halothane v/v			
Range	0–5.0	0–5.0	0.5
Increments	0.5	0.25 (0–0.5) 0.5 (0.5–5.0)	0.2 (0–1) 0.5 (1–5)
Weight (kg)	6.3	7.2	7.0
Dimensions			
Width (mm)	135	105	114
Depth (mm)	145	145	197
Height (mm)	205	225	237
Temperature-compensated (ambient and cooling effect)	Yes	Yes	Yes
Pressure-compensated	Yes	Yes	Yes
Keyed filler option	Yes	Yes	Yes
Selectatec mounting option	Yes	Standard	Standard
Non-spill	No	Yes	Yes
Allowable tilt	90°	180°	180°
Integral interlock	No	Yes	Yes
Safety 'lock-on' facility	No	Yes	Yes
Safety 'off/ isolation' facility	No	Yes	Yes
Resistance to gas flow Vaporizer 'off'			
(kPa)	0.49	Not applicable for TECs 4 & 5	
(cmH₂O)	5	Not applicable for TECs 4 & 5	
Vaporizer 'on' Carrier gas O₂ @ 5 litres/min @ 21°C			
(kPa)	2.06–2.84	2.06–2.84	1.47–1.96
(cmH2O)	21–29	21–29	15–20

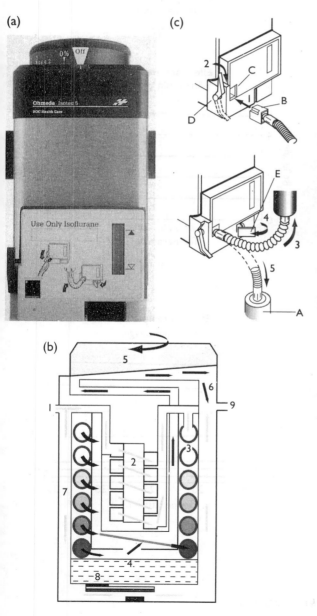

(a)

(c)

(b)

Figure 5.14 (a) The TEC 5 vaporizer. (b) Working principles. 1, Inlet; 2, elongated passage that prevents 'pumping effect'; 3, helical wick; 4, base of vaporizing chamber; 5, rotary valve for metering vapour saturated carrier gas; 6, mixing chamber; 7, bypass; 8, temperature-compensating device; 9, outlet. (c) Filling the vaporizer. 1, Insertion of keyed filler B into vaporizer filling port C; 2, applying the lock D to make the filler/vaporizer connection secure; 3, inverting and raising the bottle of agent to create a filling pressure; 4, opening the chamber lock E to fill the chamber; 5, lowering the bottle below the vaporizer to empty the chamber if required.

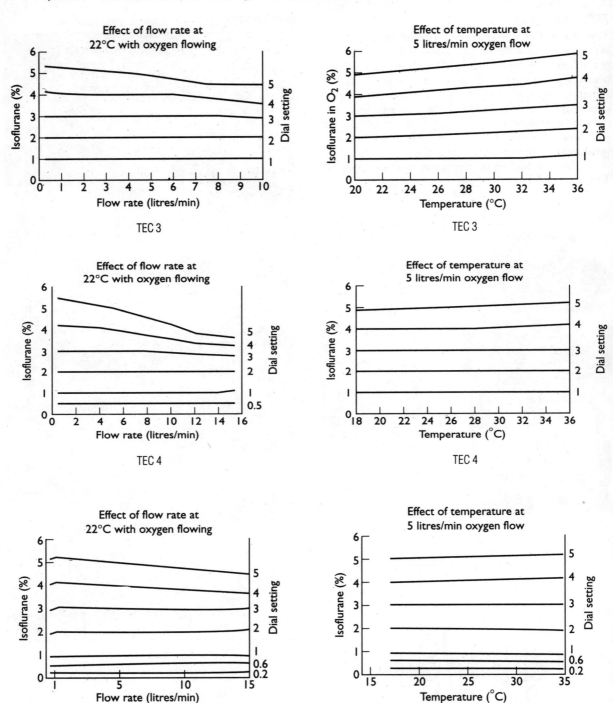

Performance of TEC 3, TEC 4 and TEC 5, as influenced by changes in flow rate and temperature.

Blease Datum

This fulfils all the criteria for a temperature-compensated vaporizer. It has:

- a heat sink;
- a thermal compensating device (see Fig. 5.6c,d);
- a large surface area for vaporization;
- an elongated inlet to minimize the damping effect.

The wick is made from a long tube of PTFE (Teflon) mesh that is supported internally by a wire coil (8). This is wound into a spiral to create a large surface area for contact with carrier gas that passes through the tube. At the base of the spiral, the Teflon is made to drape into the liquid reservoir (6). The material has a high capillarity to ensure that the wick is saturated at all times even when the reservoir is low (liquid level compensation).

In the OFF position, there is a 'zero lock' (3) on the dial that isolates the vaporization chamber so that all the patient-designated gas travels through the bypass. In the ON position this gas is split into two flows. One passes through the elongated wick (8) collecting vapour (the elongated passage behaving as a damping device to counteract the pumping effect). From here, the gas which is now saturated with anaesthetic vapour travels through to the vapour control valve (10) operated by the control dial (2). It then joins the remainder of the gas in the bypass. A thermal compensator rod (4), which is sensitive to the temperature of the vaporizing chamber, alters the flow through the bypass (12) to accommodate changes in vapour production.

Figure 5.15 shows a vaporizer, a schematic diagram and performance curves.

(a)

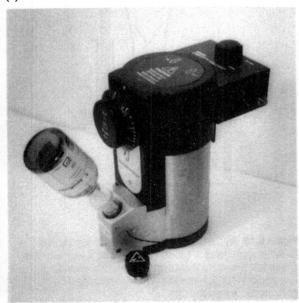

(b)

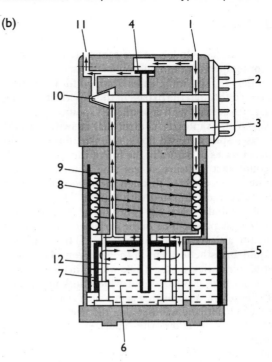

(c)

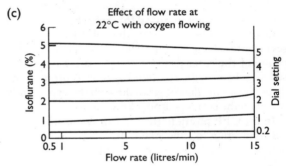

Effect of flow rate at 22°C with oxygen flowing

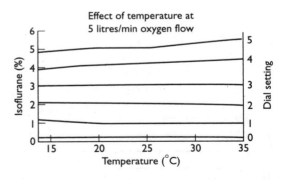

Effect of temperature at 5 litres/min oxygen flow

Figure 5.15 (a) The Blease Datum vaporizer with agent-specific filler for sevoflurane. (b) Working principles. 1, Fresh gas input; 2, control dial; 3, zero lock; 4, thermal compensator rod; 5, filler block for agent-specific device; 6, agent reservoir; 7 & 9, wick extension; 8, elongated Teflon wick; 10, vapour control valve; 11 combined gas and vapour output; 12, variable resistance bypass valve. (c) Performance characteristics for variations in temperature and flow.

Dräger 'Vapor' 19 Series of Vaporizers

Figure 5.16 shows a vaporizer, a flow diagram and performance curves. Models in the range are all compensated for temperature and pumping effects.

In the OFF position, gases destined for the patient are directed through the bypass in the vaporizer without coming into contact with anaesthetic vapour.

When the vaporizer control dial is switched ON, these gases split into two flows; one part flows initially through a series of baffles in the top of the vaporizer (1) that counteract pressure surges (the pumping effect). From here, it is directed through the vaporizing system where it becomes saturated with vapour. This takes the form of a tubular wick (2) coiled in a spiral through which the gas passes. The outer surface of the spiral is attached to a sleeve of similar material (3) that dips into the liquid anaesthetic agent in the reservoir (4) so as to keep the spiral wick soaked. (The wick is made of a material with a high capillarity but which does not absorb agent. Therefore, a stabilizing agent such as thymol that is added to halothane will not clog the wick and reduce its efficiency. This allows the vaporizer to be used for prolonged periods between services.)

From the vaporizing chamber, the saturated gases pass to a conical control valve (5) whose aperture is adjusted by the calibration dial (6). From here they pass to a mixing chamber (7) where they blend with bypass gases prior to leaving the vaporizer. If the operating temperature of the latter drops, a compensating device (8) based on a bi-metallic rod (see Fig 5.6c,d) proportionately decreases the flow of gases through the bypass so as to maintain the correct output of the vaporizer.

In the OFF position, the vaporizing chamber has a small connection to atmosphere that allows some gas to escape when liquid agent is added. This makes the filling process easier.

(a)

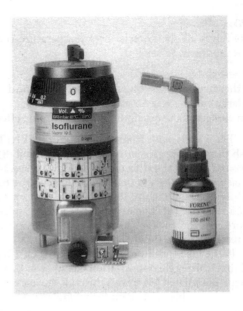

(b)

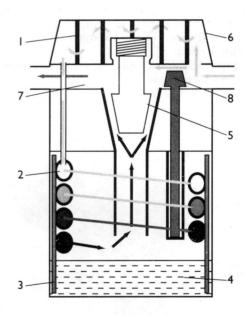

(c)

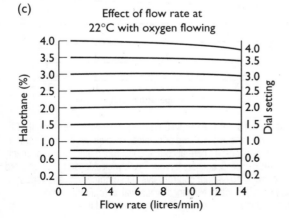

Effect of flow rate at 22°C with oxygen flowing

Halothane (%) / Dial setting: 4.0, 3.5, 3.0, 2.5, 2.0, 1.5, 1.0, 0.6, 0.2

Flow rate (litres/min): 0, 2, 4, 6, 8, 10, 12, 14

Figure 5.16 (a) The Dräger Vapor with an agent-specific filler. (b) Working principles. 1, baffles; 2, tubular wick; 3, wick extension; 4, reservoir; 5, concentration control valve; 6, calibration dial; 7, mixing chamber; 8, temperature-compensating device. (c) Performance characteristics.

Penlon Sigma Elite Vaporizer

The Penlon Sigma Elite shown in Fig. 5.17 includes all the features of a modern Plenum vaporizer.

In the OFF position, gases destined for the patient are directed through the bypass (1). A closing mechanism (2) prevents any gases from coming into contact with anaesthetic vapour in the vaporizer.

When the control knob is turned on, the closing mechanism is released and a second channel is opened that ducts a portion of these gases through the vaporizing system. These pass initially through a helical damping coil (3) that prevents saturated vapour tracking back through the vaporizer and contaminating other gases in the back bar (the pumping effect). From here they pass into the vaporizing chamber (4) and around the wick (5). The latter is novel in that it is made of sintered polyethylene (1 m long) that is held in close proximity to a copper backing plate. The two are then coiled into a spiral, the top and bottom of which are made gas-tight. The carrier gases therefore have to pass around the spiral, coming into contact with the whole surface area of the wick so that they become saturated. The wick assembly is designed as a cartridge for ease of removal and cleaning, and has a long service life.

Gases saturated with anaesthetic vapour leave the chamber and pass through an orifice whose aperture is varied by a needle valve (6) attached to the control knob (7). The latter, therefore, controls the amount of vapour flowing through the device to mix with the bypass gases.

A bi-metallic temperature-compensating element (8) (see also Fig. 5.6c,d) is placed in the vaporizing chamber so that its base is immersed in the vaporizing liquid.

Its top impinges into the bypass and is arranged so that it increases the resistance to gas flow when the vaporizer chamber cools. This diverts more gas through the vaporizer chamber pathway in order to maintain the accuracy of the vaporizer output.

(a)

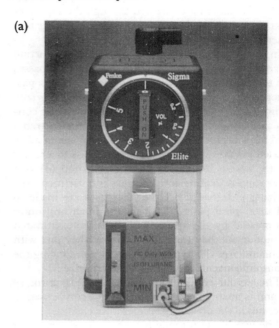

(b)

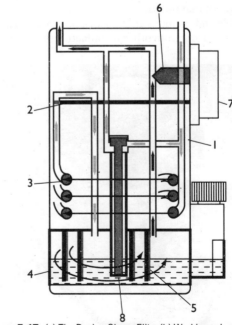

(c)

Effect of flow rate at 22°C with oxygen flowing

Output (%) vs *Flow rate (litres/min)* — *Dial setting*

Effect of temperature at 5 litres/min oxygen flow

Output (%) vs *Temperature (°C)* — *Dial setting*

Figure 5.17 (a) The Penlon Sigma Elite. (b) Working principles. 1, The bypass; 2, the closing mechanism; 3, the helical damping coil; 4, the vaporizing chamber; 5, the wick; 6, the needle valve; 7, the control knob; 8, the bimetallic temperature-compensating element. (c) Performance characteristics.

M&IE Vapamasta Vaporizer 5 & 6

As another example of a temperature-compensated vaporizer, Fig. 5.18b shows the working principles and temperature-compensating valve operation of the Vapamasta 5 (M&IE). In the OFF position, gases destined for the patient are directed through the vaporizer bypass (1) (which is always open) without coming into contact with anaesthetic vapour.

In the ON position this flow splits so that a portion enters the vaporizing system. En route, it first passes into a temperature-compensating device (2) that is part submerged in liquid agent in the base of the vaporizer. (Within this device is an ether-filled bellows that contracts as the vaporizer cools.) This movement is transmitted via a piston to a leaf valve which opens to allow increased gas flow. From here, the gases pass to a rotary valve (3) inside the calibrated control knob (4) that further adjusts the flow into the next compartment, the vaporizing chamber (5). Here, the gases are made to travel in a spiral path (6) within the inner and outer wicks created by the spacer and so become saturated with vapour. As they leave this chamber they mix with the remainder of the bypass gases before producing the final output concentration leaving the vaporizer.

The vapour concentration is adjusted by a rotary valve and is maintained accurately by the compensating device should the operating temperature change.

The Vapamasta 6 range is technically similar with the exception that the back bar mount is now 'Selectatec' compatible and includes an interlocking device that will disable vaporizers from other manufacturers.

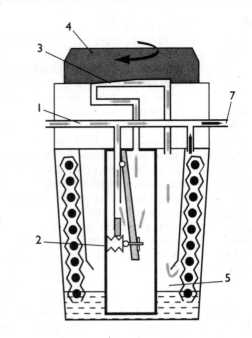

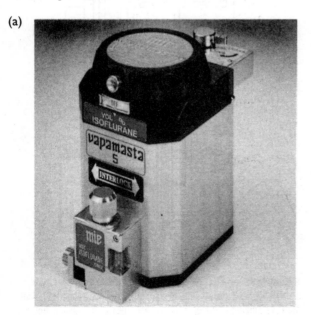

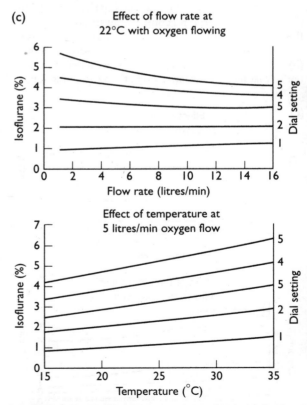

Figure 5.18 (a) The M&IE Vapamasta. (b) Diagram of the vaporizer in the ON position. 1, Bypass; 2, temperature-compensating device; 3, rotary valve; 4, calibrated dial that operates the rotary valve; 5, vaporizing chamber; 6, inner and outer cloth wicks separated by a helical spacer; 7, vaporizer outlet. (c) Performance characteristics.

Draw-over Vaporizers

All the Plenum vaporizers described above offer resistance to gas flow. For this reason the gases have to be driven through them and it is not, therefore, possible to install them in a breathing system. However, pressurized gas sources are not always available in some countries or in certain situations. Draw-over vaporizers, with their low-resistance gas pathways, can be installed in a breathing system and are therefore a useful alternative to Plenum systems despite not being as accurate. Fig 5.19 illustrates various breathing systems in which a draw-over vaporizer has been installed. In systems a–d, exhaled gases are vented to the atmosphere (suitably scavenged where appropriate). However, in system e, the patient's exhaled gases are recirculated through the vaporizer. This is of importance since not only will the concentration of volatile agents be increased by the repeated passage of the gases through the vaporizer, but the latter must be of a type without cloth wicks, since these could become saturated with water condensed from the expired air and so cease to function.

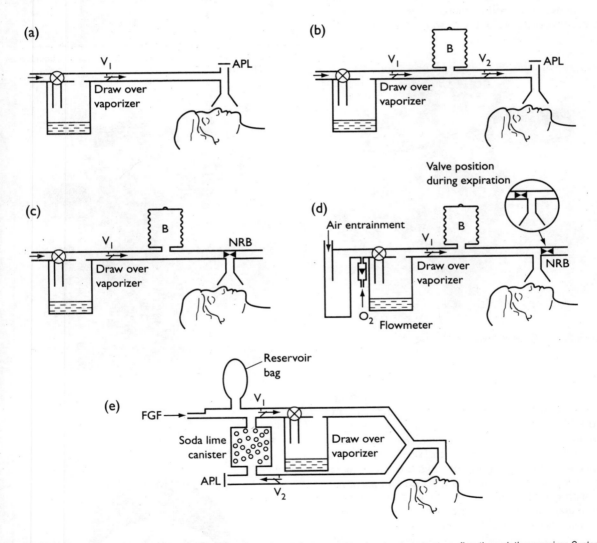

Figure 5.19 Draw-over anaesthetic systems. Note that they all contain non-return valves to prevent reverse flow through the vaporizer. System a is used for spontaneous respiration. System b incorporates a bellows and therefore requires a second non-return valve (V_2). If this is used for controlled ventilation (system c), a non-return valve is often substituted for the APL valve. If the former is of a design which has a tendency to jam, the second valve V_2 is either removed, or in the case of the Oxford Inflating Bellows, held open by a magnet. In system d an oxygen flowmeter has been added. During the expiratory phase, the continuing supply of oxygen flows into the reservoir and is stored for use in subsequent breaths. In system e the vaporizer has been placed in a circle breathing system. A vaporizer in this position is often referred to as a VIC (vaporizer in circle).

Typical examples of draw-over vaporizers are described below.

The Goldman vaporizer (Fig. 5.20), although no longer produced, is a small, simple and inexpensive vaporizer which is still used in parts of the world for potent agents such halothane in relatively low concentrations, when it is introduced as an adjuvant to nitrous oxide and oxygen anaesthesia. It is neither temperature nor level compensated and its output is somewhat influenced by the gas flow rate. Since the resistance to gas flow is small, this vaporizer may be used within the breathing system. Typical performance figures are shown in Table 5.3, although these will be increased when it is used in recirculating systems, for the reasons stated above.

Table 5.3 The Goldman vaporizer

Drum position*	Gas flow rate (litres/min)		
	2	8	30
Halothane			
1	0.03	0.03	0.03
2	0.41	0.74	0.92
3	0.73	2.21	1.31
On	0.74	2.08	1.21
Trichloroethylene			
1	0.01	nil	0.01
2	0.16	0.44	0.35
3	0.47	0.68	0.52
On	0.45	0.70	0.45

* Halothane and trichloroethylene percentages by volume, liquid levels 20 ml at 21°C after 1 min.

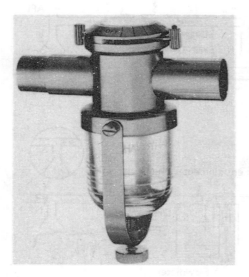

Figure 5.20 The Goldman halothane vaporizer.

(a)

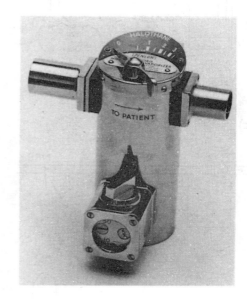

The Oxford Miniature Vaporizer (Fig 5.21) is primarily used with portable anaesthetic equipment and has the advantage that it may be drained of one anaesthetic agent and charged with another. Detachable scales are available for several agents. It is very simple to use and needs little in the way of servicing. It is not temperature compensated, but there is a sealed compartment, filled with water plus antifreeze, which acts as a heat sink to minimize changes of temperature. The 'Triservice' version is described in Chapter 30.

(b)

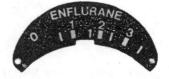

Figure 5.21 The Oxford Miniature vaporizer. Note that the direction of flow is indicated. On some models the flow to the patient is from right to left. Note also that the scale is fixed by two screws and is detachable. It may be replaced by scales for other agents, shown in (b).

(c)

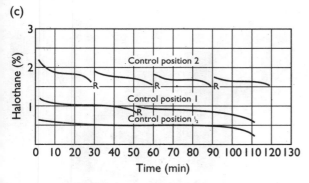

(d)

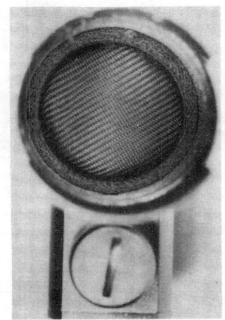

(a)

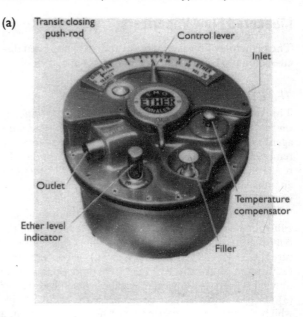

(b)

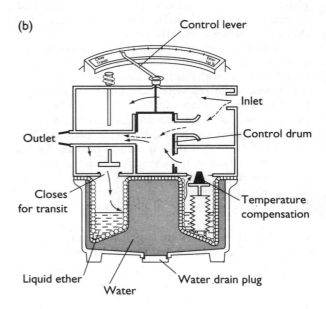

Figure 5.21 (continued) (c) Performance characteristics. Note that there is no temperature compensation, but a mass of water in the base of the vaporizer acts as a heat sink and reduces temperature changes during use. The letter R indicates refilling of the vaporizer. (d) The wick within the vaporizer is constructed of wire gauze and may therefore be cleaned by rinsing the vaporizer with ether, draining it, and then blowing air or other gases through it until all the ether has been eluted.

The EMO (Epstein, Macintosh, Oxford) vaporizer, or EMO ether inhaler (Fig. 5.22), has been deservedly the most popular draw-over vaporizer for the administration of ether, and is still widely used throughout the world. For spontaneous respiration it is often used in conjunction with the OMV (Oxford Miniature vaporizer). The latter is usually filled with halothane to provide smooth and rapid induction of anaesthesia, which is then continued by ether from the EMO. Both vaporizers may be used in conjunction with a self-inflating bellows for techniques employing controlled ventilation.

Figure 5.22 (a) The EMO ether inhaler. This is a low-resistance vaporizer which is both temperature and level compensated. (b) Working principles. Note that there is a mass of water, which provides a heat sink. When the control lever is put to the 'close for transit' position, the ether chamber is sealed off to prevent spillage.

Measured Flow Vaporizers

The principle of measured flow vaporizers has been discussed on p. 51 and illustrated in Fig. 5.4 a, b.

TEC 6 (Desflurane)

This vaporizer (Fig. 5.23) has been designed specifically for the recently introduced volatile agent desflurane. This agent is unusual in that its boiling point is around room temperature and so it would not remain as a liquid in the reservoir of a conventional vaporizer. It therefore requires an unusual design which dispenses with most of the conventional compensating devices mentioned above.

The reservoir of the TEC 6 has two thermostatically controlled electric heating elements (1) which raise the temperature of the desflurane to 39°C. At this temperature the SVP is 194 kPa (1500 mmHg). When vapour is required, a shut-off valve (2) opens and pure vapour under pressure is allowed to escape from the reservoir (3). It passes to an electronic pressure regulator (4) which reduces the pressure to that normally found in a Plenum vaporizer (1–2.5 kPa) and then to a calibrated concentration selection dial (5) from where it is fed into the carrier gas flow leaving the vaporizer (6).

Fresh gas flow into the vaporizer (7) has to pass through a narrow constriction (8) so that its pressure (which increases with flow) matches that normally found in a Plenum vaporizer. With increasing flows, two independent sensors (9) in the pathway detect the pressure rise and instruct the desflurane pressure regulator to increase proportionately the desflurane pressure (and flow) to the selection dial, so as to maintain the set vapour concentration. If the readings from the two sensors are not similar, the shut-off valve closes and isolates the vaporizing chamber.

The vaporizer has several other features:

- The vaporizer heaters are switched on automatically when the unit is connected to the electricity supply. However, a 5–10 min warm-up time is required to reach operating temperature. During this time the concentration dial cannot be turned on.
- There are two more electric heaters in the upper part of the vaporizer to prevent vapour condensation.
- The concentration dial has graduations of 1% but from 10 to 18% these are increased to 2%. There is an interim stop at 12% which can be manually overridden to access the higher concentrations.
- The front panel has five lights (light emitting diodes, LEDs). From top to bottom they are: Operational LED to indicate that the unit is ready to be used; No Output LED for when the agent drops below minimum operating level; Low Agent LED to indicate that

(a)

(b)

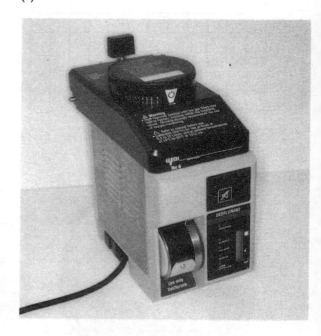

Figure 5.23 (a) The TEC 6 vaporizer. (b) Working principles. 1, Heater in the vapour chamber; 2, shut-off valve; 3, reservoir; 4, electronic pressure regulator; 5, concentration dial; 6, vaporizer outflow; 7, fresh gas flow; 8, restrictor; 9, differential pressure sensors.

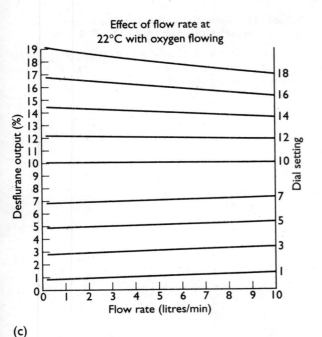

Effect of flow rate at
22°C with oxygen flowing

(c)

Figure 5.23 (continued) (c) Performance characteristics of TEC 6 vaporizer.

refilling is required; Warm-Up LED (see below); and Alarm Battery Low LED for when the back-up alarm power is either low or disconnected. The latter consists of a 9 V alkaline battery which requires changing annually. The front panel also houses an LCD (liquid crystal display) of 20 vertically mounted bars that receives electronically processed signals from a sensor in the reservoir. The bars gradually disappear as the vaporizer empties, at which point the heaters are switched off and the low agent LED flashes. There are three symbols displayed on the side of the LCD. The uppermost (equivalent to all 20 bars showing) indicates that the reservoir is full (390 ml). The middle, a mark, indicates that a 240 ml refill is possible (a whole bottle) and the lowest indicates that the reservoir has only 60 ml left.

- At the beginning of the warm-up time the vaporizer begins a self-testing sequence. The warning alarm sounds for 1 s and all the LEDs flash. When operating temperature is reached the warm-up light (amber) extinguishes, the operational light glows (green) and the concentration dial unlocks.
- There is a detector that shuts off the vaporizer if it senses more than a 15° tilt from the vertical axis.
- The filler port accepts only the specific filler nozzle (SAF-T-FIT), which is crimped onto the supply bottle for desflurane. To fill the vaporizer, the filler nozzle is pushed into a spring-loaded aperture in the filler port, which is then rotated upwards by inverting the bottle. The contents of the bottle will then decant

into the vaporizer reservoir. If the latter is filled only when the LCD bars fall below the 240 ml refill mark, then it will accept the whole bottle. When empty, the bottle may be returned to the starting position at which point the spring in the filler port will eject the filler nozzle. The filling process may be carried out even when the vaporizer is in use. (As the bottle is pressurized, it is coated in plastic to prevent the glass splintering in the event of damage.) Overfilling is prevented in normal circumstances by placing the outlet from the reservoir above the level attained by the bottle in its filling position. However, should the vaporizer be tilted (and this can only happen if the vaporizer is not in use and not attached to the back bar), overfilling can occur although liquid will be prevented from leaving the reservoir by the shut-off valve. When the vaporizer is next commissioned a small amount of liquid might leave the reservoir but would rapidly vaporize.

Measured Flow Vaporizers Built into Anaesthetic Machines

The Engström ELSA and PhysioFlex anaesthetic machines have electronically controlled measured flow vaporizers. A description of these can be found in the relevant parts of Chapter 7.

FURTHER READING

Vaporizer Performance

Cole JR (1966) The use of ventilators and vaporizer performance. *British Journal of Anaesthesia* 38: 646–651.

Graham S (1994) The desflurane TEC 6 vaporizer. *British Journal of Anaesthesia* 72: 470–473.

Gray WM (1988) Dependence of the output of a halothane vaporizer on thymol concentration. *Anaesthesia* 43: 1047–1049.

Henegan CPH (1986) Vapour output and gas driven ventilators. *British Journal of Anaesthesia* 58: 932.

James MFM, White JF (1984) Anesthetic considerations at moderate altitude. *Anesthesia & Analgesia* 63: 1097–1105.

Kopriva CJ, Lowenstein E (1969) An anesthetic accident: cardiovascular collapse from liquid halothane delivery. *Anesthesiology* 30: 246–247.

Leigh JM (1985) Variations on a theme splitting ratio. *Anaesthesia* 40: 7072.

Palayiwa E, Hahn CEW (1995) Overfill testing of anaesthetic vaporizers. *British Journal of Anaesthesia* 74: 100–103.

Palayiwa E, Hahn CEW, Sugg BR (1985) Nitrous oxide solubility in halothane and its effect on the output of vaporizers. *Anaesthesia* **40**: 415–419.

Satterfield JM, Russell GB, Graybeal JM, Richard RB (1989). Anaesthetic vaporizers accurately deliver isoflurane in hyperbaric conditions. *Anesthesiology* **71**: A360.

Schaefer HG, Farman IV (1984) Anaesthetic vapour concentrations in the EMO system. *Anaesthesia* **39**: 171–180.

Scott DM (1991) Performance of BOC Ohmeda TEC3 and TEC4 vaporizers following tipping. *Anaesthesia and Intensive Care* **19**: 441–443.

— 6 —

THE CONTINUOUS FLOW ANAESTHETIC MACHINE

Contents

INTRODUCTION

Inhalational anaesthesia is still the most commonly used technique worldwide. Where compressed gases are available, this is usually achieved by the use of the continuous flow anaesthetic machine (Fig. 6.1). A typical machine would consist of:

- a rigid metal framework on wheels. Attached to this is a source of compressed gas consisting of a pipeline system and/or metal cylinders containing the relevant gases;
- pressure regulators for reducing the high pressures in the attached cylinders to machine working pressures of approximately 420 kPa (60 psi) or 310 kPa (45 psi) in some countries. (The British Standard stipulates 420 kPa which is 61.3 psi. For convenience this has been rounded off to 60 psi.)
- secondary regulators (see below);
- pressure gauges to show pipeline and cylinder pressures;
- a method of metering (flowmeters), using adjustable valves for proportioning and mixing the various gases;
- a system for attaching vaporizing chambers (vaporizers) to the anaesthetic machine for the addition of volatile anaesthetic agents to the gas mixture;

- a safety mechanism to warn of the failure of the oxygen supply and to prevent hypoxic mixtures of gas/vapour reaching the patient (oxygen failure warning device);
- a safety mechanism for releasing high-pressure build-up of gases (back bar pressure relief valve) should a fault occur in the machine;
- a system that bypasses the flowmeter for the administration of a high flow of pure oxygen in an emergency;
- a single outlet for delivering the gases and vapours into an attached breathing system (the common gas outlet).

However, the basic design described above has been gradually evolving. Many of the mechanisms regulating the flow of anaesthetic gases to the patient have traditionally been mechanically and/or pneumatically controlled. Some newer anaesthetic machines have replaced the latter with electronic devices. These are discussed in greater detail in Chapter 7.

MACHINE FRAMEWORK

The machine framework consists of box-shaped sections of either welded steel or aluminium, which provides both strength and ease of assembly. The design usually allows for upgrading from a simple model to one with

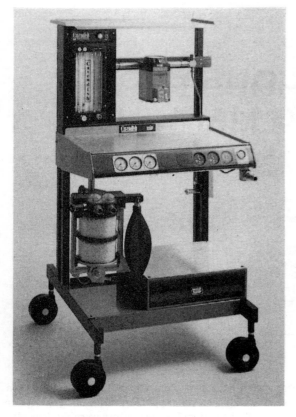

Figure 6.1 A continuous flow anaesthetic machine.

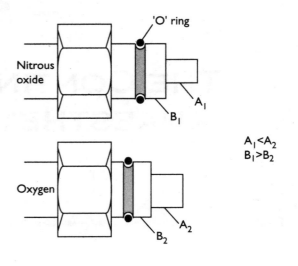

$$A_1 < A_2$$
$$B_1 > B_2$$

	Dimensions of male NIST fittings	
	Forward shaft (A)	Second shaft (B)
Nitrous oxide	9.5 mm	15.5 mm
Oxygen	11.5 mm	13.5 mm
Vacuum	12.5 mm	12.5 mm
Air	9.0 mm	16.0 mm

Figure 6.2 Male section of NIST pipeline union.

integral monitoring and a ventilator. The machine is usually mounted on wheels with antistatic tyres. These conduct away any static electricity which may affect flowmeter performance and which also presents a risk of ignition of flammable anaesthetic agents (in parts of the world where these may still be used).

THE COMPRESSED GAS ATTACHMENTS

Pipelines

Each pipeline source is attached to the machine via a gas-specific connection. The latter consists of:

- a body (attached to the machine);
- a nipple;
- a screw-threaded nut (attached to the machine end of the pipeline hose).

In the UK this is called a NIST (non-interchangeable screw-threaded) connection. The non-interchangeability of this connection is effected by the nipple (Fig. 6.2; see also Fig. 3.10), which is stepped to produce two different diameters along its shaft and which includes a slot for a rubber sealing washer ('O' ring). The two diameters are specific to each gas service and should fit only the equivalent female recesses in the body. The nipple is inserted into its matching body and the connection is made gas tight by securing the nut on the thread provided on the outer surface of the body. The nut is the same size and uses the same thread diameter for all NIST connections (Fig. 6.3). Hence, the term *non-interchangeable screw-threaded connection* is somewhat misleading, as it implies that the screw threads for each connection are different, which is not the case. The incompatibility is created by the individual shape of the body and nipple for each gas.

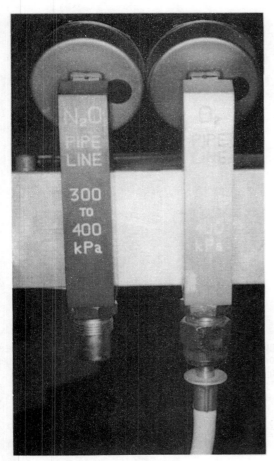

Figure 6.3 Oxygen NIST pipeline connection to the anaesthetic machine.

In the USA a similar system is employed called DISS (diameter indexed safety system). However, the diameters of the nipples and bodies for the various connections are smaller and not compatible with the NIST system. Also, there are further differences in the oxygen and vacuum systems. The oxygen nipple has a small single diameter shaft and a smaller than standard securing nut. The vacuum nipple also has a single (large) diameter nipple, but a standard diameter securing nut that is longer than the others.

The pipeline union block usually contains a metal gauze filter and also a one-way spring-loaded check valve to prevent retrograde gas leaks should the relevant system be disconnected.

Cylinders

The cylinders are clamped on to the machine by a yoke arrangement and secured tightly using a wing-nut (Fig.

6.4a). To prevent installation of the wrong gas cylinder to a yoke, the cylinder heads are coded with appropriately positioned holes that match pins on the machine yoke (Fig. 6.4a). This is called a *pin index system*, for which there is an internationally agreed standard (ISO 2407) for those countries that wish to comply (Fig. 6.4b). The yokes are permanently and legibly marked (BS 1319 in the UK) for the appropriate gas. A thin neoprene and aluminium washer (Bodok seal) or other non-combustible washer is interposed between the cylinder head and yoke to provide a gas-tight seal when the two are clamped together.

Cylinder yokes are also fitted with filters and one-way spring-loaded non-return (check) valves (Fig. 6.5a). These one-way valves prevent retrograde leaks where two cylinder yokes are connected in parallel and one does not have a cylinder attached.

A leak of not more than 15 ml/min through an open yoke is acceptable in new machines. However, in older machines the non-return valve is not as efficient owing either to the design (valve not spring loaded) or to wear and tear, and could result in greater than acceptable back-pressure leaks. These leaks, when occurring unexpectedly, have been shown to alter the composition of the gas leaving the flowmeter block and have resulted in the delivery of a hypoxic gas mixture to an attached breathing system (see section on flowmeters). Blanking plugs (dummy cylinder heads) are available and should be inserted into all empty yokes to overcome this problem (Fig. 6.6).

Pressure (Contents) Gauges

The pressure in cylinders and pipelines is measured by Bourdon-type gauges (see Fig. 4.6, p. 38) that are usually fitted adjacent to the yokes and the pipeline connections. The gas entry to the pressure gauge has a constriction so as to smooth out surges in pressure that could damage the gauge, as well as to prevent total and rapid loss of gas should a gauge rupture. The gauges are labelled and colour coded (BS 1319C, UK) for each gas, according to the standards for each country. They are also calibrated for each gas used on the machine. The scale on the gauge extends to a pressure at least 33% greater than either the filling pressure of the cylinder or pipeline pressure as well as the 'full' indicated position (at a temperature of 20°C). Each cylinder yoke is fitted with a gauge, although this has not always been the case in the past. In modern machines a single-cast brass block is often used to house the NIST/DISS pipeline connection, cylinder yoke, pressure regulator and housings for the pressure gauges in order to minimize the number of connections and potential leaks (see Fig. 6.7).

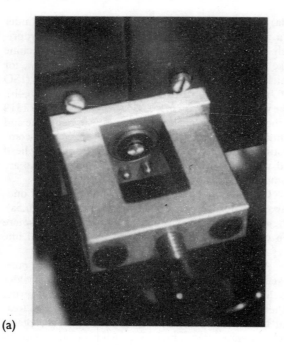

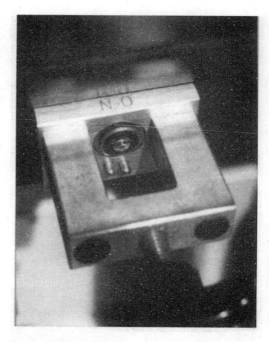

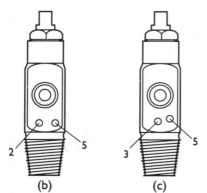

(a)

(b)   (c)

Figure 6.4 (a) Oxygen (left) and nitrous oxide (right) cylinder yokes showing securing screw, Bodok seal and pin index systems. Pin index configuration: (b) oxygen (O_2); (c) nitrous oxide (NO_2); (d) Entonox (50% N_2O + 50% O_2); (e) carbon dioxide (CO_2).

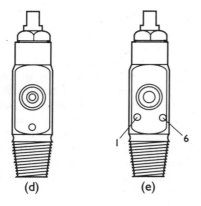

(d)   (e)

Pressure Regulators (Reducing Valves)

Pressure regulators are used on anaesthetic machines for three main reasons:

- The pressure delivered from a cylinder is far too high to be used with safety in apparatus where a sudden surge of pressure might accidentally be delivered to the patient.
- If the pressure were not reduced, flow-control (fine-adjustment) valves, tubing and various other parts of the apparatus would have to be very much more robust, and a fine and accurate control of gas flow would be difficult to achieve. There would also be a danger of pressure building up and damaging other components of the apparatus.
- As the contents of a cylinder are exhausted, the pressure within the cylinder falls. If there were no regulating mechanism to maintain a constant reduced pressure, continual adjustment would have to be made of the flow-control valve in order to maintain a constant flow rate.

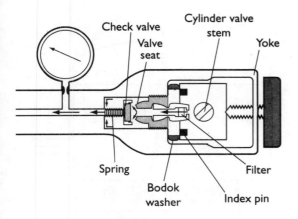

Figure 6.5 Position of valves and gauge when one oxygen cylinder is turned on in a double-yoke assembly.

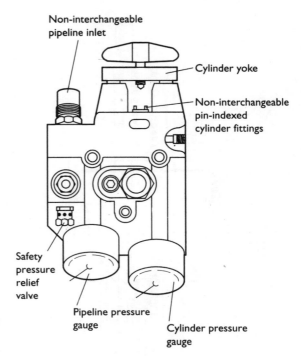

Figure 6.7 Single-cast gas block.

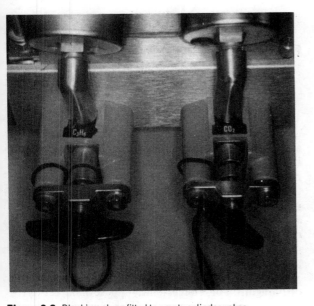

Figure 6.6 Blanking plugs fitted to empty cylinder yokes.

Not only is the pressure reduced, but it is also kept constant, and for this reason the correct term for this type of valve is a *pressure regulator*.

Working Principles

In Fig. 6.8, the chamber C is enclosed on one side by the diaphragm D. As gas enters the chamber through the valve V, the pressure in the chamber is increased and the diaphragm is distended against its own elastic recoil plus

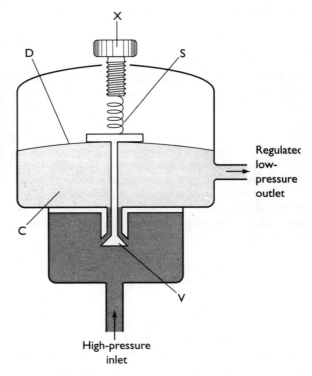

Figure 6.8 A simple pressure regulator. D, diaphragm; S, spring; C, low-pressure chamber; V, valve seating; X, adjustment screw.

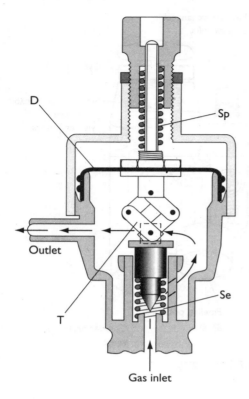

Figure 6.9 The Adams regulator. D, diaphragm; Sp, spring; Se, seat; T, toggle levers.

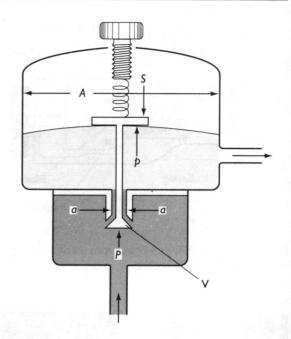

Figure 6.10 Forces acting in a simple regulator.

the tension in the spring S. Eventually the pressure rises so much and the diaphragm moves so far that valve V is closed. The pressure at which this occurs may be varied by adjusting the screw X so as to alter the tension in the spring S. If gas is allowed to escape from the outlet of the chamber, the pressure falls and valve V reopens. When the regulator is in use a steady pressure is maintained in the chamber by the partial opening of valve V.

In another form of regulator (Adams valve), the push-rod is replaced by a 'lazy tongs' toggle arrangement (Fig. 6.9), which reverses the direction of the thrust transmitted from the diaphragm.

The Accuracy of Regulators

Let us consider (Fig. 6.10) that the push-rod is pushed downward by two forces: the tension in the spring and the elastic recoil of the diaphragm. Let these be added together and represented by S. The force that opposes S consists of two parts: the high pressure (P) of the gas pushing on the valve V over an area of a; and the low pressure (p) acting on the diaphragm over an area A, so:

$$S = Pa + pA$$

Thus if S remains constant, as P falls, p rises so that as the cylinder empties, the regulated pressure increases. In fact, as P falls, the valve V will have to open further to permit the same flow rate. The spring expands and therefore the tension in it is reduced, and in the same way the tension in the diaphragm is reduced. Therefore as P falls, there is a small reduction in S, which partially reverses the effect shown here.

In the Adams valve (Fig. 6.11), it will be seen that the pressure P exerted by the high-pressure gas on the valve V to open it is assisted by the spring and the recoil of the diaphragm S. These forces jointly oppose the force exerted by the low-pressure gas on the diaphragm, so:

$$Pa + S = pA$$

Now as P falls, so does p; therefore the regulated pressure falls slightly as the cylinder pressure drops. At the same time the valve V opens slightly and this, by allowing the spring to *expand*, reduces S, which slightly accentuates the fall in p. The fall of p can be minimized by making S great compared with Pa.

There are several types of pressure regulator available, the choice being dependent on:

- the maximum flow rate required;
- the regulated pressure to which it is to be set;
- the maximum input pressure that it is to handle.

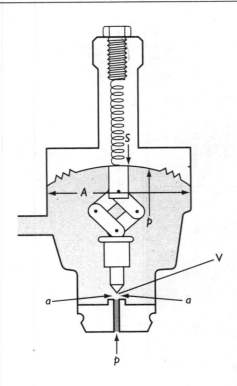

Figure 6.11 Forces acting in an Adams regulator.

Common Faults in Regulators

- Damage to the soft seating of valves may occur as a result of the presence of grit or dust, usually from a dirty cylinder. This may cause a steady build-up of pressure in the apparatus when the cylinder is left turned on but with no gas flowing.
- A hissing noise may indicate a leaking or burst diaphragm. The regulator will need replacing or repairing by the manufacturer or service engineer.
- Adams valves sometimes develop a fault that causes continual 'jumping' of the flowmeter bobbin, indicating an intermittent change of pressure and flow rate. This is usually due to the 'lazy tongs' sticking as a result of wear, but it may also be caused by small particles of grit or metal in the lazy tongs or the valve seating.

On older versions of the Adams valve there were fins on the nitrous oxide regulator to conduct heat from the surrounding air to prevent excessive cooling of the valve. Prior to this, it was not uncommon for the nitrous oxide to contain a significant quantity of water vapour as an impurity, and this condensed upon the valve seating and then froze, jamming the valve. The extra heat conducted by the fins was sufficient to prevent this freezing.

Relief Valves on Regulators

Safety blow-off valves are often fitted on the downstream side of regulators to allow the escape of gas if, by accident, the regulators fail and allow a high-output pressure. With a regulator designed to give a pressure of 420 kPa (60 psi), the relief valve may be set at 525 kPa (70 psi). These valves may be spring loaded, in which case they close when the pressure falls again, or they may operate by rupture, in which case they remain open until repaired.

Primary Pressure Regulators

Modern anaesthetic machines may have several pressure regulators (primary and secondary) for each gas. Primary regulators are used mainly to reduce high cylinder pressures (potentially dangerous) to lower machine working pressure (typically 420 kPa (60 psi)).

Table 6.1 shows the range of pressures employed within the anaesthetic machine and the variation between manufacturers and different countries. Some manufacturers adjust their cylinder regulators to just below 420 kPa (60 psi) (i.e. 375 kPa (45 psi)). This allows the anaesthetic machine to use pipeline gas preferentially when the reserve cylinders have been accidentally left turned on, so reducing the potential for premature emptying of these cylinders. However, even with this

For low-pressure regulators, the diaphragms are frequently made of rubber or neoprene, whereas in those for higher pressures the diaphragm is made of metal. Adjustments to alter the regulated pressure should be made only by service engineers, On some anaesthetic machines 'universal' regulators are used. These operate equally well from an input of 420 kPa (60 psi) from the pipeline, as from a maximum of 14 000 kPa (2000 psi) from cylinders and are of the Adams type. The British Standard stipulates a pressure of 420 kPa (61.3 psi). This has been rounded off in the text to 60 psi. The term 'universal' is also used in a different context (see below).

Interchangeability of Regulators

Pressure regulators used to be labelled and coded for specific gases. This is because a special alloy was required in the valve seating for some gases (e.g. nitrous oxide) in order to prevent corrosion. However, modern regulators are designed to be compatible with all anaesthetic gases. This is achieved by using materials such as PTFE coatings on the diaphragms and Nitrile valve seats and chrome-plated brass for the regulator body. These too are called 'universal' by their manufacturers.

Table 6.1 Pressures of the various gases within the anaesthetic machine

Cylinder pressures¹:
- O_2: UK 13700 kPa/1980 psi; USA 15170 kPa/2200 psi
- N_2O: UK 4400 kPa/640 psi; USA 5690 kPa/825 psi
- $CO_2$²: UK 4980 kPa/723 psi; USA 5690 kPa/825 psi

Pipeline:
- O_2: UK 420 kPa/60 psi (approx.); USA 345 kPa/50 psi (approx.)
- N_2O: France 310 kPa/45 psi (approx.)

Manufacturer		1st stage regulator O_2, N_2O, CO_2	2nd stage regulator O_2	N_2O	CO_2	Back bar pressure relief valve activated at:	Oxygen failure Alarm activation pressure	Flow from:
M & IE Ltd	UK	410 kPa/60 psi	Not fitted			42 kPa/6 psi	240 kPa/35 psi	35 litres/min minimum
M & IE Ltd	USA	310/45 psi					205 kPa/30 psi	
Ohmeda	UK	410 kPa/60 psi	140 kPa/16 psi	265 kPa/30 psi	265 kPa/30 psi [1]	42 kPa/6 psi	172 kPa/25 psi	35–75 litres/min
Ohmeda	USA	310/45 psi						
Penlon Ltd	UK	375 kPa/55 psi	270 kPa/40 psi	Not fitted		30 kPa/4.5 psi	205 kPa/30 psi	30–70 litres/min
Penlon Ltd	USA	310 kPa/45 psi	250 kPa/37 psi					
Penlon Ltd	France	270 kPa/40 psi						

*Not a standard fitting.

¹Nitrous oxide and carbon dioxide are stored in cylinders as liquids under pressure. Therefore cylinder pressures only reflect their saturated vapour pressure at the temperature at which the cylinders are filled and not their content.

²Some slight discrepancies in converting kPa to psi are due to the rounding off of psi values.

differential, many regulators are known to 'weep', i.e. gradually empty their contents. Reserve cylinders should therefore always be turned off after testing until required.

Secondary Pressure Regulators

Several factors cause the machine working pressure (420 kPa in the UK) to fluctuate by up to 20%. For example, at times of peak demand in a hospital, pipeline pressures may well drop by this amount. Similarly, if an auxiliary outlet on the anaesthetic machine is used to drive a ventilator with a very high sudden and intermittent gas demand, a similar pressure drop will occur before the pipeline or cylinder is able to restore the supply. These pressure fluctuations produce parallel fluctuations in flowmeter performance. A second (secondary) regulator set below the anticipated pressure drop smoothes out the supply, minimizing these fluctuations. This is important in machines incorporating mechanically linked anti-hypoxia systems attached to the flowmeter bank (see below) as these systems assume that the oxygen supply pressure is constant in order to achieve an accurate flow of gas. A mechanically linked system would not be able to detect altered gas flow rates caused by changing pressures. Furthermore, secondary regulators also prolong the accurate supply of oxygen to the flowmeter if there is a gradual failure of the oxygen supply (i.e. cylinder emptying) prior to the oxygen failure warning device being activated.

Regulators have to meet stringent criteria before being installed. They are required to withstand pressure of 30 mPa (megaPascals) without disruption and their output should not vary more than 10% across a wide flow range (100 ml/min to 12 litres/min). They should also be fitted with a pressure relief valve that opens at a pressure not exceeding 800 kPa (UK).

As mentioned above, primary regulators can be incorporated into single block castings of both cylinder yokes and NIST/DISS connections (e.g. Ohmeda). However, older machines needed to employ heavy-duty metal pipework to connect the cylinder yokes to the regulators so as to cope with potential high pressure surges when cylinders are turned on.

Flow Restrictors

Although no longer used, it was an occasional practice to omit regulators from the pipeline supply (420 kPa (60 psi)) in older anaesthetic machines. Sudden pressure surges at the patient end of the anaesthetic machine were prevented by flow restrictors. These consist of constrictions in the regulated pressure pipework upstream of the flowmeters. The disadvantage of using flow restrictors

without regulators is that changes in pipeline pressure are reflected in changes of flow rate, which makes re-adjustment of the flow control valves necessary. Also, there is a danger that if there is an obstruction at the outlet from the anaesthetic machine, pressure could build up in the vaporizers and cause damage. This is normally prevented by the inclusion of a 'blow-off' safety valve (see section on backbar below). Flow restrictors do not normally require any maintenance.

TYPES OF GAS-TIGHT CONNECTIONS WITHIN THE MACHINE

The various components within the anaesthetic machine are joined to each other by a series of pipes of either metal or synthetic material.

Permanent Joints in Metal Tubing

Two metal pipes may be joined by one of two methods:

- In the first method, one pipe has a slightly larger diameter than the other so that they overlap (Fig. 6.12a).
- Where the diameters are similar, both ends are inserted into a sleeve of metal (Fig. 6.12b).

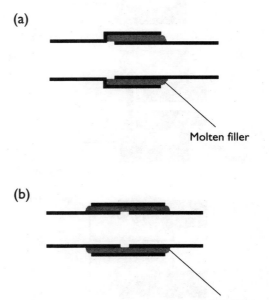

(a)

Molten filler

(b)

Molten filler

Figure 6.12 Permanent metal joints in anaesthetic machines. (a) A brazed overlapping joint; (b) a sleeved joint.

The adjacent surfaces are then bonded together by brazing (applying a molten filler alloy whose melting temperature is above 430°C) or hard soldering (a similar principle using an alloy with a lower melting point). After making such a joint it is important that all traces of flux are removed. Flux is a material applied to the surfaces to be bonded, allowing the molten filler to spread more evenly. More recently, a system of brazing copper pipes and brass fittings without flux has been evolved. This is used particularly for medical gas pipeline installations.

Detachable Joints in Metal Tubing

Where provision has to be made for the subsequent disconnection and reconnection of the joint, a *union* is used. This consists of two parts held together in a gas-tight manner, usually by a nut or cap, which screws onto a parallel male thread. Figure 6.13a shows a ball and cone (or cone seated) union, in which the seating is by direct metal to metal contact. A flange (or flat seated) union (Fig. 6.13b) requires a washer to complete the seal. With pipes carrying oxygen, this washer should be of non-flammable material.

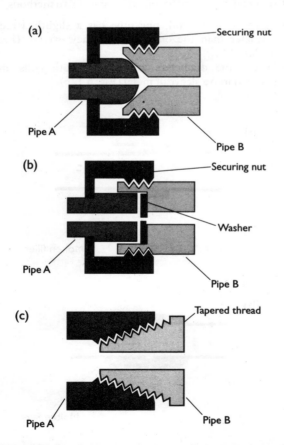

(a)

Securing nut

Pipe A

Pipe B

(b)

Securing nut

Washer

Pipe A

Pipe B

(c)

Tapered thread

Pipe A

Pipe B

Figure 6.13 Detachable metal joints in anaesthetic machines. (a) A ball and cone union; (b) a flat seated union; (c) a tapered union.

For some other purposes tapered threads (Fig. 6.13c) may be used and the seal made either by screwing them down extremely tightly or by interposing a sealing compound such as PTFE (polytetrafluoroethylene/Teflon) in the form of a tape. The joint between the valve block and the body of the cylinder is sealed by a metal foil between two tapered threads.

Other Detachable Joints

The metal pipework (420 kPa (60 psi)) of an anaesthetic machine has always been joined by one of the methods described above. However, more recently, high-density nylon tubing, connected by metal junctions, has been used to convey gas through the machine pipework. Joints are made gas-tight by an 'O'-ring (see Fig. 6.14) fitted between the components. This consists of a simple ring made to a fine tolerance out of a material such as neoprene. It is housed in a recess in the larger component to stop it becoming dislodged.

In the joint described, the nylon tube is pushed firmly into the junction where it is gripped by an 'O'-ring and a folding spring. The folding spring has backward pointing barbs which grip the tube, preventing its removal. When removal of the tube is required (for maintenance purposes), the barbs of the spring can be retracted by applying pressure to the pushing ring situated on the inlet of the junction. This pushes a bush (leading bush) against the barbs, forcing them away from the nylon tube. Each gas service may have its own unique diameter of tubing and junctions so as to prevent cross-connection.

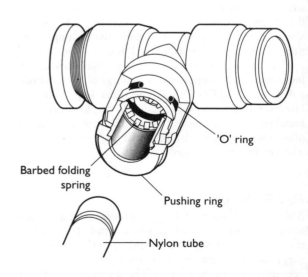

'O' ring

Barbed folding spring

Pushing ring

Nylon tube

Figure 6.14 A cut-away showing a high-density nylon tube joined to a metal junction using an 'O'-ring and a retractable barbed spring.

Valve Glands

Where a valve spindle passes from an area of high pressure to one of low pressure, provision must be made to prevent the leak of gases along the line of the spindle. This is achieved by means of a gland (Fig. 6.15). If the valve spindle is turned counter-clockwise (by convention) to open the valve, gas is permitted to enter the latter. However, it could do so by one of two routes either through the outlet as intended or along the line of the spindle (S) and casing (C) and past the nut (N). The latter course is prevented by the packing (P) in the gland. The nut (N) must be screwed down sufficiently tightly to

dle S and the casing C are suitably designed, an 'O'-ring is all that is required to prevent leakage at this point. 'O'-rings can withstand remarkably high pressures and yet cause very little friction between the spindle and the casing.

FLOWMETERS (ROTAMETERS)

Gas from either a pipeline supply or cylinder, at a suitably regulated pressure, is passed through a flowmeter, which accurately controls the flow of that gas through the anaesthetic machine. The anaesthetic machine conventionally has a bank of flowmeters for the various gases used (Fig. 6.16). Flowmeters are described briefly here, but more detailed information can be found in Chapter 4.

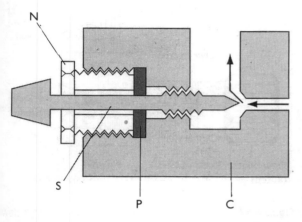

Figure 6.15 A valve gland. The packing (P) is compressed by screwing down the nut (N) until it is applied sufficiently tightly around the spindle (S) to prevent the gas from leaking.

ensure that the packing is applied so closely to the spindle that no gas can escape by this route. There is provision for the nut to be tightened down further to prevent leaks as the packing wears.

The principle can be used for a high-pressure gland, such as that of an oxygen cylinder (see Chapter 3), or in a low-pressure gland, such as that in a flowmeter (Fig. 6.17, see below). In the case of high-pressure valves, a special type of leather or long fibre asbestos was at one time used for the packing, but modern glands are filled with specially shaped nylon. Those in low-pressure flow control valves may be filled with rubber, nylon, neoprene or cotton.

O-rings

In certain circumstances the packing of a stuffing box may be replaced by an 'O'-ring (*see* Fig. 6.14). If the valve spin-

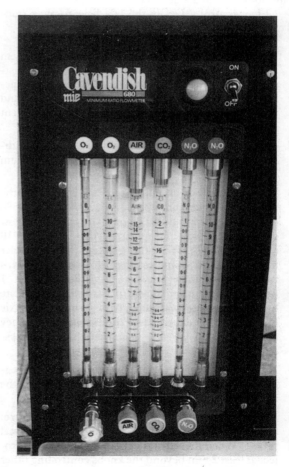

Figure 6.16 A flowmeter bank. Note the 'cascade' flowmeters for oxygen and nitrous oxide, the protrusion of the oxygen flow control valve and the on/off master switch.

A typical flowmeter assembly (Fig. 6.17) consists of:

- a needle valve;
- a valve seat;
- a conically tapered and calibrated gas sight tube which contains a bobbin.

Gas entering the sight tube pushes the bobbin up it in proportion to the gas flow. The bobbin floats and rotates inside the sight tube, without touching the sides, giving an accurate indication of the gas flow. The sight tube is made leak-proof at the top and bottom of the flowmeter block by 'O' rings, neoprene sockets or washers. The glass sight tubes, with their own bobbins, are individually calibrated (in litres/min) for their specific gases at a temperature of 20°C and an ambient pressure of 101.3 kPa and are non-interchangeable. Misconnection is made physically impossible by constructing the glass sight tubes of different diameters and/or lengths or by using a pin index system at each end.

Flow control valves in the UK have to meet standards set down BS 4272 which stipulate that:

1. The torque (twisting force) required to operate them must be high enough to minimize accidental readjustment (this torque can be adjusted by the manufacturer by varying the degree of tightness of the gland nut, although these may work loose during frequent use).
2. Values must be accurate to within 10% of the indicated flow (between 10 and 80% of the maximum indicated flow).
3. When axial push or pull forces are applied to the valve spindle without rotation (at a flow rate 25% of the maximum indicated flow), the maximum flow change must not be greater than 10% or 10 ml/min, whichever is the greater. (Several older machines have spindles that do not meet this requirement. Axial pressures at a flow rate of 1 litre/min have been shown to change the flow rate by 50% in these machines, with resultant hypoxic mixtures being delivered to the patient, when they are used with a low-flow anaesthetic breathing system.)
4. Each flow control valve must be permanently and legibly marked indicating the gas it controls (using the name or chemical symbol).
5. As well as conforming to (4), the oxygen flow control knob (Fig. 6.17) must have an individual octagonal profile. When the valve is closed the knob must project at least 2 mm beyond the knobs controlling other gases at all flow rates. Its diameter must also be greater than the maximum diameter of the flow control knobs for other gases.

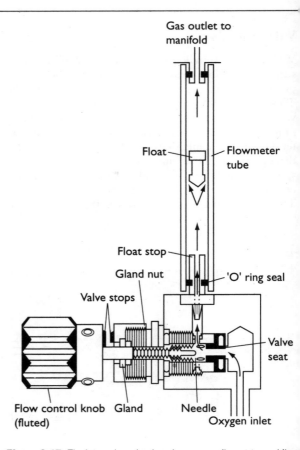

Figure 6.17 The internal mechanics of an oxygen flowmeter and flow control valve.

The Flowmeter Block

In the UK and many other countries, the flowmeters are traditionally arranged in a block with the oxygen flowmeter on the extreme left, the nitrous oxide on the extreme right and those for compressed air and carbon dioxide (where fitted) in between these. However, some machines such as those manufactured by Ohmeda and Acoma incorporate a system that delivers a minimum concentration of oxygen such as 25%, and requires the oxygen and nitrous oxide flow control valves to be adjacent, as they are linked by a sprocket and chain.

The flowmeters are mounted vertically, and usually next to each other, in such a way that their upper (downstream) ends discharge into a manifold. Traditionally, this was unfortunately arranged in such a way that if there were a leak in, say, the central tube, oxygen would be lost rather than nitrous oxide. As a result, a hypoxic mixture might be delivered to the patient (Fig. 6.18a). In most modern machines, oxygen is the last gas to flow into the manifold so that a leak would not lead to such a hypoxic mixture (Fig. 6.18b). As a solution to the same problem, in some countries such as the USA and Canada, the order of the flowmeters in the block has been reversed, with oxygen on the right. However, this too has led to patients receiving a hypoxic mixture because anaesthetists have not been made aware of the transposition.

The practice of removing carbon dioxide cylinders (and in the past cyclopropane) from their yokes has exposed a further hazard in older machines. Oxygen can be lost via a retrograde leak through a carbon dioxide (or cyclopropane) flowmeter, even when intact, if the corresponding needle valves are inadvertently left open. Gas can track back from the manifold via the flowmeter and open needle valve to the unblocked cylinder yoke and escape. The one-way (check) valves fitted to cylinder yokes in some machines were never intended to provide a perfect gas-tight seal under all conditions (see above). They were not spring loaded because they were designed to work against high back-pressures rather than the relatively low back-pressures produced in the retrograde leak mentioned. This leak may be increased by adding an extra resistance to flow downstream of the flowmeter block (i.e. some types of minute volume divider ventilator or high-resistance vaporizer), which effectively increases the gas pressure in the flowmeter block. All empty cylinder yokes for air, carbon dioxide and cyclopropane (where these still exist) should be fitted with blanking plugs (Fig. 6.6) so as to prevent this problem.

Recent increased interest in low-flow anaesthesia systems has created a demand for flowmeters that can more accurately measure flows below 1 litre/min. This is achieved by the use of two flowmeter tubes for the same gas. The first is a long thin tube accurate for flows from 0 to 1000 ml/min that complements the second conventional tube calibrated for higher flows (1–10 litres/min or more). Both are activated from the same flow control valve. These 'cascade' flowmeter tubes for a specific gas are arranged sequentially so that when the flow control valve is opened the low-flow tube is seen to register first.

Carbon Dioxide Flowmeters

The provision of carbon dioxide on anaesthetic machines is somewhat controversial, as several deaths have occurred owing to the inadvertent and excessive use of the gas. Typically, in these accidents, the flowmeter valve had been left fully open, either during a check procedure or at the end of a previous case, and the bobbin was not readily noticed at the top of the flowmeter tube. The next patient then received in excess of 2 litres/min of carbon dioxide.

Manufacturers have responded by producing flowmeters calibrated either for maximum flows of 600 ml/min, or by introducing a flow restrictor that limits the flow into a standard flowmeter to 600 ml/min. Also, flowmeters have been introduced that do not have a bezel at the top of the tube which can hide the flowmeter bobbin.

Anti-hypoxia Devices

Most manufacturers have progressed one stage further in minimizing the availability of potentially hypoxic gas mixtures. They have designed systems whereby it is physically impossible to set the nitrous oxide and oxygen flow rates in which an oxygen concentration can be less than 25%.

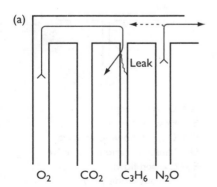
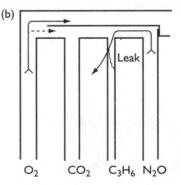

Figure 6.18 Diagram to show the effect of a leak from one of the Rotameter tubes. (a) A leak from the cyclopropane tube in the traditional form of flowmeter block would result in back-pressure from the nitrous oxide, causing oxygen to escape through the leak. The patient would therefore receive an anoxic mixture. (b) A rearrangement whereby the oxygen is the last gas to enter the mixed gas flow and nitrous oxide rather than oxygen would be expelled through a leak. This would not lead to the patient receiving an anoxic mixture.

Mechanical Devices e.g. 'Link 25' System (Ohmeda)

This device (Fig. 6.19) incorporates a chain that links the flow control valves for nitrous oxide and oxygen. There is a fixed sprocket (cog) on the nitrous oxide spindle that relays its movement to a larger cog on the oxygen flowmeter spindle via a 'bicycle chain'. The oxygen cog moves along a static, hollow worm gear, through which the oxygen flowmeter spindle passes. As the nitrous oxide flowmeter control is turned counter-clockwise (increasing the nitrous oxide flow), the chain link moves this larger cog nearer to the oxygen flowmeter control so that, when a 25% oxygen mixture is reached, it locks on to the oxygen control knob and moves it synchronously with any further increase in nitrous oxide flow. The oxygen flow control can of course be independently opened further but cannot be closed below a setting that if nitrous oxide is flowing, will produce less than 25% oxygen in the mixture. Other manufacturers use inter-linking gears to achieve the same effect. This type of mechanical link, however, has some limitations:

- It takes no account of other gases in the flowmeter block (air and carbon dioxide) that could potentially dilute the mixture below a 25% oxygen concentration.
- On its own it will not recognize and compensate for variations in gas supply pressure that affect flowmeter performance.

However, these systems include secondary pressure regulators in both the oxygen and nitrous oxide systems, the purpose of which is to prevent variations in gas supply pressure from affecting flowmeter performance.

A further safety feature of this system includes a mechanical stop fitted to the oxygen flowmeter control valve, ensuring that a minimum standing flow of 175–250 ml/min of oxygen is maintained even when the valve is fully closed. This flow, of course, can occur only when the machine master switch for all the gases is switched on.

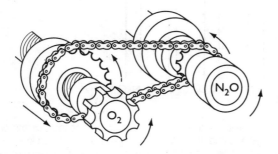

Figure 6.19 The Ohmeda Link 25 antihypoxia system.

Pneumatic Devices e.g. Minimum Ratio Gas System (M&IE)

This system relies on a ratio mixer valve (Fig. 6.20) to ensure that the oxygen concentration leaving the flowmeter block never drops below 25% of the nitrous oxide concentration. When the machine master switch is turned on, a basal flow rate of 200–300 ml/min of oxygen is established. This is independent of, and bypasses, the ratio mixer valve. Oxygen supplied to the ratio mixer valve exerts a pressure on one side of a diaphragm, which is opposed by the pressure of the nitrous oxide supplied on the other side. Any increase in the flow of nitrous oxide results in an increase in pressure on that side of the diaphragm, causing the latter to move towards the compartment containing oxygen. This increases the pressure on the oxygen contained in its compartment and therefore increases the flow rate of oxygen through the ratio

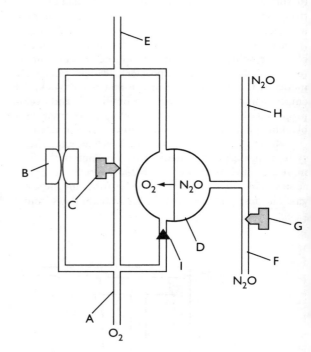

A = Oxygen supply
B = Flow restrictor
C = Oxygen flowmeter valve
D = Minimum ratio mixer valve
E = Oxygen flowmeter
F = Nitrous oxide supply
G = Nitrous oxide flowmeter valve
H = Nitrous oxide flowmeter
I = One way valve

Figure 6.20 Minimum gas ratio system.

mixer valve to the flowmeter tube. The diaphragm is so constructed that it will increase the oxygen flow rate by a ratio of 25% of any increase in the nitrous oxide flow rate. This increased oxygen flow is independent of the main oxygen flow control valve that bypasses the ratio mixer valve and, of course, can be adjusted independently. The ratio mixer valve ingeniously does not work in reverse; that is, if the nitrous oxide flow rates are reduced, the oxygen flows remain as set. This is because the nitrous oxide side of the ratio mixer valve diaphragm is connected downstream of the nitrous oxide flow control valve and does not have access to an unrestricted flow of gas (nitrous oxide) as the oxygen delivery system does.

Electronically Controlled Anti-hypoxia Devices (Penlon Ltd)

In this system, a paramagnetic oxygen analyser is used to sample continuously the mixture of gases leaving the flowmeter bank. If the oxygen concentration in these gases falls below 25%, a battery-powered electronic device sounds an audible alarm and the nitrous oxide supply is cut off. This results in an increase in the oxygen concentration and, as a result, the nitrous oxide supply is temporarily restored. If the oxygen flow rate has not been increased, the nitrous oxide disabling system is reactivated and the alarm will again sound. The whole process is repeated, thus providing an intermittent oxygen failure alarm and at the same time assuring a breathing mixture with more than 25% oxygen (although the total flow rate will be lower than intended).

If the oxygen supply fails completely, there is a continuous audible alarm. The power is provided by a maintenance-free lead-acid battery that is kept charged by the mains electricity supply while the machine is in use and will continue to operate in the absence of a mains supply for 1.5 h. If the audible alarm is activated during this period it will sound for 20 min, after which a visual and audible 'low battery' warning is given. If for some reason the lead-acid battery is not adequately charged at the beginning of an anaesthetic session, the nitrous oxide supply (as well as medical air in US versions) is disabled and cannot be used. However, under no circumstances is the oxygen supply interrupted. This alarm is in addition to the standard oxygen failure warning device (Ritchie Whistle, see below).

THE BACK BAR

Strictly speaking, the term 'back bar' describes the horizontal part of the frame of the machine, which supports the flowmeter block, the vaporizers and some other components. However, it is often used loosely to include also those components and the gaseous pathways interconnecting them. In fact, in modern machines the latter are often housed within the framework. The vaporizers are mounted, either singly or in series, along the back bar, downstream from the flowmeter block.

Traditionally, vaporizers were bolted on to the back bar and linked to each other by tapered fittings. The various manufacturers employed different sizes of tapers and mounting positions but these have been superseded by the provisions of BS 3849 (UK), which recommends 23 mm 'cagemount' tapers. (The term cagemount originally refers to a type and *size* of tapered connection for a reservoir or rebreathing bag that has a small wire cage fitted to its inlet to prevent the neck of the bag from being obstructed, when the latter is empty and collapsed.)

Currently, the trend is towards vaporizers that may easily be removed from the back bar and replaced by those for another agent. Thus, the back bar provides mounting blocks as described below.

The Penlon 'Back Entry' System (Fig. 6.21)

The vaporizer is attached to the back bar by a fixing bolt protruding through the rear panel of the machine.

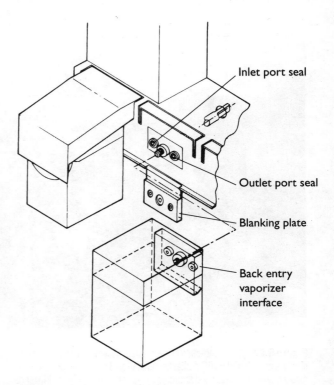

Inlet port seal

Outlet port seal

Blanking plate

Back entry vaporizer interface

Figure 6.21 The Penlon back-entry system.

(a)

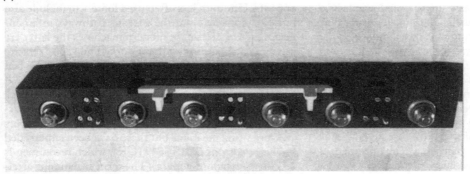

(b)

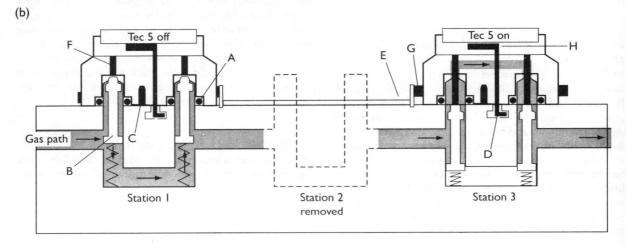

(c)

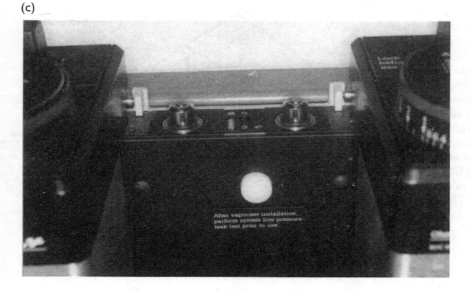

Figure 6.22 (a) A three-station 'Selectatec' back bar. (b) Schematic diagram showing a TEC 5 vaporizer attached at station 1 and switched OFF, an empty station 2 and a TEC 5 attached at station 3 but switched ON. A, 'O'-ring seal; B, valve; C, TEC 3 lock-out pin; D, recess for vaporizer lock; E, safety interlock; F, recessed spindles in the vaporizer; G, immobilizer rod; H, back bar lock. (c) A three-station back bar showing the safety interlock mechanism.

Protruding pegs and seals on the back bar automatically locate and seal the inlet and outlet connections to the vaporizer. The fixing bolt is tightened using a gas cylinder key to produce a leak-proof seal. Three entry systems can be mounted in series along the back bar. Each system incorporates a cover which, when closed, shuts two valves in the back bar, effectively sealing the inlet and outlet ports on that back bar entry position and diverting the gases across that portion of the back bar. However, if the cover is inadvertently lifted without a vaporizer present, a leak will occur, and therefore the fitment of a blanking plate to effect a gas-tight seal is essential.

The Ohmeda 'Selectatec' System

Each Selectatec station on the back bar (Fig. 6.22b) has two vertically mounted male valve ports (inlet and outlet) between which is an accessory pin (see below) and a locking recess (see station 1). The matching vaporizer assembly has two female ports between which there is a key assembly. The vaporizer is lowered on to the male valve ports and the key is turned to lock it into the recess on the back bar (see station 1). 'O'-rings on the male valve ports ensure a gas-tight fit. The two female ports on the vaporizer have recessed spindles (TEC 4, 5 and 6) that, when the vaporizer is switched on, protrude through the gas-tight seals of the male valve ports on the back bar. The ball valves (which provide the seals) in the male ports are displaced downwards occluding the back bar and gas from the back bar diverted into the vaporizer (see station 3). TEC 3 vaporizers have fixed spindles that automatically depress the ball valves in the male valve ports when the vaporizer is lowered on to the back bar assembly. Gas, therefore, passes through the head of the vaporizer even when it is not switched on or even locked on. This arrangement obviously increases the potential for a gas leak and has been modified by the recessable spindle assembly on the TEC 4, 5 and 6.

All three models also incorporate a 'safety interlock'. This consists of an extension rod that protrudes sideways from a vaporizer as it is turned on, and immobilizes the equivalent pin on the vaporizer beside it, preventing the latter from being switched on. On a three-station backbar, there is a plastic lever (see Fig 6.22a) linking stations 1 and 3. Should station 2 be empty, the lever links the extension rods between vaporizers 1 and 3 to ensure that only one of them can be in use at any one time.

Current versions of the Selectatec back bar are also fitted with an accessory pin (see Fig. 6.22a) sited between the male valve ports at each vaporizer station to prevent TEC 3 vaporizers from being attached. The latter have no safety interlock mechanism (see below) and so cannot inactivate other vaporizers mounted on the back bar. The absence of this mechanism allows two vaporizers to be used simultaneously (which is generally thought to be inadvisable).

Dräger Interlock

The mounting system is similar to the 'Selectatec' version although the dimensions are different and unique (Fig. 6.23).

Systems in which vaporizers may be detached are generally regarded as an advance over the permanent cagemount system. Ease of removal has resulted in a greater flexibility in the choice and use of vaporizers (especially with newer agents becoming available), and also ensure that anaesthetic machines do not have to be taken out of use to allow the servicing of the vaporizers.

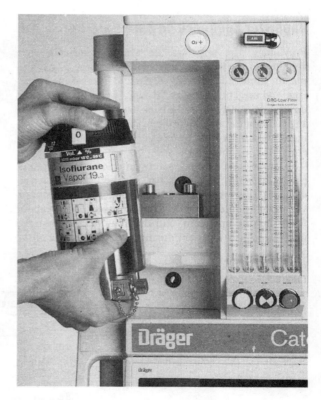

Figure 6.23 Dräger interlock vaporizer and backbar.

Problems with Detachable Vaporizer Systems

Removable vaporizer systems generate their own specific problems:

- As mentioned above, there is a greater potential for leaks.
- The vaporizer may be accidentally dropped and damaged in transit to or from the back bar.
- Tipping of older models of vaporizer in transit could result in liquid agent entering the bypass system causing either liquid or high concentrations of vapour to be present in the breathing system.
- Also, in countries where trichloroethylene is still used, a vaporizer containing this agent may accidentally be attached to a back bar station in a position that results in the vapour being passed into a breathing system containing soda lime. Trichloroethylene is known to react with warm soda lime to produce substances that are neurotoxic if inhaled.

Vaporizer Sequence on Back Bars

Previously, the sequence in which vaporizers were attached to the back bar was very important. For example, on some older machines, a trichloroethylene vaporizer, where fitted, was always permanently sited downstream of a tap on the back bar. This diverted gas to a specific outlet to which the breathing system containing soda lime could be connected without trichloroethylene contamination.

Vaporizers without safety interlock mechanisms, placed in series on a back bar, can be used simultaneously. If this were allowed to occur, the downstream vaporizer would become contaminated with vapour from the one upstream, and this may be administered inadvertently to a patient during a subsequent use of the machine. At one time it was recommended that the vaporizer for the more volatile agent in use should be mounted upstream. Later, when the danger of halothane contaminating a vaporizer for trichloroethylene was pointed out, it was considered prudent to mount the vaporizer for the more volatile agent downstream. The rationale for this is that if an upstream vaporizer for halothane were turned 'on' at the same time as a downstream one for trichloroethylene, halothane could be dissolved in (or absorbed by) the liquid trichloroethylene. When the trichloroethylene vaporizer was next used a high concentration of halothane could be given off (the saturated vapour pressure of halothane being 30% at room temperature). Bearing in mind the advent of other agents, perhaps one should consider the ratio between the saturated and the highest clinically safe vapour concentrations and mount the vaporizer for the agent with the lowest ratio upstream and that with the highest ratio, downstream. As mentioned previously, this situation is now remedied with newer vaporizer systems, which have interlocking devices that disable all other vaporizers not intended to be in use on the back bar.

Back Bar Working Pressures

The flowmeter tubes in the flowmeter bank have, as a rule, been calibrated for gas flows assuming no downstream resistance. In a traditional back bar (23 mm internal diameter system) with the vaporizers switched off, the wide bore of the gas passages offers minimal flow resistance and so the back bar pressure developed at conventional flow rates (5–10 litres/min) is marginally above atmospheric pressure. However, many modern

Table 6.2 Selectatec back bar working pressures

Recorded gas pressures in a two station back bar		Nominal flow rates at atmospheric pressure		*Percentage change in flowmeter sight readings at	
		5 litres	10 litres	5 litres	10 litres
Beginning of back bar (no vaporizers in situ)		1.18 kPa (12 cmH$_2$O)	4.2 kPa (43 cmH$_2$O)	None	Minimal
At 2nd vaporizer station (no vaporizers in situ)		0.78 kPa (8 cmH$_2$O)	2.45 kPa (25 cmH$_2$O)	None	Minimal
Beginning of back bar with TEC 4 vaporizer at 2nd station delivering different concentrations	0%	1.18 kPa (12 cmH$_2$O)	4.2 kPa (43 cmH$_2$O)	None	Minimal
	1%	3.23 kPa (33 cmH$_2$O)	8.5 kPa (87 cmH$_2$O)	None	<5%
	5%	2.74 kPa (28 cmH$_2$O)	7.74 kPa (79 cmH$_2$O)	None	<5%
Total occlusion of common gas outlet		30.5 kPa (312 cmH$_2$O)		20%	20%

*This column shows the percentage change in sight readings, in a flowmeter initially calibrated at atmospheric pressure caused by the various resistances to flow seen in a 'Selectatec' back bar and TEC 4 vaporizer.

back bars have narrow bore (8 mm) gas passages, which increase flow resistance and thus back-pressure on the flowmeters.

The addition of high-resistance vaporizers and minute volume divider ventilators, which cause a build-up of pressure in the fresh gas flow (see Chapter 12), increases back bar pressures. Table 6.2 shows typical back bar pressures developed and percentage changes in flowmeter settings with the 'Selectatec' back bar with and without a high-resistance vaporizer fitted. It should be noted that the small decreases in the flowmeter indications produced does not mean a decrease in the flow of gas to a patient. It is merely that the gas is compressed at the higher pressures and subsequently re-expands downstream when the various resistances have been overcome. Readjustment of the flowmeters to the original settings following an induced pressure rise would therefore be inappropriate.

SAFETY FEATURES

Several safety features are installed either on or downstream of the back bar:

- Intermittent back-pressure surges from certain minute volume divider ventilators can adversely affect vaporizer performance (see Chapter 5), and so most machines employ a spring-loaded non-return valve in the system to prevent these surges reaching the vaporizers.
- Since high pressure build-up in the back bar can damage flowmeter and vaporizer components, a pressure relief valve (commonly set at 30–40 kPa) is fitted. This is often fitted in the same housing as the non-return valve (Fig. 6.24).

Emergency Oxygen

A flowmeter bypass valve for an emergency oxygen supply is now fitted as standard (BS 4272, UK) near the common gas outlet so that, when activated, it preferentially supplies oxygen at a rate of not less than 30 litres/min into an attached breathing system. In earlier anaesthetic machines this bypass for oxygen was fitted near the flowmeter block. When it was operated, this resulted in an initial surge of gas and vapour to the patient prior to the pure oxygen being delivered.

This valve should no longer have a locking facility since this is regarded as dangerous and has resulted in cases of barotrauma when it has been switched on accidentally. Furthermore, there have been cases where the locking facility was in use and unnoticed, which caused a

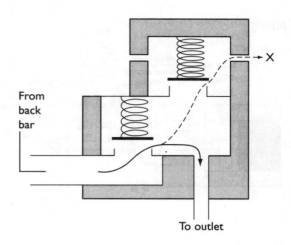

Figure 6.24 Combined non-return and pressure-relief valve at the end of the back bar. If the outlet is obstructed, the gases escape at X, so protecting the back bar from overpressure. A low-pressure relief valve is also available to protect the patient.

substantial dilution of anaesthetic agents resulting in patients becoming conscious during anaesthesia. The valve knob should also be recessed to minimize the chances of its inadvertent operation.

Oxygen Failure Warning Devices

These were first introduced in the 1950s as a response to the problems of unobserved emptying of oxygen cylinders. However, early models could be unreliable as the battery powered part of the alarm could be switched off or the battery could be exhausted or missing! The gas powered part, which relied on nitrous oxide, could also be switched off or fail simultaneously with the oxygen (in which case the alarm would also not work).

The Ritchie Whistle

The Ritchie whistle was introduced in the mid-1960s and now forms the basis for most current alarms. It was the first device to rely exclusively on the failing oxygen supply for its power. Figure 6.25 shows an oxygen failure warning device incorporating a Ritchie whistle marketed at one time by Ohmeda and is still present on older machines in service.

The alarm is powered by an oxygen supply at a pressure of 420 kPa (60 psi) in the UK, which is tapped from the oxygen pipework upstream of the flowmeter block. This enters the alarm inlet valve and pressurizes the

(a)

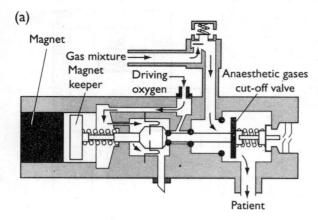

(b)

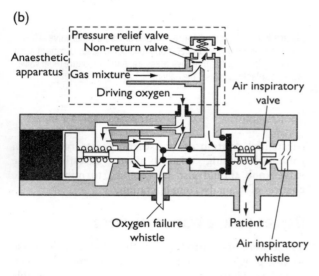

Figure 6.25 Oxygen failure warning device: (a) normal operation; (b) operation during oxygen failure.

rolling diaphragm, opening the anaesthetic cut-off valve, and closing the air inspiratory valve and the port to the oxygen failure whistle. Anaesthetic gases may then pass freely through this device, which is now at standby.

When the oxygen pressure supplying the flowmeter block drops below 260 kPa (38 psi), a spring causes the anaesthetic gases cut-off valve to begin to close and the oxygen failure whistle valve to open, permitting a flow of oxygen (via the restrictor) to operate the oxygen failure whistle. The whistle sounds continuously until the oxygen pressure has fallen to approximately 40.5 kPa (6 psi).

At a pressure of approximately 200 kPa (30 psi) the force of the magnet keeper return spring and the magnet causes the anaesthetic gases cut-off valve to be closed,

cutting off the supply of anaesthetic gases to the patient. At the same time the spring load on the air inspiratory valve is released, allowing the patient to inspire room air. Whenever the patient inhales, the inspiratory air whistle sounds.

With the anaesthetic gases cut-off valve closed, the now potentially hypoxic gas from the flowmeter block vents to the atmosphere through the pressure-relief valve on the back bar.

Current Oxygen Failure Warning Devices

British Standard 4272 Part 3 specifies the criteria required for oxygen failure warning devices fitted to current anaesthetic machines.

1. The alarm shall be auditory, shall be of at least 7 s duration and shall have a noise level of at least 60 dB measured at 1 m from the front of the anaesthetic machine.
2. The energy required to operate the alarm shall be derived solely from the oxygen supply pressure in the machine gas piping and the alarm shall be activated when this pressure falls to approximately 200 kPa.
3. The alarm shall be of a design that cannot be switched off or reset without initially restoring the oxygen supply pressure.
4. The alarm shall be linked to a gas shut-off device that performs at least one of the following functions:

   (i) It shall cut off the supply of all gases other than oxygen (and air, where fitted) to the common gas outlet.
   (ii) It shall progressively reduce the flow of all other gases while maintaining the preset oxygen flow or proportion of oxygen until the supply of oxygen finally fails, at which point the supply of all other gases shall be shut off.
   (iii) Where an air supply is fitted, it shall progressively reduce the flow of all other gases except air while maintaining the preset oxygen flow or proportion of oxygen until the supply of oxygen fails, at which point the supply of all other gases, except air, shall be shut off.
   (iv) It shall establish a pathway between the machine gas delivery system and the atmosphere.
   (v) The gas cut-off device shall not be activated before the oxygen failure alarm is activated.
   (vi) It shall not be possible to re-set the gas cut-off device without prior restoration of the oxygen supply pressure to above the pressure of approximately 200 kPa.

A schematic diagram of such a device is shown in Fig. 6.26.

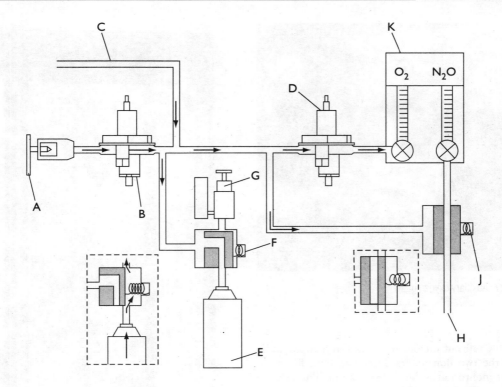

Figure 6.26 A schematic diagram of a current oxygen failure warning device. A, Cylinder yoke for oxygen; B, primary regulator for oxygen (137 000 kPa → 420 kPa); C, pipeline oxygen supply; D, secondary regulator for oxygen (420 kPa → 140 kPa); E, reservoir of oxygen required to power the Ritchie Whistle for a minimum of 6 s; F, spring-loaded regulator. When oxygen supply pressure drops to 200 kPa reservoir E is connected to the Ritchie Whistle; G, Ritchie Whistle; H, nitrous oxide supply; J, spring-loaded shut-off valve to nitrous oxide supply activated when oxygen supply pressure drops below 200 kPa; K, flowmeter bank.

COMMON GAS OUTLET

The various medical gases and vapours exit the machine via a 22 mm male / 15 mm female conically tapered outlet (BS 3849, UK). This common gas outlet may be fixed, or swivelled through 90° (Cardiff Swivel), and should be strong enough to withstand a bending moment of force of up to 10 Nm applied to its axis, since heavy equipment is often attached. BS 4272 (UK), recommends that this outlet is fitted with an anti-disconnect device. Some outlets include a male thread for securing heavy devices such as a fuel cell oxygen analyser or other equipment.

AUXILIARY GAS SOCKETS

Anaesthetic machines may now be fitted with mini-Schrader gas sockets (Fig. 6.27), but only for air or oxy-gen. These are used to power several devices such as ventilators for low-flow anaesthesia systems, venturi systems for bronchoscopy, and suction units. The sockets should be permanently and legibly marked for their specific gases (air or oxygen) and their working pressure of 400 kPa approximately (in the UK). They should also carry a warning symbol consisting of an exclamation mark within a triangle.

QUANTIFLEX MACHINES

These were one of the earliest commercial attempts to embody safety devices to prevent the administration of potentially hypoxic mixtures of gases amount of oxygen. The Quantiflex MDM (Fig. 6.28) is described below. Note that the oxygen flowmeter is usually on the right and nitrous oxide flowmeter is on the left.

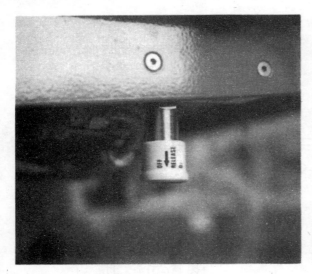

Figure 6.27 Auxiliary oxygen outlet.

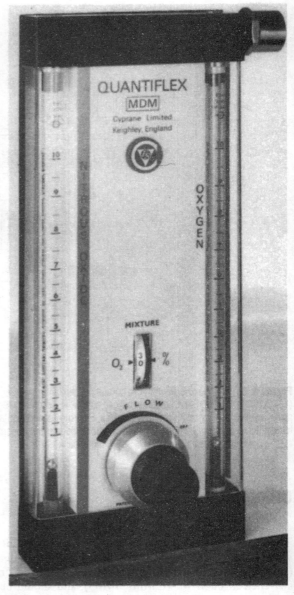

Figure 6.28 The Quantiflex MDM anaesthetic machine. The lower knob controls the flow rate and the wheel above it adjusts the percentage of oxygen. Notice that 30% is the minimum amount of oxygen in the mixed gas flow. Note also that the nitrous oxide and oxygen flowmeters are in the reverse sequence to that which is customary in the UK.

The flow rates of nitrous oxide and oxygen are indicated by the two flowmeters. However, both flows are adjusted synchronously by a single knob. The relative percentages of nitrous oxide and oxygen are determined by the mixture control wheel, which is calibrated in steps of 10% from 30% to 100% oxygen. Thus, never more than 70% nitrous oxide can be given. This device was incorporated in some anaesthetic machines but is currently fitted only to equipment dispensing nitrous oxide/oxygen mixtures in the dental operatory (*see* Chapter 15).

MAINTENANCE OF ANAESTHETIC MACHINES

In the UK it is recommended that all anaesthetic machines are serviced by competent engineers according to the manufacture's advice. This has usually been four times a year, with ventilators being serviced every 6 months. This service consists of:

- cleaning all parts of the machine, including the flowmeter tubes;
- checking of flowmeters, regulators and all other parts such as corrugated tubing and breathing bags;
- the cleaning of circle absorbers, etc. as appropriate.

It does not, however, usually include attention to the temperature-compensated vaporizers, which are serviced by the manufacturer or a specialist subcontractor.

Service intervals for these depend on the model and the agent used. Thymol, a normal constituent of halothane, tends to collect in vaporizers, and most manufacturers advise that temperature-compensated vaporizers be returned to their factory once a year for an overhaul. It is usually possible to obtain a service exchange or other vaporizer on temporary loan while the original is away at the factory.

Besides maintenance by service engineers, it is wise for anaesthetists to carry out their own checks (see Appendix IV).

The Medical Devices Directorate in the UK has issued guidelines to hospitals (*HEI 98*, Nov. 1990) on the management of medical equipment (which includes anaesthetic machines and ventilators). These guidelines include the keeping of a record book (log book) that is kept permanently with each item of equipment. It should contain the following information:

- The commissioning into service of that item by an appropriately qualified person.
- The provision of a record of all repairs, modifications, routine inspections and servicing, and that the latter were performed on the due date.
- A method of drawing attention to any unreliability (that may be indictated by frequent breakdown).
- An indication that a user check has been performed following a service.
- An indication that a functional check has been performed on the equipment before it is used on a patient.
- A record of any minor faults that develop during use so that these can be brought to the attention of the service engineer at the next routine service.

The procedures for record keeping in the log book should be clearly established and documented, and should include dates and signatures. The books should be examined regularly by a designated person to ensure that the above guidelines are being followed.

The guideline *HEI 98* is under revision and a new version is expected sometime in 1997.

FURTHER READING

British Standards Institution (1989) *Anaesthetic and Analgesic Machines, Part 3: Specifications for Continuous Flow Anaesthetic Machines*, BS 4272. Milton Keynes, Bucks, UK: British Standards Institution.

Editorial (1990) Carbon dioxide cylinders on anaesthetic apparatus. *British Journal of Anaesthesia* 65: 155–156.

McQuillan PJ, Jackson JB (1987) Potential leaks from anaesthetic machines. *Anaesthesia* 42: 1301–1312.

Ritchie JR (1974) A simple and reliable warning device for failing oxygen pressure. *British Journal of Anaesthesia*, 46: 323.

Schreiber P (1985) *Safety Guidelines: Anaesthesia Systems.* Telford, Penn., USA: North American Drager.

– 7 –

ELECTRONICS IN THE ANAESTHETIC MACHINE

Contents

INTRODUCTION

The modern anaesthetic machine has, not surprisingly, been invaded by electronics. This invasion has taken place, or will take place, in several ways, namely:

1. Integral physiological monitoring equipment.
2. Electronic monitoring of a conventional pneumatic anaesthetic machine.
3. Electronic control of gases and vapours in an entirely new form of pneumatic circuit.
4. Servo-control of gases and vapours.
5. Servo-control of depth-of-anaesthesia.

Monitoring of physiological variables is dealt with in Chapter 18 and the monitoring of gas composition and flow is dealt with in Chapter 19.

Over the last decade the invasion of electronics has proceeded relentlessly. Anaesthetic machines now vary from basic pneumatic Boyle's machines (Chapter 6) to machines that would previously be completely unrecognizable as anaesthetic machines. This does not mean that the totally pneumatic machine is now redundant. There are many merits in these basic machines, including their being easy to understand, cheaper to purchase, reliability, and they are easy to maintain. There are many merits in the KISS principle (Keep It Simple, Stupid)!

ERGONOMICS

Ergonomics is the study of the efficiency of persons in their working environment and *human factors engineering* is the design and development of equipment to improve the ergonomics of a task. This has the effect of making the working environment not only more pleasant but less tiring and less stressful, which should lead to increased safety. The conventional pneumatic anaesthetic machine 'just grew' and there has been little attempt in the past to consider ergonomics. For example, when considering the fresh gas output of the anaesthetic machine, the anaesthetist has in mind a minute volume or fresh gas flow rate and an inspired oxygen percentage in either air or nitrous oxide. To acquire this output he or she has to select a flow rate for each of the component gases, add the flow rates mentally, and calculate the proportions of the constituents. It would be much more convenient to him or her if it was possible to select:

- the combination: oxygen/nitrous oxide or air/oxygen;
- the required total flow in litres/min;
- the percentage of oxygen.

Consideration also needs to be given to the display of any information, composition of gases, flow rates, airway pressure, etc. In order to make such changes to the ergonomics of the anaesthetic machine it is necessary to start from scratch, firstly asking what is required (as above) and then using new technologies to implement these goals. The ultimate goal is to increase safety in anaesthesia. However, it is equally important that it is possible to learn how to use any new anaesthetic machine quickly; unfortunately, this is not the case with many machines. In this day and age when junior doctors move from hospital to hospital regularly and locum anaesthetists are frequently engaged, this is a very important factor.

THE CRITICAL INCIDENT

The *critical incident* as elucidated by Schreiber occurs when one or more of the components of the control loop (Fig. 7.1) behaves unpredictably, be it the machinery, the patient or the anaesthetist. The time course of a critical incident is shown in Fig. 7.2.

When an adverse condition begins, the danger of injury to the patient increases with time, as shown. There is a time delay before the problem is noticed by

the anaesthetist and identified. Another delay occurs before the problem is corrected, after which there should be a recovery to safe conditions if the correction is made early enough. Excessive delay in noticing the problem or in its correction will lead to permanent injury.

The reliability of the human for constant vigilance over long periods of time is questionable and the ability to make decisions when bombarded with multiple sensory inputs is sorely put to the test. Monitoring during anaesthesia should not be limited to electronic surveillance of the patient's physiology but should also include monitoring of the equipment's performance and of the anaesthetist. Monitoring of the anaesthetist's performance may be done with automatic generation of the anaesthetic record chart, which may also form part of a medical audit.

Research shows that alarm systems should be designed to make as long as possible the time available to correct a problem before injury begins. Examination of Fig. 7.2 shows that this may be accomplished by minimizing the pre-alarm period and making it as clear as possible to the anaesthetist what the problem is and its level of urgency.

Schreiber has also pointed out that the further along the system from the gas and electricity supplies to the patient that a parameter is monitored (Fig. 7.3), the greater the delay before the alarm is sounded and the greater the number of possible causes of that particular problem. For example, if the oxygen supply fails, the oxygen supply alarm would sound immediately. Some seconds later, depending on the fresh gas flow into the breathing attachment, the inspired oxygen monitor alarm would become active. However, it may be more

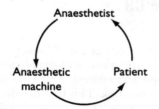

Figure 7.1 Anaesthetic 'control loop'.

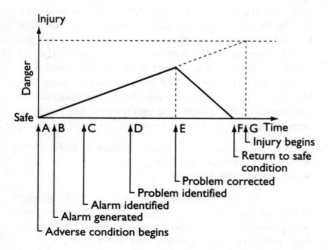

Figure 7.2 Diagram of Schreiber's time course of a critical incident as it would occur in anaesthetic practice.

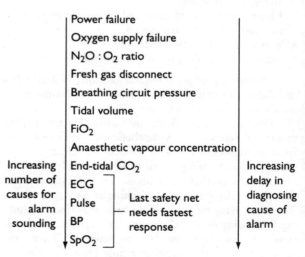

Figure 7.3 The further along the system from the supplies to the patient that a parameter is monitored, the greater the delay before the problem is corrected.

than a minute before the saturation as indicated by a pulse oximeter would fall below the critical level. Furthermore, the causes of a drop in SpO_2 are numerous compared with the causes of the sounding of the oxygen supply pressure alarm.

Alarms do not necessarily refer to emergencies but may indicate abnormal situations that may or may not have the potential to become emergencies. The ideal monitoring system should differentiate between advisory (requiring awareness), caution (requiring a prompt response) and warning (requiring immediate response). Ideally an audible warning differentiating between these three levels should draw the anaesthetist's attention to a visual indication of what the problem is. Figure 7.4 shows a conventional anaesthetic machine with monitoring equipment mounted on it. Regularly, during an anaesthetic, the anaesthetist must scan all the visual displays indicated and when a crisis occurs he or she must not only differentiate the alarm sounds but must then locate the appropriate display before making a decision

as to the cause and then correcting it. The anaesthetic machine shown in Fig. 7.5 was developed to minimize the delay between the onset of an adverse condition and its detection and correction. Extensive use of 'human factors engineering' has led to a machine with a structured alarm system with centralized displays for alarms and data, a centralized control panel for functions that apply to the entire system, a centralized connection panel for the physiological monitoring and a centralized power supply with automatic battery back-up in case of power failure.

The advantage of this integrated system is that information from each of the monitoring systems may be prioritized by a computer before any alarm is sounded. The data may be displayed in the most convenient fashion for easy and quick assimilation and may also be printed to provide a permanent record. However, this type of anaesthetic machine is still only the electronic monitoring of a conventional pneumatic circuit.

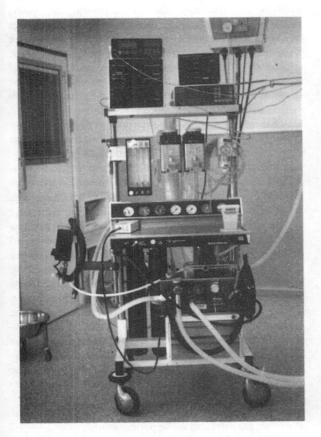

Figure 7.4 Conventional anaesthetic machine with monitoring equipment. Note the wide and random distribution of the individual displays. Compare this with Fig. 7.5.

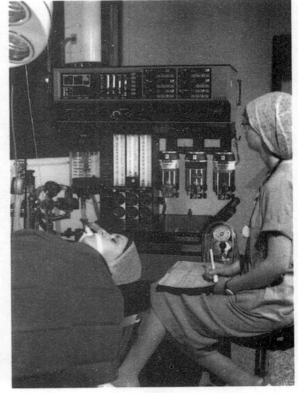

Figure 7.5 Dräger Narkomed III anaesthetic machine with integrated monitoring and alarms.

ELECTRONIC CONTROL OF THE BREATHING SYSTEM

The next step in the progression integrates the control of the breathing system. An example of this is the Dräger Cato anaesthetic machine (Fig. 7.6). In this case the selection of breathing system is electronically selected by a single control button for:

- spontaneous respiration using a circle system;
- intermittent positive pressure ventilation;
- synchronized intermittent mandatory ventilation.

The Cato is able to ventilate patients requiring tidal volumes from 20 ml to 1400 ml; positive end-expiratory pressure (PEEP) is also available.

The gas circuit is conventional from gas supplies to the output of the conventional vaporizer (Fig. 7.7). Although this is recognizable, there are some important differences from the basic circle system. Pressure and flow are continuously measured and in the intermittent positive pressure ventilation (IPPV) and synchronized intermittent mandatory ventilation (SIMV) modes the stroke volume of the piston ventilator is continuously adjusted to maintain the required tidal volume despite changes in lung compliance and the rate of fresh gas flow into the circle. There is a very sensitive pressure monitoring system such that it is not possible to cause barotrauma to a baby even if the selected tidal volume is for an adult. The sensors are also sensitive enough to allow the SIMV mode. Before applying the breathing tubes to the patient, the Y-connector is occluded and the internal computer calculates the compliance of the entire gas circuit. Allowances are then made during all modes of breathing so that the indicated values are more accurate than on a simple anaesthetic machine with add-on monitoring. The gases and volatile anaesthetic agent are measured both before and in the circle.

During controlled respiration, in the inspiratory phase, the excess gas outlet valve and the fresh gas shut-off valve are closed and gas streams from the piston pump to the patient. The expiratory phase is initiated by the opening of the fresh gas shut-off valve. Gas from the patient then streams into the breathing bag, which serves as a reservoir, and also into the retracting piston pump. The excess gas outlet valve remains closed unless there is excess gas in the system as would occur when greater than basal fresh gas flow is entering the circuit. Unlike conventional semi-closed breathing systems, the valve opening time for discharging excess gas is controlled as required; the valve remains open during the expiratory phase for longer the higher the fresh gas flow. If the fresh gas flow chosen by the anaesthetist is too low this is detected by the pressure sensor in the circuit, which detects the patient's end expiratory pressure has fallen below −0.5 mbar causing the piston pump to stop extracting gas and sounding an alarm.

Gas composition is continuously monitored both at the fresh gas inlet and at the patient connection.

This machine may also have integrated blood pressure and electrocardiogram (ECG) monitoring and pulse oximetry.

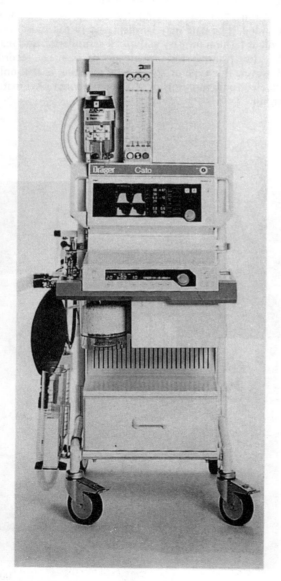

Figure 7.6 Dräger Cato anaesthetic machine with electronic control and monitoring of the breathing system.

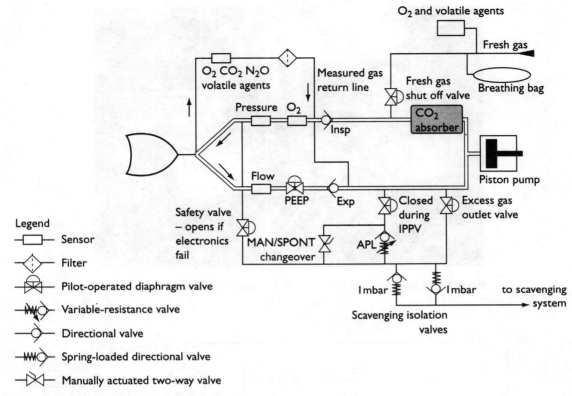

Figure 7.7 Diagram of the gas circuit of the Cato anaesthetic machine.

THE NEXT STAGE IN THE PROGRESSION

The Engström ELSA illustrates many of the principles of the anaesthetic machine of the future (Fig. 7.8). It has been developed with ergonomics and safety as prime considerations. A simplified description of the ELSA is given below.

The ELSA is divided into two sections, namely a lower anaesthetic delivery unit and an upper monitoring unit; although this layout is used for ergonomic reasons, the two units are fully integrated.

The supply pressures of oxygen, nitrous oxide and air are monitored electronically by semiconductor pressure transducers; the oxygen supply also has a conventional pneumatic alarm whistle. The pressure-regulated gases then pass to the gas mixer (Fig. 7.9).

Familiar controls are provided for oxygen, nitrous oxide and air, which operate conventional needle valves. These control knobs have pointers associated with them that give an approximate indication of the relevant flow rate so that a fresh gas flow can be maintained in the event of a power failure. The actual value of flow set is measured by an electronic thermistor mass-flow sensor and displayed electronically as a bar-graph. Flows down to 200 ml/min can be selected accurately by observing the bar-graph as the needle valve is adjusted. The mixer provides a minimum flow of 200 ml/min continuously, for safety, corresponding to the basic adult metabolic requirement. An oxygen-flush facility enables an emergency oxygen flow of about 50 litres/min to pass directly to the fresh gas outlet or the circle system. As an extra check on the function of the gas mixing valves, the total measured flow of the mixed gases is compared internally with the individual gas flows.

If a breathing gas mixture containing less than 21% oxygen is set and not corrected, the nitrous oxide flow is automatically shut off after 5 s. Simultaneous delivery of air and nitrous oxide is not possible.

The Vaporizer

The volatile anaesthetic agent is delivered directly into the fresh gas mixture as very small boluses of 100% vapour by a vaporizer that is unlike the conventional manually operated type (Fig. 7.10). There are three

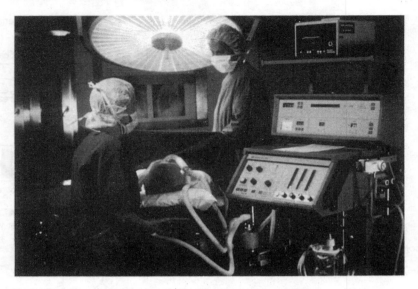

Figure 7.8 Engström ELSA electronically controlled anaesthetic machine.

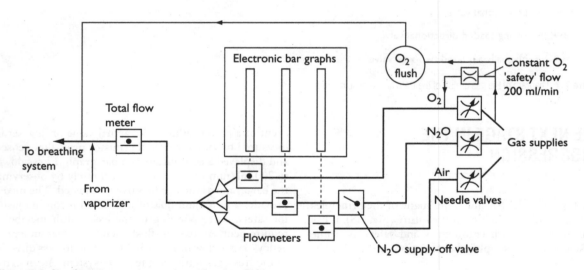

Figure 7.9 Simplified diagram of a gas mixer of Engström ELSA.

separate vaporizers, one for each of the agents: halothane, enflurane and isoflurane. The supply of volatile agent is stored on the machine in its original bottle, which is attached to the vaporizer assembly with a non-interchangeable adaptor. A pressure of 0.4 bar of oxygen is applied to the contents of the bottle to drive the liquid as required into the vaporizing chamber. A capacitive electronic sensor is used to measure the remaining contents of the supply bottle. This level is indicated on a bar-graph display on the front of the machine. The liquid then passes to the vaporizing

chamber, which is electrically heated. The temperature at the top of the chamber is maintained at 75°C in the case of the halothane and isoflurane vaporizers, and 80°C in the case of enflurane. This falls to a temperature of about 45°C at the bottom of the chamber where the liquid enters. Thus the upper part of the chamber contains 100% anaesthetic vapour whilst the lower part contains the liquid form. One millilitre boluses of this 100% vapour are then allowed to join the gases from the gas mixer by the opening, for short periods, of an electro-magnetically controlled valve at the top of the chamber.

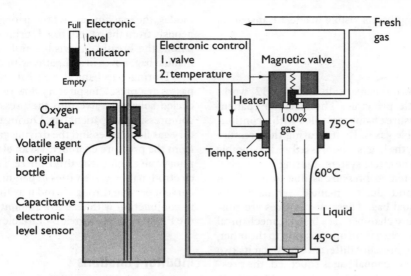

Figure 7.10 Simplified diagram of a vaporizer – Engström ELSA.

The frequency with which these 1-ml boluses of vapour are allowed into the fresh gas flow is automatically varied so that the dialled vapour concentration is maintained irrespective of the fresh gas flow rate.

The Breathing Systems

The fresh gas supply, with or without added volatile agent, is passed either to a fresh gas outlet for the addition of standard breathing systems, or to an integral circle absorber system with a built-in ventilator. The circle system is shown diagramatically in Fig. 7.11. The gas flow is conventional but the parts shown within the boxed area may be removed as a single unit and autoclaved. Both the inspiratory and expiratory gas flows are measured using venturi flowmeters as described in Chapter 5. The airway pressure is monitored electronically and also displayed using a conventional mechanical aneroid pressure gauge. A safety inlet valve allows ingress of air if there is insufficient gas in the

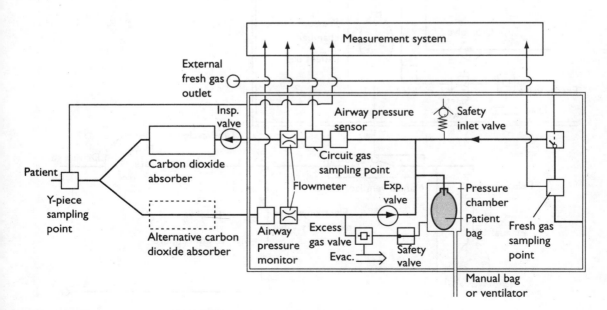

Figure 7.11 Simplified diagram of the breathing system of Engström ELSA.

circle. The breathing bag is visible inside a transparent pressure chamber.

The Ventilator

The ventilator, shown schematically in Fig. 7.12, works on the bag-in-bottle principle. The reservoir (patient bag) inside the pressure chamber is filled with a continuous flow of respirable gases. By increasing the pressure inside the chamber, the bag is compressed and respirable gas is pushed into the circle system. During mechanical ventilation, the increased pressure is due to flow from the driving gas, and during manual ventilation by squeezing the manual bag. These two sources are connected to the pressure chamber via a bistable mechanical valve. This valve switches from one position to the other, depending upon the pressure difference between its two inputs. Whenever the manual bag is squeezed, the pressure increase automatically switches the bistable valve to connect the manual bag to the pressure chamber. To allow rapid adjustment of the gas volume in the manual bag, there is a filling valve that allows oxygen into the system. During the induction and spontaneous ventilation modes, the machine allows the patient to breath spontaneously from the patient bag. During spontaneous ventilation, the breaths are visible and may be 'felt' as the manual bag moves in sympathy with the patient bag.

During mechanical ventilation, the driving gas passes at a preset 'inspiratory flow rate', through a time-cycled solenoid valve into the pressure chamber, thus compressing the patient bag. During exhalation, inspiratory gas flow ceases and the driving gas is allowed to pass from the pressure chamber, via an electrodynamic expiratory valve, out to the atmosphere. This flow through an electrodynamic valve varies depending upon the electric current passing through it and may therefore be adjusted in conjunction with an extra amount of driving gas (via the PEEP valve) to provide a variable amount of PEEP.

Monitor Functions

Transducers convert the following variables into electrical signals:

- gas supply pressures;
- airway pressure;

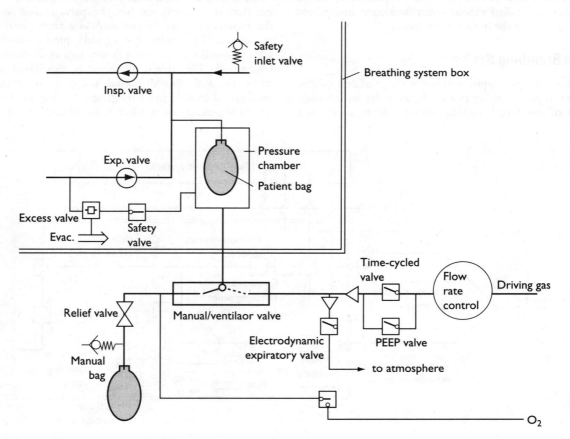

Figure 7.12 Simplified diagram of the ventilator of Engström ELSA.

- inspired and expired breathing gas volumes;
- fresh gas flows, individually and total;
- fresh gas temperatures;
- vaporizer temperatures;
- volatile agent liquid levels;
- oxygen concentration (paramagnetic);
- carbon dioxide (infrared);
- volatile agents (infrared).

The analogue signals from these transducers are all converted to digital format and two microprocessors, one for the ventilator and the other for all other functions, use the signals for control and safety monitoring of the machine function. Control messages and alarms are clearly displayed on the monitoring panel.

The control and safety functions of the microprocessors are fully integrated and will protect the patient from: gas supply failure; electrical supply failure; hypoxic mixtures; disconnections; soda-lime exhaustion; hypercapnoea; sum of fresh gas flows different from total fresh gas flow; vaporizer set too high; excessive airway pressure; exhaled minute volume outside preset limits; measured oxygen or volatile agents outside preset limits; measured end-tidal carbon dioxide outside preset limit and technical failure.

Use of microprocessor technology in an anaesthetic machine in this way also means that automatic intervention can be made to occur under certain alarm conditions.

- Oxygen supply failure automatically shuts off the nitrous oxide supply.
- A delivered hypoxic fresh gas mixture instantly initiates an alarm, and if it is not corrected within 5 s the nitrous oxide is shut off.
- Nitrous oxide is automatically shut off if air flow is opened.
- If an excessive airway pressure occurs, it is automatically relieved.
- Vaporizer malfunction causes automatic shut-off and depressurization of the supply bottles.
- Anaesthetic agent concentration above a preset level in the circle system causes the vaporizer to shut off.

Most importantly, all of these conditions cause an alarm to sound and the nature of the fault condition to be displayed in words in the centre of the monitor panel.

A COMPLETE REDEVELOPMENT – THE PHYSIOFLEX

The PhysioFlex, shown in Fig. 7.13, fully exploits the advantages of the closed circuit system but at the same time avoids the disadvantages. The main disadvantage of conventional closed circuits is the limited possibility to create a feedback-controlled closed circuit ventilator. The principles are shown in Fig. 7.14. The ventilator consists of four chambers, each of which is divided into two chambers by a highly flexible diaphragm; for simplicity, this is shown as a single chamber in Fig. 7.14. One or more of the four chambers are used in parallel depending upon the required tidal volume and the size of the patient. During the inspiratory phase, driving gas passes into the non-patient-gas half of the chamber causing the diaphragm to be deflected, increasing the pressure in the circle and inflating the patient's lungs. The movement of the diaphragm is monitored by a displacement sensor. The circle has no valves in it. To ensure that there is no rebreathing of gas that has not had its carbon dioxide removed, a continuous unidirectional gas flow of 70 litres/min around the circle is maintained by an electrically powered circulator pump. As there are no valves, there is therefore a very low resistance to the patient.

There is continuous gas analysis. A paramagnetic oxygen analyser monitors the oxygen concentration in the circulating gases. A sample of gas from close to the

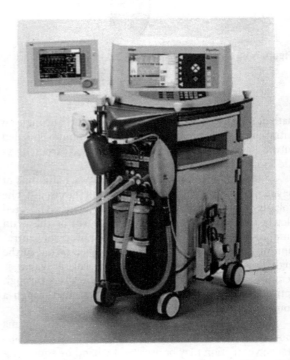

Figure 7.13 The PhysioFlex anaesthetic machine (Physio BV, The Netherlands).

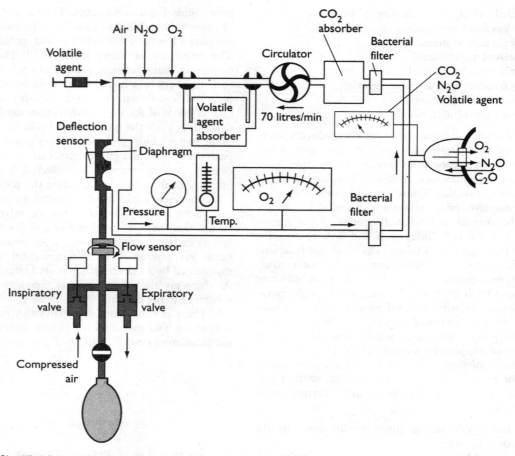

Figure 7.14 Simplified diagram of the PhysioFlex anaesthetic machine.

patient's airway is continuously drawn off through an infrared absorption spectrometer to monitor inhaled nitrous oxide, and both inhaled and exhaled carbon dioxide and the volatile anaesthetic agents.

Through small injection nozzles, exact amounts of oxygen, nitrous oxide or air are added to the circuit. The volatile anaesthetic agent in liquid form is injected slowly into the circuit under the control of the main computer at a rate to maintain the required concentration in the circuit. It is rapidly vaporized owing to the high flow of circulating gas. Excess volatile agent is removed when necessary, by passing the gases through activated charcoal. Excess gases are let out through a control valve to a vacuum system.

During spontaneous respiration the diaphrams move freely and the breathing bag expands and contracts; ventilation may be assisted by hand by squeezing the bag. During controlled ventilation, compressed air is used to deflect the diaphragms to inflate the lungs. Tidal

volume is monitored by a flow sensor in the control gas circuit; pressure and temperature of the gases in the circuit are also continuously monitored.

All these transduced measurands are used to control the flow of oxygen, nitrous oxide, air and anaesthetic agent into the circuit, release of waste gases to the vacuum system and also to control the ventilator.

SERVO-CONTROLLED ANAESTHESIA

There is currently much debate about the possibility of 'closing the loop' to servo-control the administration of anaesthesia. Figure 7.15a shows a commonly used servo-control loop for the control of blood pressure with vasoactive drug infusions. In essence this is once again the control loop of Fig. 1.11. Even with this simple

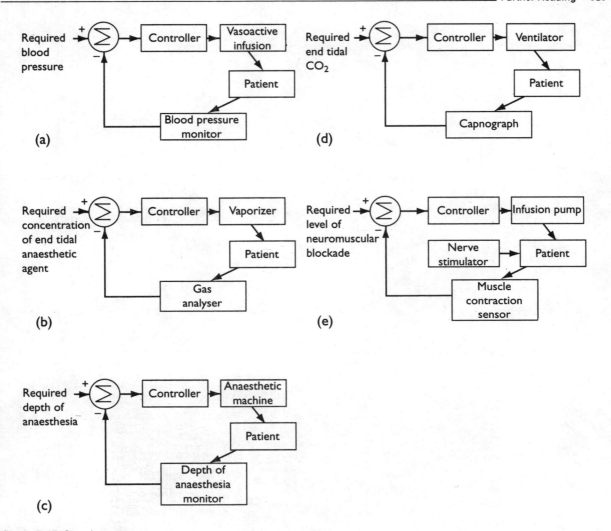

Figure 7.15 Servo loops.

system, complications are introduced, as there is a variable delay between the change in infusion rate and the change in blood pressure, and this delay is not constant in time or between patients. Also, as a closed-loop system is used to control more and more powerful drugs, safety becomes an even greater priority, with the necessity of one microprocessor system controlling a loop whilst an independent microprocessor monitors the loop for safety. Possible examples for future closed loop control are shown in Fig. 7.15b–e.

FURTHER READING

Schreiber P (1985) *Safety Guidelines: Anesthesia Systems.* Telford, Penn., USA: North American Dräger.

Schreiber P, Schreiber J (1987) *Anesthesia System Risk Analysis and Risk Reduction.* Telford, Penn., USA: North American Dräger.

The Anesthesia Work Station (1994) *Journal of Clinical Monitoring* 10: no. 5.

Verkaaik APK, Van Dijk G (1994) High flow closed circuit anaesthesia. *Anaesthesia and Intensive Care* 22: 426–434.

– 8 –

BREATHING SYSTEMS AND THEIR COMPONENTS

Contents

INTRODUCTION

The definition and classification of methods in which inhalation agents are delivered to a patient have undergone several changes since the beginnings of anaesthesia. Most current anaesthetic literature uses the following definitions and classifications.

DEFINITIONS

Breathing systems. A breathing system (not a circuit) now describes both the mode of operation and the apparatus by which inhalation agents are delivered to the patient, i.e. a Mapleson A type breathing system (generic terminology) would describe the mode of operation of a Magill breathing system (specific terminology).

Rebreathing. Rebreathing in anaesthetic systems now conventionally refers to the rebreathing of some or all of the previously exhaled gases, including carbon dioxide and water vapour. (Rebreathing apparatus in other spheres, e.g. fire fighting and underwater diving, has always referred to the recirculation of expired gas

suitably purified and with the oxygen content restored or increased.)

Apparatus dead space. This refers to that volume within the apparatus which may contain exhaled patient gas and which will be rebreathed at the beginning of a subsequent inspiratory breath (Fig. 8.1).

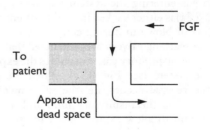

Figure 8.1 Apparatus dead space in a breathing system. FGF, fresh gas flow.

Functional dead space. Some systems may well have a smaller 'functional' dead space owing to the flushing effect of a continuous fresh gas stream at the end of expiration replacing exhaled gas in the apparatus dead space (Fig. 8.2).

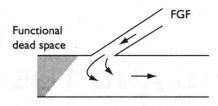

Figure 8.2 Functional dead space in a breathing system with an angled FGF inlet. FGF, fresh gas flow.

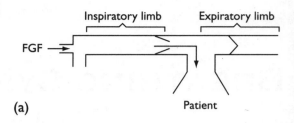

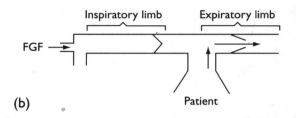

Figure 8.3 Non-rebreathing valve: (a) inspiration; (b) exhalation. FGF, fresh gas flow.

CLASSIFICATION OF BREATHING SYSTEMS

These may be classified according to function:

- non-rebreathing systems (using non-rebreathing valves);
- systems where some rebreathing of previously exhaled gas is possible, but normally prevented by the flow of fresh gas through the system;
- non-rebreathing systems using carbon dioxide absorption
  (a) unidirectional (circle) systems
  (b) bi-directional (to-and-fro) systems.

Non-rebreathing Systems

The simplest way to deliver a consistent fresh gas supply to a patient is with a system that includes a non-rebreathing valve (or valves).

Fresh gas entering the system via the inspiratory limb (Fig. 8.3a) is either sucked in by the patient's inspiratory effort or blown in during controlled ventilation. The non-rebreathing valve is so constructed that when it opens to admit inspiratory gas, it occludes the expiratory limb of the system (see Fig. 8.3a). When the patient exhales, the reverse occurs, i.e. the valve mechanism moves to occlude the inspiratory limb and opens the expiratory limb to allow expired gases to escape (Fig. 8.3b).

The inspiratory limb usually includes a distensible neoprene or rubber bag (2-litre capacity) which acts as a reservoir for fresh gas. This reservoir contains enough gas to cope with the intermittent high demand that occurs in inspiration. For example, a patient breathing normally (with a minute volume of 7 litres) may well have a tidal volume of 500 ml inhaled over approximately 1 s. This produces an average inspiratory flow rate (not peak flow rate) of 30 litres/min. Without this reservoir in the system, the fresh gas flow rate would have to at least match this figure (probably more, to match the patient's

peak inspiratory flow rate) in order to avoid respiratory embarrassment.

The reservoir bag is refilled with fresh gas during the expiratory phase. It can also be compressed manually to provide assisted or controlled respiration since the non-rebreathing valve works equally effectively in this mode as it does for spontaneous respiration.

In the non-rebreathing system described, the fresh gas flow rate *must not be less than* the minute volume required by the patient.

Systems Where Rebreathing is Possible

A miscellany of breathing systems was developed by early pioneers (largely intuitively) that allowed the to-and-fro movement of inspiratory and expiratory gases within the breathing system. Carbon dioxide elimination was achieved by the flushing action of fresh gas introduced into this breathing system, rather than by separation of the inspiratory and expiratory gas mixtures by a non-rebreathing valve described above. As it is mainly the flushing effect of fresh gas that eliminates carbon dioxide, these systems retain the potential for rebreathing of carbon dioxide when fresh gas flow rates are reduced.

Mapleson (1954) classified these systems (A to E) according to their efficiency in eliminating carbon dioxide during spontaneous respiration. An F system, the Jackson Rees modification of system E (Ayre's T-piece), was later added to the classification by Willis (1975) (see below).

Mapleson's Classification of Breathing Systems

Figure 8.4 illustrates a modified Mapleson classification of breathing systems. These all contain similar components but are assembled in different sequences so that they may be used more conveniently in specific circumstances. However, the efficiency of each system is different. They are catalogued in order (A, B, C, D, E, F) of increased requirement of fresh gas flow to prevent rebreathing during spontaneous respiration. System A requires 0.8–1 times the patient's minute ventilation, B and C require 1.5–2 times the patient's minute ventilation and systems D, E and F (functionally similar) require 2–4 times the patient's minute ventilation to prevent rebreathing during spontaneous respiration.

WORKING PRINCIPLES OF BREATHING SYSTEMS

Mapleson A Breathing System (Fig. 8.5)

The Mapleson A system illustrated is the Magill arrangement (or attachment) as popularized by Sir Ivan Magill in the 1920s. It consists of the following:

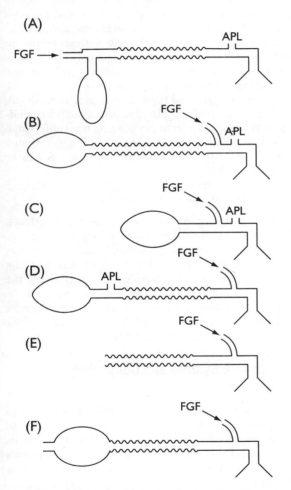

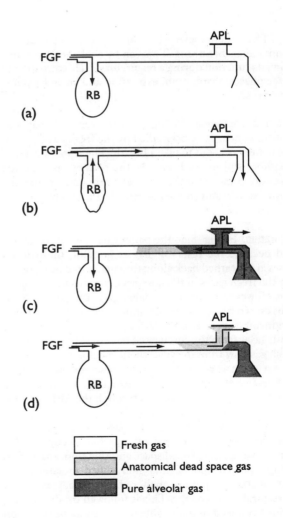

Figure 8.4 A modified Mapleson classification of breathing systems in which there is potential for rebreathing. System (A) houses the gas reservoir in the afferent limb and is alternatively referred to as an afferent reservoir system. The fresh gas flow (FGF) need only be at or just below the patient's minute ventilation without functional rebreathing occurring. Systems (B) and (C) (junctional reservoir systems) require FGF of 1.5 times the minute ventilation to avoid rebreathing. Systems (D), (E) and (F) (efferent reservoir systems) require 2–3 times the minute ventilation to avoid rebreathing.

Figure 8.5 The Mapleson A system used with spontaneous breathing (see text). FGF, fresh gas flow; APL, adjustable pressure-limiting (expiratory) valve; RB, reservoir bag.

- at one end, an inlet for fresh gas linked to a 2-litre distensible rubber reservoir bag. (Not a rebreathing bag, as the patient's exhaled gases should never be allowed to pass back into it.) This is attached to:
- a length of corrugated breathing hose (minimum length 110 cm with an internal volume of 550 ml). This represents slightly more than the average tidal volume in an anaesthetized adult breathing spontaneously. This volume is important as it minimizes the backtracking of exhaled alveolar gas back to the reservoir bag (see below). This is in turn connected to:
- a variable tension, spring-loaded flap valve for venting of exhaled gases. This valve should be attached at the opposite end of the system from the reservoir bag and as close to the patient as possible. It will be subsequently referred to as an APL (adjustable pressure limiting) valve.

The system makes efficient use of fresh gas during spontaneous breathing. This can be explained by examining its function during a respiratory cycle consisting of three phases: inspiration, expiration and an end-expiratory pause.

The first inspiration. In Fig. 8.5a the reservoir bag and breathing hose have been filled by the fresh gas flow and the patient is about to take a breath. The whole system is therefore full of fresh gas. As the patient inspires, the gases are drawn into the lungs at a rate greater than the fresh gas flow and so the reservoir bag partially empties, as shown in Fig. 8.5b.

Expiration. In Fig. 8.5c the patient has begun to exhale, and because the reservoir bag is not full, the exhaled gases are breathed back along the corrugated hose, pushing the fresh gases in the hose back towards the reservoir bag. However, before the exhaled gases can pass as far as the reservoir bag (hence the importance of the length of the inspiratory hose), the latter has been refilled by the fresh gases from the corrugated hose plus the continuing fresh gas flow from the anaesthetic machine.

A point is reached when the reservoir bag is again full and as the patient is still exhaling, the remaining exhaled gases have to pass out through the APL (expiratory) valve, which now opens.

The first portion of exhaled gases to pass up the corrugated hose from the patient was that occupying the patient's anatomical dead space and therefore apart from being warmed and slightly humidified (a satisfactory state of affairs), they are unaltered, having not taken part in respiratory exchange. This is followed by alveolar gas (with a reduced oxygen content, and containing carbon dioxide), some of which enters the corrugated hose, and some which is expelled through the APL valve when the reservoir bag is full.

End-expiratory pause. The next stage is the end-expiratory pause. The fresh gas flow entering the system now drives those exhaled gases, or some of them that had tracked back along the corrugated hose, out through the APL valve. It will be seen that the expiratory pause is important because it prevents the patient's rebreathing of exhaled alveolar gases contained in the hose at the end of expiration (Fig. 8.5d).

During the end-expiratory pause, all the alveolar gases and some of the dead-space gases are expelled from the corrugated hose through the APL valve by the continuing fresh gas flow. Thus, during the next inspiratory phase, the gas inspired may well initially contain some of the remaining dead-space gases from the previous breath, along with fresh gas. As explained above, these dead-space gases may be re-inspired without detriment to the patient. The fresh gas flow rate may therefore be rather less than the patient's minute volume and rebreathing of alveolar gas is prevented.

In theory, provided there is no mixing of fresh gas, dead-space gas and alveolar gas, and a sufficient end-expiratory pause, the fresh gas flow rate need only match alveolar ventilation (approximately 66% of the minute volume), as in this situation only alveolar gas will be vented through the APL valve.

In practice, however, several factors dictate a higher fresh gas flow rate (70–90%), for instance:

- There is mixing of the various gaseous interfaces, which reduces the theoretical efficiency of the system.
- Occasionally, larger than expected tidal volumes may well be exhaled and therefore reach the reservoir bag, in which case carbon dioxide will contaminate the reservoir bag and the subsequent inspiratory gases.
- Rapid respiratory rates will reduce or even eliminate an end-expiratory pause and reduce the potential for carbon dioxide elimination that this pause allows.

Mapleson A System and Controlled Ventilation

The mechanical aspects of the Mapleson A (Fig. 8.6) (Magill attachment) system as described above relate to its use in spontaneous respiration. However, if controlled or assisted ventilation is used, with the patient's lungs inflated by means of squeezing the reservoir bag, a different state of affairs occurs:

- *Inspiratory phase*. The APL valve has to be kept almost closed so that sufficient pressure can develop in the system to inflate the lungs. During the first inspiratory phase with the anaesthetist squeezing the bag, it is fresh gases that are blown out of the valve.
- *Expiratory phase*. At the end of inspiration, the reservoir bag may be almost empty, and as soon as the anaesthetist relaxes pressure on it, the patient exhales

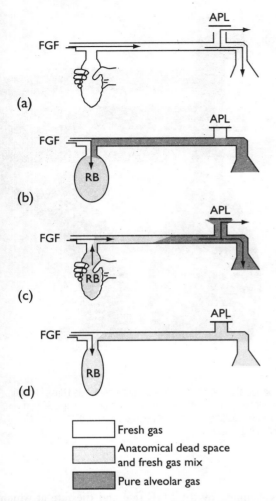

(a)

(b)

(c)

(d)

▢ Fresh gas

▨ Anatomical dead space
and fresh gas mix

▨ Pure alveolar gas

Figure 8.6 Mapleson A system with assisted or controlled ventilation: (a) at the end of inspiration; (b) at the end of expiration; (c) during subsequent inspiration; (d) at the end of the subsequent inspiration. Note that much rebreathing takes place (see text). FGF, fresh gas flow; APL, adjustable pressure-limiting (expiratory) valve; RB, reservoir bag.

into the corrugated hose. The exhaled dead space and alveolar gases may then pass right back into the reservoir bag. (The capacity of the standard 110-cm corrugated hose is about 550 ml.)

There is a natural tendency to allow little or no expiratory pause, so that when the anaesthetist squeezes the bag again, the first gases to enter the patient's lungs will be the previously exhaled alveolar gases. The volume of gases escaping via the APL valve during this second inspiratory phase is initially small (the valve being almost closed) but gradually increases as the pressure in the system rises towards the maximum inspiration. Therefore, the greatest amount of gas will be dumped late in the

cycle and will consist mainly of fresh gas. Under these circumstances there is considerable rebreathing (Fig. 8.6). Furthermore, as alveolar gas will have entered the reservoir bag, there will always be carbon dioxide contamination in any subsequent inspirate. In order to prevent this and thereby minimize the potential for rebreathing alveolar gas, a high fresh gas flow rate is required. This is usually of the order of two times the patient's minute ventilation. This situation is highly wasteful of fresh gas and also increases the potential for pollution.

Other Mapleson A Breathing Systems

Lack Co-axial Breathing System (Fig. 8.7a)
The traditional layout of a Magill system sites the APL valve as close to the patient as possible. However, this:

- reduces the access to the valve in head and neck surgery and
- increases the drag on the mask or endotracheal tube when the valve is shrouded and connected to scavenging tubing.

The Lack system overcomes these two problems. The original version was constructed with a co-axial arrangement of breathing hoses. Exhaled gases passed through the orifice of the inner hose sited at the patient end of the system and then back towards the APL valve, which is now sited on the reservoir bag mount. The valve is thus conveniently sited for adjustment by the anaesthetist and its weight, and that of any additional scavenging attachment, is now supported by the anaesthetic machine (see Fig. 8.7). The system still functions as a Mapleson A system. The co-axial hosing on early models was criticized as being too narrow and having too high a flow resistance. In later models, the inner and outer breathing hose diameters were subsequently both increased, to 15 and 30 mm respectively, to overcome this problem. Another problem was that the tubing was heavy and stiff, putting a stress on the connection to the facepiece or endotracheal connection.

Lack Parallel Breathing System (Fig. 8.7b)
Co-axial breathing systems have not found universal favour. If the inner hose were to become disconnected or to split, as has been the case, the leak may pass unnoticed. It drastically alters the efficiency of the system in eliminating carbon dioxide and is therefore potentially very dangerous. A version of the Lack system with parallel hoses is now available (see Fig. 8.7b).

Mapleson B and C Systems

These place both the fresh gas supply, reservoir bag and APL valve closer to the patient, allowing the anaesthetist

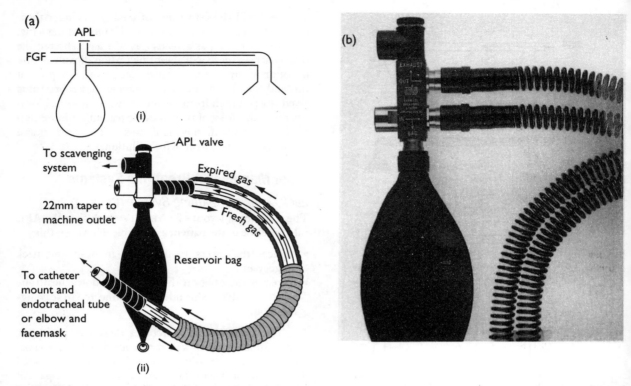

Figure 8.7 (a) The Lack co-axial breathing system. (i) Working principles. (ii) The actual assembly. Note that the outer corrugated hose is partly transparent so that the inner tube may be seen to be intact. The adjustable pressure-limiting valve (APL) is fitted with a shroud having a 30 mm outlet so that it may be attached to a scavenging system. (b) The Lack parallel breathing attachment. The inner (expiratory) limb of the co-axial arrangement has been replaced by one that is parallel to the inspiratory limb. FGF, fresh gas flow.

easy access to the latter two, whilst at the same time allowing the fresh gas source to be sited at a distance if necessary. However, as mentioned above neither is as economical as the A system for spontaneous respiration. The reasons are outlined below for the B system:

- *The first inspiration.* The system is initially assumed to be full of fresh gas so that during the first inspiration the patient breathes only fresh gas.
- *Expiration.* During expiration, the exhaled gases (initially dead space gas and then the first part of the alveolar gas), mixed with the fresh gas flow (FGF) pass to the reservoir bag. When the latter has been refilled, the remainder of the exhaled gases (the rest of the alveolar gas) and the FGF are voided via the APL valve (expiratory valve).
- *End-expiratory pause.* During this phase, it is fresh gas that escapes from the APL valve as this is closer to the valve than the bag.
- *The next inspiration.* This will be supplied by the contents of the bag, which has a mixture of fresh, dead space and alveolar gas, the proportion of which will be

determined by the FGF rate and the rate at which exhalation occurred. If the FGF is high and the exhalation rate was slow, there will be a greater amount of fresh gas in the inspirate.

Mapleson D System

Mapleson D System with Spontaneous Respiration
The system is best explained if, again, the three phases of the respiratory cycle are considered inspiration, expiration and end-expiratory pause:

- *The first inspiration.* The system is initially assumed to be full of fresh gas so that during the first inspiration the patient breathes only fresh gas (Fig. 8.8a).
- *Expiration.* During expiration, the exhaled gases, mixed with the FGF, pass down the corrugated hose to the reservoir bag (Fig. 8.8b); when this has been refilled the remainder of the exhaled gases and the FGF are voided via the APL valve (expiratory valve). Of the expired gases it is those from the dead space that are voided first, followed by alveolar gases.

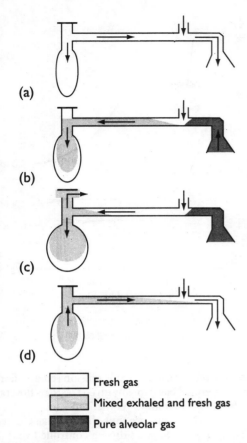

(a)

(b)

(c)

(d)

	Fresh gas
	Mixed exhaled and fresh gas
	Pure alveolar gas

Figure 8.8 The Mapleson D system with spontaneous ventilation (see text). FGF, fresh gas flow; APL, adjustable pressure-limiting (expiratory) valve.

- *End-expiratory pause*. During the end-expiratory pause the FGF passes down the corrugated hose, displacing some of the mixture of exhaled gas and FGF, which is now vented out through the APL valve (Fig. 8.8c). The amount of fresh gas occupying and thus stored in the patient end of the corrugated hose at the end of expiration depends on the FGF rate, the duration of the end-expiratory pause and the degree of mixing (due to turbulence) of the various gaseous interfaces within the corrugated hose.
- *At the next inspiration* the inhaled gases consist initially of this stored fresh gas followed then by the mixture of exhaled gases and FGF that remain in the tube (Fig. 8.8d).

However, there are practical problems with this concept, since the expiratory pause may be short, or absent (especially in infants) during spontaneous breathing (when volatile anaesthetics only are used without opioid supplement). In this case the FGF needs to be sufficiently high to flush the exhaled gases downstream prior to the next inspiration. In fact, rebreathing of exhaled alveolar gas occurs unless the FGF is at least two times and possibly up to four times the patient's minute ventilation.

It is worthy of note that the Mapleson D system is functionally similar to a T-piece (Mapleson E). However, with a T-piece, the limb through which the ventilation occurs, if used without a reservoir bag, must be of such a length that the volume of gas in it when augmented by the volume of the FGF being delivered during inspiration is no less than that of the patient's tidal volume, otherwise dilution of anaesthetic by entrained air will occur.

Mapleson D System with Controlled or Assisted Ventilation

- *The first inspiration*. As the bag is squeezed, the FGF entering the system as well as fresh gases stored in the wide-bore breathing hose pass to the patient. At the same time some gases from the reservoir bag are lost through the partially open APL (expiratory) valve (Fig. 8.9a).
- *Expiration*. A mixture of the FGF and exhaled gases passes along the hose, eventually entering the now deflated reservoir bag, causing it to refill (Fig. 8.9b).
- *Expiratory pause*. At this point, provided that there is an expiratory pause, the fresh gas supply continues to flow down the hose to replace and drive the mixed gases out via the APL valve. A longer expiratory pause allows a greater amount of fresh gas to enter the breathing hose (Fig. 8.9c).
- *The next inspiration*. At the next squeeze of the reservoir bag (Fig. 8.9d), the continuing FGF plus the fresh gas now stored in the breathing hose plus any previously expired gases that may remain in the hose pass to the patient, while some of the mixed gases within the bag escape via the APL valve. The cycle then repeats itself.

Thus to prevent rebreathing in the Mapleson D system during both spontaneous and controlled ventilation, the FGF must be sufficiently high enough to:

- purge the breathing hose of exhaled gases;
- supplement the stored fresh gas in this breathing hose so that any mixed gas in the reservoir bag is prevented from entering the hose and reaching the patient. The amount of fresh gas required will always be greater than the patient's minute volume and will depend largely on the expiratory pause. The longer the pause, the more effective will be the ability of the fresh gas to purge the breathing hose of expired gas.

However, during controlled ventilation, *deliberate use is often made of functional rebreathing*. Theoretically, if slow

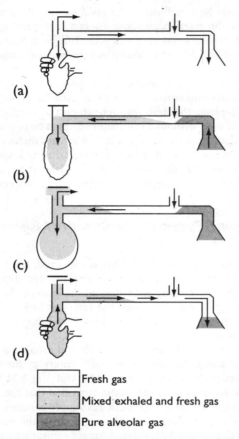

Fresh gas

Mixed exhaled and fresh gas

Pure alveolar gas

Figure 8.9 Mapleson D system with manual ventilation. (a) The first inspiration; note that the APL valve is forced open. (b) Early exhalation; the APL valve is closed and the partially collapsed reservoir bag is filling. (c) Late exhalation/expiratory pause; mixed gas is vented from the system. (d) Subsequent inspiration.

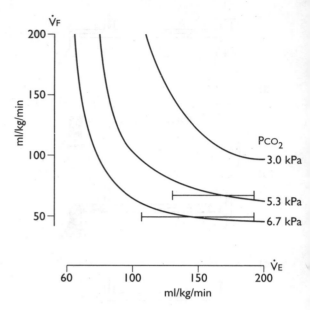

Figure 8.10 Isopleths showing the relationship between fresh gas flow ($\dot{V}_F$), minute ventilation ($\dot{V}_E$) and alveolar carbon dioxide tension.

ventilation rates (with long expiratory pauses) and large tidal volumes are chosen, then sufficient expiratory time will elapse to allow a modest FGF to fill the proximal part of the system with sufficient fresh gas to provide alveolar ventilation. This will enter the lungs first, followed by a mixture of previously expired gases (from the machine end of the system), which will then occupy anatomical dead space. Hence, theoretically, it should be possible to reduce the FGF to the volume required for alveolar ventilation.

In practice, there is turbulent mixing of the various gaseous interfaces so that alveolar gas is widely distributed (and diluted). Even so, provided a *sufficiently large controlled minute ventilation* is delivered so that most of the FGF reaches the alveoli, adequate alveolar ventilation will occur with FGF rates of 70% of the anticipated minute ventilation since, as mentioned above, some rebreathing is acceptable. Figure 8.10 demonstrates this, as well as the

fact that the arterial carbon dioxide tension remains fairly constant (horizontal bars) for any given fresh gas flow rate despite alterations in minute ventilation.

Mapleson D systems are thus able to make efficient use of fresh anaesthetic gases during controlled ventilation and could have considerable cost-saving benefits. Figure 8.11 shows how the Mapleson D system may be employed with an automatic ventilator. The reservoir bag is removed and replaced with a standard length of corrugated hose of sufficient capacity to accommodate the air or oxygen that is delivered by the ventilator, and which prevents it reaching the patient in place of the intended anaesthetic gases.

The Bain System

The Bain breathing system (Fig. 8.12) is similar in function to the Mapleson D system. The only difference is that the FGF is carried by a tube within the corrugated hose (a co-axial arrangement). In the earlier models in particular, there was a risk that the inner tube could become disconnected at the machine end; if this happened a very big dead space was introduced. It could also become kinked, so cutting off the supply of fresh gases.

Hybrid Systems

Several breathing systems have been described that, by means of a lever switch, can convert the system from a Mapleson A to a Mapleson D or E, allowing a system to be

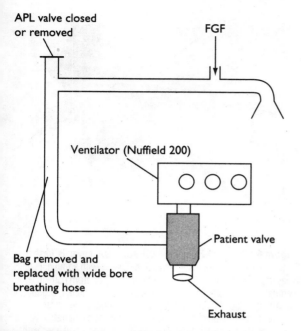

APL valve closed or removed

FGF

Ventilator (Nuffield 200)

Patient valve

Bag removed and replaced with wide bore breathing hose

Exhaust

Figure 8.11 Controlled ventilation with a Mapleson D system using a ventilator. Note that with the employment of a ventilator that operates as a 'gas piston', the former must be separated from the breathing system by a suitably long piece of breathing hose (with an internal volume of at least 500 ml). This prevents the driving gas from reaching the patient and diluting the anaesthetic mixture. APL, adjustable pressure-limiting valve; FGF, fresh gas flow.

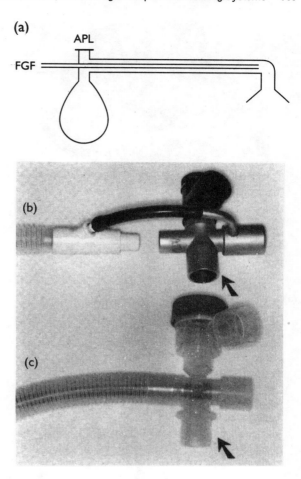

(a)

APL

FGF

(b)

(c)

Figure 8.12 The Bain breathing system. (a) Working principle; (b) and (c) show two different arrangements of the FGF bypassing the bag mount (arrow). They are functionally identical. FGF, fresh gas flow; APL, adjustable pressure-limiting (expiratory) valve.

chosen and used in its most efficient mode (i.e. system A, spontaneous respiration; system E, controlled respiration). The Humphrey ADE system (M&IE and Anaequip UK) seems to be the most popular version (Fig. 8.13).

With the lever switch in the A mode (Fig. 8.13b), the reservoir bag on the ADE block is connected to the inspiratory pathway as in a Mapleson A system. The breathing hose connecting the block to the patient is now designated as the inspiratory limb. However, expired gas is ducted down a separate limb back to an APL valve mounted on the block, which is shrouded to facilitate scavenging. In practice it appears to function more efficiently than a traditional Magill attachment. The improved efficiency is thought to relate to the geometrical arrangement of the components at the patient end of the system. Towards the end of exhalation in the Magill attachment, the exhaled dead-space gas that has passed up the breathing hose is now returned towards the APL valve by the flushing action of the FGF entering the system. At the APL valve, it meets and mixes with alveolar gas in a turbulent fashion, and a mixture of both is discharged from the valve. However, in the Humphrey (and Lack) systems alveolar gas is diverted in a more laminar

fashion into a physically separate expiratory limb, which minimizes any potential for mixing of the two gas phases in question. This arrangement, and the removal of the APL valve assembly away from the patient end of the system, also reduces apparatus dead space, so that with further modification (see below) it may be suitable for infants and neonates.

With the lever in the D/E mode (Fig. 8.13c), the reservoir bag and APL valve are isolated from the breathing system. What was the 'inspiratory' limb in A mode is now a gas delivery tube to the patient end of the system as in T-piece (see below). The breathing hose returning gas to the ADE block now functions as the reservoir limb of a T-piece. This hose is opened to the atmosphere via a port adjacent to the bag mount. As this mode does not incorporate a reservoir bag, it is strictly a Mapleson E system.

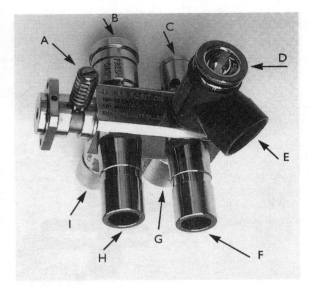

(a)

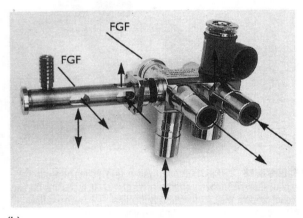

(b)

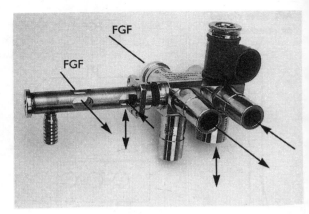

(c)

Figure 8.13 (a) The Humphrey ADE system. A, Lever; B, fresh gas input; C, overpressure relief valve; D, APL valve with spindle; E, scavenging shroud; F, 22 mm breathing hose port from patient; G, ventilator port; H, 22 mm breathing hose port to patient; I, bag mount. (b) An exploded diagram; with the lever set upright, the system functions in its Mapleson A mode for spontaneous respiration with a recommended fresh gas flow (FGF) of 70 ml/kg or less if used with capnography. Manual ventilation is easily instituted by pressing on the spindle to close the valve during inspiration and releasing it during exhalation. (c) For mechanical ventilation the lever is positioned downwards, converting the breathing system to the Mapleson E mode by isolating the reservoir bag and APL valve but incorporating the ventilator port. The fresh gas flow may be kept the same.

The port described above is usually connected to a ventilator of the 'bag-squeezer' type, so that the system is used in its most efficient mode for controlled ventilation. If a reservoir bag and APL valve were to be attached to this port, it would function as a D system. However, this is not recommended because it may encourage the system to be used uneconomically for spontaneous respiration, as a high FGF is required to prevent rebreathing.

The Anaequip version is supplied with 15-mm smooth-bore non-kinking breathing hose and a unique APL valve (see later in chapter). Interestingly, the use of this smooth bore hose reduces turbulence in the range of flows seen in quietly breathing adults, so that its performance is little different from that of 22-mm corrugated hose. The narrower bore hose also reduces the internal volume of the system to an extent that it is now also suitable for use with infants. A low internal volume is important in a paediatric breathing system in order that:

- during controlled ventilation, the small tidal volumes required are delivered more efficiently; and
- during spontaneous respiration, the energy expended by the patient in overcoming the inertia of the gas present in the system is reduced, especially as with high respiratory rates the direction of gas flow is reversed very frequently.

Mapleson E and F Systems

The T-piece System

However efficient an expiratory valve may be, it is bound to offer some resistance to exhalation, which may not be acceptable in certain anaesthetic techniques such as those used for neonatal and infant anaesthesia. To avoid this resistance, the T-piece system may be used. In Fig. 8.14 the fresh gases are supplied via a small-bore tube to the side arm of an Ayre's T-piece. The main body of the T-piece is within the breathing system and must, therefore, be of adequate diameter. One end of the body is connected by the shortest possible means to the patient.

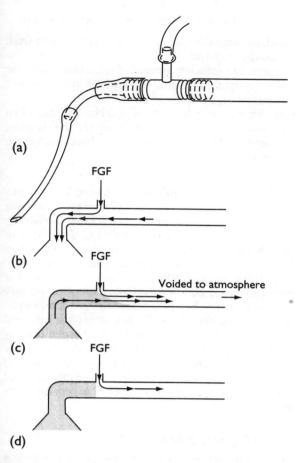

(a)

FGF

(b)   FGF

Voided to atmosphere

(c)   FGF

(d)

Figure 8.14 (a) The Ayre's T-piece connected to an endotracheal tube; (b) during spontaneous inspiration; (c) during expiration; (d) during the expiratory pause. FGF, fresh gas flow.

(The volume of this limb makes up apparatus dead space.) The other end is connected to a length of tubing that acts as a reservoir.

In the case of spontaneous ventilation, the FGF rate must be high. During inspiration the peak inspiratory flow rate is higher than the FGF, so some gases are drawn from the reservoir limb. During expiration both the exhaled air and the fresh gases, which continue to flow, pass into the reservoir limb and are expelled to the atmosphere. During the end-expiratory pause the FGF flushes out and refills the reservoir limb. The dimensions of the reservoir limb and the FGF rate are governed by the following considerations:

- The diameter of the reservoir limb must be sufficient to present the lowest possible resistance (not more than 0.07 kPa (0.75 cmH$_2$O) for a neonate and not more than 0.2 kPa (2 cmH$_2$O) for an adult at the appropriate flow rates).

- The volume of the expiratory limb should be not less than the patient's tidal volume. Too great a volume would matter only in that the greater length would lead to increased resistance. Too great a diameter would lead to mixing of the fresh gases with alveolar gas and to inefficiency of the system. For an adult a standard 110 cm length of corrugated hose is satisfactory.

- The optimum FGF rate depends not only on the patient's minute volume and respiratory rate but also on the capacity of the reservoir limb. If the latter is at least that of the patient's tidal volume, then a rate of 2.5 times the patient's minute volume is sufficient. This is the most satisfactory arrangement. However, if the capacity of the reservoir is reduced, the flow rate must be increased. If the capacity of the reservoir is reduced to zero, the flow rate must be in excess of the peak inspiratory flow rate so as to reduce the possibility of ingress of air.

The shape of the T-piece is also important. Normally the side arm is at right angles to the body. If it is at an angle pointing towards the patient, there is continuous positive pressure applied, which would act as a resistance during expiration; similarly, if the gases were directed towards the reservoir, a subatmospheric pressure would be caused by a venturi effect. As mentioned previously this continuous positive airways pressure is thought to be beneficial in minimizing the fall in functional residual capacity (FRC), especially in neonates.

Controlled Ventilation with the T-piece
Controlled ventilation may be effected by intermittently occluding the end of the reservoir limb with the thumb. This should be done with care, since when the outlet is occluded the full pressure supplied by the anaesthetic machine is applied to the patient. It would seem prudent to include, in infant systems at least, a blow-off valve set to about 4 kPa (40 cmH$_2$O) pressure, but this is seldom done. A limitation in its use arises from the fact that the peak inspiratory flow rate is limited to that of the FGF. This is overcome in the Rees T-piece, described below.

The T-piece system is particularly suited to neonates and infants, where an expiratory valve would produce a significant resistance. The scaling down of a system suitable for adults may be quite inappropriate for use with small children.

The Rees T-piece (Mapleson F System)
A great improvement to the T-piece was made by Rees, who added a small double-ended bag to the end of the reservoir limb (Fig. 8.15).

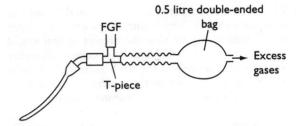

Figure 8.15 The Rees T-piece. FGF, fresh gas flow.

However, the tubular portion of the limb should still approximate to the patient's tidal volume, or rebreathing could occur as a result of the mixing of expired and fresh gases. During spontaneous ventilation small movements of the semi-collapsed bag demonstrate the patient's breathing. During the inspiratory phase of manual ventilation, the bag is squeezed with the open end of the bag partially or totally occluded by the anaesthetist. During exhalation, the open end is released to allow the gas in the system to escape. This simple method is extremely efficient for infants and small children. Several mechanical devices are available that can be placed in the tail of the bag so as to provide a variable restriction similar to that described above. However, these may all be accidentally turned off, occluding the expiratory limb completely. As the system does not contain an over-pressure safety valve, a dangerously high pressure could build up which could damage the lungs of any infant connected to it. These devices cannot therefore be recommended.

Other paediatric breathing systems are described in Chapter 14.

Alternative Classification for Mapleson-Type Systems

An alternative nomenclature has recently been proposed for the systems described above, which relates to the position of the reservoir bag within the breathing system. The Mapleson A system in which the reservoir bag stores fresh gas is described as an *afferent reservoir system*. System D, in which the reservoir bag stores mixed expired gases, is described as an *efferent reservoir system*, and systems B and C, in which the reservoir bag stores mixed inspired and expired gases, are called *junctional reservoir systems*.

Non-rebreathing Systems with a Facility for Carbon Dioxide Absorption

High flows of inhalation anaesthetic agents (i.e. at least approximately equal to the patient's minute ventilation) are regularly used with most breathing systems at the beginning of an anaesthetic for the following reasons:

- both to purge the system of air and to fill it with fresh anaesthetic agents;
- to provide a sufficient amount of inhalational agent for alveolar uptake (which is initially high at the onset of anaesthesia);
- to eliminate exhaled carbon dioxide. (As described previously, the efficiency with which this is done depends on the characteristics of the breathing system chosen.)
- to eliminate body nitrogen.

However, when equilibrium between the patient's blood and inspired concentration of anaesthetic has been reached, this inspired concentration is exhaled relatively unchanged, and so the main function of high FGFs in most breathing systems is the elimination of carbon dioxide (whilst at the same time providing oxygen!).

Thus to continue a high FGF after equilibrium has been achieved is both wasteful and expensive and may increase theatre pollution. This exhaled gas at near equilibrium can be reused in suitable systems if it is purged of exhaled carbon dioxide, and has the oxygen concentration restored (oxygen is always removed from the inspiratory mixture by the lungs at a rate between 120 and 250 ml/min). The reutilization of suitably modified exhaled gases can thus reduce the FGF to very low levels (see below).

Carbon Dioxide Absorption

Carbon dioxide can be removed from exhaled gases by a chemical reaction with various metallic bases (hydroxides). This reaction requires the presence of water in order that these bases and carbon dioxide (as carbonic acid) can exist in ionic form. There are two types of commercial preparation of these metallic bases:

1. *Soda lime*. This is made up of approximately 80% calcium hydroxide, 4% sodium hydroxide and 14–20% added water content. The sodium hydroxide is included both to improve the reactivity of the mixture and for its hygroscopic properties (binding the necessary added water in the mixture). The addition of hardeners (silica and kieselguhr, a clay) to help form the required granule size in soda lime is no longer required in modern manufacturing processes. Similarly, potassium hydroxide, which was thought to improve the activity of soda lime when cold, is no longer added.
2. *Barium lime*. Barium lime is made up of 80% calcium hydroxide and 20% barium hydroxide (octahydrate). The barium hydroxide has its own naturally occurring 'water of crystallization' and in combination with calcium hydroxide has never required additional hardeners. The main chemical reaction is:

$$CO_2 + H_2O = H^+ + HCO_3$$

Carbon   Water   Carbonic acid
dioxide

$$Ca(OH)_2 + H^+ + HCO_3 = CaCO_3 + 2H_2O$$

Calcium   Carbonic Calcium   Water
hydroxide   acid   carbonate

The reaction is interesting in that:

- it produces heat energy (it is an exothermic reaction);
- it changes the pH of the soda lime, which allows the use of indicator dyes to show when the soda lime is exhausted; and
- it produces more water than that used up in the reaction.

The size of the granules is important. Too large a granule size produces large gaps in a canister of stacked granules, leading to poor contact with gases passing through, with a consequent inefficient absorption of carbon dioxide. Too small a granule may provide an unacceptably high resistance to gas flow along with the increased possibility of dust formation. The optimum size of granule is thought to be between 1.5 and 5 mm in diameter. The product is sieved through various meshes to retain sizes between these tolerances. Mesh standards differ between countries owing to variations in thickness of the wire used to construct the mesh. In the USA soda lime granules are supplied at a USP (United States Pharmacopeia) standard of between 4 and 8 Mesh (2.36–4.75 mm). In the UK the granules are supplied to a BP (British Pharmacopoeia) standard of 1.4–4.75 mm (3–10 Mesh).

The dust is caustic and can produce burns in the respiratory tract if inhaled. This was a problem with the older type of system with 'to-and-fro' absorption (Waters canister, see below), where the absorber was placed in close proximity to the patient's airway. However, circle absorbers are usually separated from the patient by at least a metre of breathing hose, which normally hangs in a loop. This allows the dust, if present, to fall out before it can get to the patient.

Absorptive Capacity of Soda Lime

Soda lime is capable of absorbing 25 litres of carbon dioxide per 100 g, and barium lime 27 litres of carbon dioxide per 100 g. However, in continuous use, the soda lime appears exhausted (as indicated by the colour change) before these capacities are reached, because the outside of the granule is exhausted before the whole granule is used up. Furthermore, the contact time between the absorbent and carbon dioxide affects the efficiency of the absorbent. Smaller canisters containing 500 g of soda lime appear exhausted at a carbon dioxide load of 10–12 litres per 100 g of absorbent. 'Jumbo' absorbers containing 2 kg of soda lime, which allow a longer contact time between the carbon dioxide and absorbent, appear exhausted at a carbon dioxide load of 17 litres per 100 g.

When the system is allowed to stand for a few hours, the soda lime appears to 'regenerate' as the surface carbonate is diluted by hydroxide ions migrating from within the granule. The colour of fresh soda lime and barium lime depends on which indicator dye is added by the manufacturer. For example M&IE (UK) markets 'Durosorb' and 'Viosorb' soda lime. Durosorb has 'Clayton yellow' added, which turns from deep pink when fresh to off-white when exhausted, whereas Viosorb contains 'ethyl violet' as the indicator dye, which changes from white when fresh to purple when exhausted.

The Exothermic Reaction

The heat and water produced by the reaction of soda lime on carbon dioxide has been considered to be beneficial in that (at low flows) they warm and partially humidify the inspiratory gas. The temperature and humidity of the inspired gas is related to several factors:

- Firstly, for example, if the FGF rate is high, the dry gas entering the system reduces both the humidity and the temperature of the recirculating gas.
- Secondly, at low FGFs, if the gas circulation time is high, the humidity and temperature rise.
- Thirdly, the longer the system is in use at low FGFs, the greater are the humidity and temperature of the circulating gas.

The heat produced, however, is not necessarily all beneficial. There is an increased chemical reaction with volatile anaesthetic agents in proportion to the temperature within the system.

Trichloroethylene can be decomposed to dichloroacetylene (which is neurotoxic) and further to phosgene, if the temperature within the soda lime exceeds 60°C. Older anaesthetic machines often incorporated a switching system on the back bar that could divert gas directly into a circle system rather than to the common gas outlet. The trichloroethylene vaporizer (where fitted) was always positioned downstream of this switch so that it could never be used with the circle absorber system.

Anaesthetic agents with the CHF_2 moiety (desflurane, enflurane and isoflurane) react with dry, warm soda lime or barium lime (Baralyme) to produce varying amounts of carbon monoxide. Dry Baralyme appears to have twice the tendency to produce carbon monoxide than does soda lime. Fresh absorbent, which has approximately a 15% water content (as water of crystallization), appears to prevent this. In fact a significant reaction occurs only when the water content drops below 2%. This problem seems to occur where the absorbent is left to dry out in breathing systems. This can occur when the breathing system is left unused for long periods or when dry gas is allowed to pass through it between cases, overnight, or at weekends. This may occur with some anaesthetic machines even if the flowmeters are turned off, if:

- they are plugged into the pipeline supply;
- they have a minimal basal flow of oxygen through the machine;
- the absorber is so constructed that fresh gas flows through the absorbent prior to entering the inspiratory limb.

This phenomenon can easily be avoided by using:

- smaller absorbers (so that the contents have to be changed regularly);
- disconnecting them when possible;
- ensuring that only designs which allow the fresh gas to bypass the absorber are used, and unplugging machines from the pipelines when not in use for extended periods.

Sevoflurane undergoes degradation (approximately 12.9%/h) within the absorber to non-toxic fluorinated metabolites in humans (mainly a sevo-olefin called 'compound A'). Levels rise, as would be expected, with increased concentration of the agent, prolonged anaesthesia, low FGFs and increased operating temperature within the absorber. However, there is no evidence of any danger to humans.

Anaesthetic Non-rebreathing Systems Which Include Carbon Dioxide Absorption

Carbon dioxide absorption can be used in two types of system:

- a 'to-and-fro' absorption system;
- a circle absorption system.

'To-and-fro' Absorption Systems

The Waters' Canister (Fig. 8.16)
Here the patient breathes in and out of a closed bag, which is connected to the facemask or endotracheal tube via a canister containing soda lime. The part of the system between the patient and the soda lime is dead space and therefore its volume must be kept to a minimum. This means that the soda lime canister must be close to the patient's head, and this leads to mechanical difficulties. A length of wide-bore tubing may, however, be interposed between the canister and rebreathing bag without detriment. The fresh gases are introduced at the

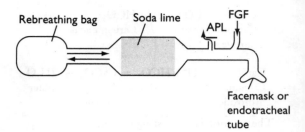

Figure 8.16 A 'to-and-fro' system incorporating a Waters' canister. FGF, fresh gas flow.

patient end of the system, and the expiratory valve is usually mounted close by, though it may equally well be put at the bag end. The canister is usually placed in the horizontal position for convenience, and it is most important that it is well packed, because if there were a space above the soda lime, 'channelling' would occur and absorption would be incomplete (Fig. 8.17). Furthermore, the soda lime at the patient end of the system becomes exhausted first and so increases the functional dead space of the system.

Canisters are available as pre-packed, disposable units. In those intended for reuse, the soda lime may conveniently be compressed to prevent gaps by the insertion of a spongy 'spacer' at one end. When the canister is closed, the sealing washer should be checked to ensure that it is in the correct position and any soda lime on the threads of the canister or the sealing washer should be carefully removed as these may cause leaks. The whole system should be tested before use.

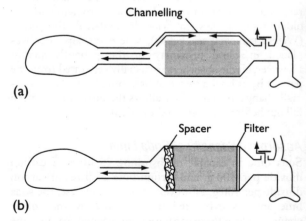

Figure 8.17 (a) Channelling in a Waters' canister. If the canister is not completely filled with soda lime and is placed in a horizontal position, the gases can pass through the void at the top and therefore fail to come into adequate contact with the soda lime. (b) The prevention of channelling by the insertion of a spacer to compress the soda lime. Note also the filter at the patient end that prevents particles of soda lime reaching the patient.

Apart from being cumbersome, the 'to-and-fro' system has the disadvantage that the patient could inhale soda lime dust. A breathing filter may be inserted in the patient end of the canister to prevent this.

Circle Absorption Systems

Here the disadvantages resulting from the soda lime canister being so close to the patient are avoided. The patient is connected to the absorber by two corrugated hoses, one inspiratory and the other expiratory, as shown in Fig. 8.18a. The one-way or 'circle' flow of gases through the system is determined by two unidirectional valves V_1, and V_2, which are accommodated in transparent domes so that their correct action may be observed.

The fresh gas port and the reservoir bag are usually sited in the inspiratory pathway close to the inspiratory valve V_1. This reduces the resistance to inspiratory effort. (Some older circle systems positioned the reservoir bag in the expiratory limb of the system downstream of the valve V_2, which required some added inspiratory effort to draw the gas through the absorber.) The APL valve is usually mounted downstream of the valve V_2 in the expiratory limb, but before gas entry into the absorber. Here, it can dump excess exhaled gas prior to entry of gas into the absorber. At one time it was considered that an APL valve could be added to the breathing system at position A for use with spontaneous respiration. This would preferentially dump alveolar gas during exhalation, thus increasing carbon dioxide elimination upstream of the absorber and conserving soda lime. However, as the scavenging hose assumed a greater importance, the inconvenience of connecting scavenging hoses to a valve in this position has limited its usefulness. Figure 8.18b,c shows two commercial versions of the system described.

The system shown in Fig. 8.19 is a disposable version. The valve V_1 is sited in the breathing hose and as close to the patient as possible. In this position it has a faster response to pressure changes caused by exhalation and closes earlier, although, as it is exhaled dead space gas that enters the system first, it is immaterial as to which limb this enters initially.

Apparatus Dead Space

The apparatus dead space is low in this system. It consists only of that volume inside the male taper at the end of the Y-piece, which joins the inspiratory and expiratory breathing hoses to the patient. However, the functional dead space of this system may vary if a fault develops in it. For example, if the unidirectional valves malfunction and do not fully close, rebreathing can occur from the expiratory limb. Furthermore, some circle systems position the APL valve just upstream of the expiratory

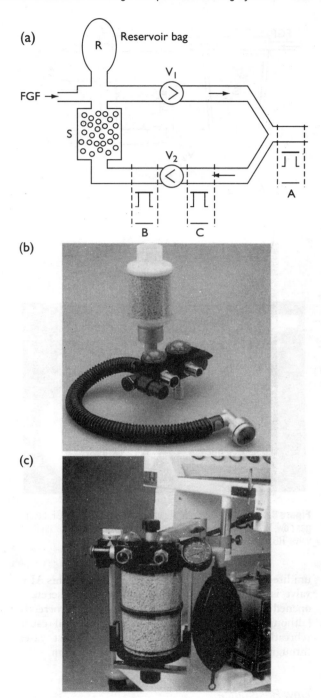

Figure 8.18 (a) Schematic diagram of a circle breathing system with absorber. FGF, Fresh gas flow; V_1 and V_2, one-way valves; R, reservoir bag; S, soda-lime canister. The diagram highlights the alternative siting of the adjustable pressure-limiting (APL) valve at points A, B or C. (b) Conventional circle-type carbon dioxide absorption system. It uses disposable and stackable soda lime canisters. (c) A 2 kg circle-type carbon dioxide absorber that uses fully autoclavable polyethersulphone canisters and valve domes.

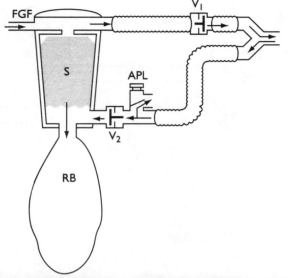

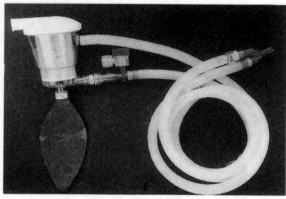

Figure 8.19 The Intersurgical disposable Circle System. FGF, fresh gas flow; V₁ and V₂, one-way valves; APL, adjustable pressure-limiting valve; RB, reservoir bag; S, soda-lime canister.

unidirectional valve (position C, Fig. 8.18). If this APL valve is mounted horizontally, and the valve screw is opened fully, the valve disc may not seat correctly (although it is supposed to do so) and will cause rebreathing due to ingress of air or exhaust gases through this valve during spontaneous respiration.

Flow Resistance

Circle systems impose a greater resistance to breathing than other commonly used breathing systems (Mapleson A–F systems), although less than co-axial arrangements of D systems (Bain system). This is largely due to the fact that there are two extra valves and a soda lime canister in the system. Several factors further influence this resistance:

- A high FGF rate will assist flow in the inspiratory side of the system, thus decreasing any inspiratory resistance, but will increase expiratory resistance through the unidirectional and APL (expiratory) valves.
- The reverse occurs with low gas flows. Low FGF rates will also increase the relative humidity and thus increase the 'stickiness' of the unidirectional valves owing to water vapour condensation, therefore further increasing flow resistance.
- Lastly, the flow rates developed by respiratory excursion (tidal volume and rate) produce the greatest swings in flow resistance (Table 8.1). These factors may not matter in healthy adults, but they can be unacceptable in young children. Several devices have been described (Revell's circulator, etc.) that reduce this problem (see later in the chapter).

Table 8.1 Flow resistance in circle breathing systems

Frequency (min)	Tidal volume (ml)	Pressure swing (cmH₂O)
12	500	−1 + ½
12	1000	−1 + 1
12	1600	−2 + 1½
24	500	−1 + 1
24	1000	−3 + 1½
44	500	−4 + 3

Reproduced from Young, T. M. Carbon dioxide absorber *Anaesthesia* vol. 26 (1971), p. 78, with permission.

Efficiency of Soda Lime Absorbers

The efficiency of carbon dioxide absorption in a canister depends on:

- the freshness of the soda lime;
- the available surface area of the granules;
- the length of time the gas to be treated is in contact with the granules.

Early canister designs contained approximately 480 g of soda lime. These required frequent changes (after approximately 2–2.5 h of continuous use at low FGFs). Many presently used absorbers are of the 'Jumbo' type, which contain 2 kg of soda lime and, since this has a large volume and surface area of granules, the expired gas is in contact with them for a relatively long period of time, so increasing the efficiency of absorption. It has been shown that a 2 kg canister lasts five times longer than a 0.5 kg canister. When a 2 kg canister is employed it usually has two chambers, one above the other. When one half appears exhausted it is refilled and then the canister is inverted so that the previously unused half now bears the brunt of absorption. Not only is the absorption thought to be more efficient in the larger absorbers, but also less frequent recharging is necessary.

With the recent introduction of routine expired carbon dioxide monitoring these last two considerations appear to be less of a problem in clinical practice, and the reintroduction of smaller absorbers (Fig. 8.18b) may well have advantages. These are easier to maintain, to use, to keep clean and have fewer leaks. The soda lime can also be supplied in disposable cartridges.

However, efficiency must also be compatible with safety and the recent concern that *carbon monoxide* may be formed in dry stale soda lime (see above) has prompted some anaesthetists to advocate the use of smaller absorbers requiring more frequent changes of absorbent.

Absorber Switch

Traditionally, an absorber bypass switch is included in a circle system. This allows expiratory gas to be channelled either through the absorption chamber or across a bypass directly into the inspiratory limb. When the switch is of the flow-splitting type, it can also proportion the flow of expiratory gas through the two channels.

Some newer European and American models omit this switch completely or make the switch to be either on or off with no intermediate flow-splitting facility. The rationale for excluding this switch involves safety reasons. Rebreathing of carbon dioxide is rendered impossible under normal operating conditions.

However, partial rebreathing during controlled respiration is an acceptable technique (see Mapleson D systems above) and this facility with a circle system is still useful with many currently used 'bag-in-bottle' ventilators whose minimum respiratory rate setting cannot be reduced below 10 breaths per minute. With these ventilators, normocarbia may sometimes be achieved only by the use of inappropriately small tidal volumes or the addition of a dead space if the facility for partial rebreathing is eliminated.

Ventilator Switch

Older absorber systems had a single outlet for connecting either a reservoir bag or the ventilator hose. Switching from one to the other was achieved by removing one manually and substituting the other. One had also to remember that when switching to the ventilator mode, the APL valve (which was often part of the absorber assembly) had also to be closed otherwise this would cause part of the intended tidal volume to be leaked during controlled or assisted ventilation. Many current absorber models (Fig. 8.20) now have a facility for connecting both the reservoir bag and the ventilator hose. Either may now be included in the breathing system by operating a switch housed on the absorber

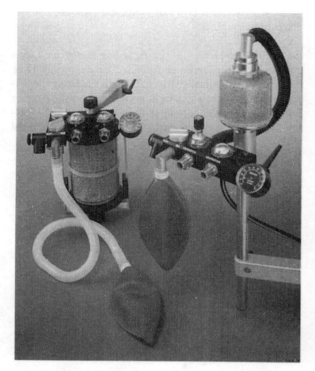

Figure 8.20 Circle absorbers with a facility to switch between ventilator and reservoir bag. (Left) 'Jumbo' absorber; (right) smaller 'Scandia' absorber. Note that this also has a modified dome over the expiratory valve that houses a PEEP valve.

assembly. The APL valve is so positioned that it is connected only to the reservoir bag and not included in the ventilator pathway. It, therefore, does not need adjusting when switching from one mode to the other and should be leak-free when using the ventilator.

The Use of Ventilators with Circle Systems

Any ventilator deemed suitable for use with a circle system must have the following features:

- It must be able to reproduce the effect of manual compression and refilling of the reservoir bag, e.g. it must have a single breathing hose inlet/outlet to allow to-and-fro movement of gas.
- It must have a valve to release excess gas in the circle system during the exhalation phase.
- It must have a power source that is independent of the fresh gas entering the circle system so that a minute ventilation can be delivered that is larger than the FGF (especially when this is set at low flows).
- If the ventilator is gas powered, this driving gas should not be able to contaminate the respirable gas reaching the patient.

There are two types of ventilator that are used to drive circle systems.

'Bag squeezer' Here, the reservoir bag is replaced by a bellows, which may be compressed mechanically (Fig. 8.21a) or pneumatically (Fig. 8.21b). In the latter the bellows is enclosed in a gas-tight container and the driving gas that enters the container then compresses the bellows but does not mix with the patient gas contained within it.

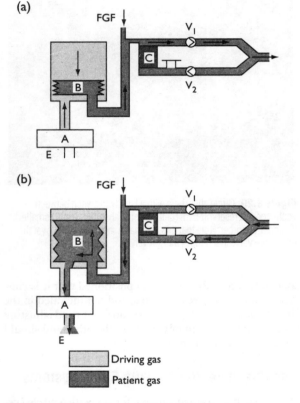

Figure 8.21 'Bag squeezer' ventilator and circle system. (a) Inspiratory phase; (b) expiratory phase. A, Ventilator; B, bellows; C, absorber; V_1 & V_2, one-way valves; E, exhaust; FGF, fresh gas flow.

'Pneumatic piston' Here, the reservoir bag is replaced by a suitably long length of breathing hose. The driving gas from the ventilator is passed through a special valve (Fig. 8.22) into the breathing hose. The latter is sufficiently long so that its internal volume is at least 1.5–2 times greater than the patient's tidal volume and prevents the driving gas from entering the circle and contaminating the patient gas. This is especially important in many circle systems where the reservoir limb is sited in the inspiratory pathway. Here, driving

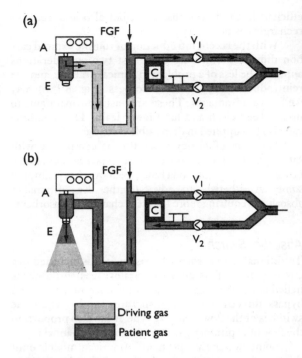

Figure 8.22 'Pneumatic piston' ventilator and circle system. (a) Inspiratory phase; (b) expiratory phase. A, Ventilator; C, absorber; V_1 & V_2, one-way valves; E, exhaust; FGF, fresh gas flow.

gas could dilute the inspiratory anaesthetic gas sufficiently to cause an inadequate level of anaesthesia to be maintained.

Mechanical Ventilation in Circle Systems

The tidal volume delivered during mechanical ventilation may be altered by the adjusting the ventilator *as well as the FGF*. Although the ventilator may be set to give a known tidal volume, when this reaches the circle it is supplemented by the fresh gas entering the system, which may significantly alter the final tidal volume. Consider the following FGF entering the circle system:

$$FGF\ 6\ litres/min = 6000\ ml/60\ s$$
$$= 100\ ml/s$$
If ventilator rate $10/min$ = 1 cycle every 6 s
If the insp./exp. ratio is $1/2$ = 2 s insp. /4 s exp.
Then inspiratory FGF in 2 s = 200 ml FGF
If ventilator setting = tidal vol. 400 ml
$$Total\ tidal\ vol. = ventilator\ tidal\ vol. \times\ insp.\ FGF$$
$$= 400 + 200$$
$$= 600\ ml$$

As the FGF is reduced, its contribution to the total tidal volume (and therefore minute ventilation) is reduced and that fraction of exhaled carbon dioxide is increased.

On some anaesthetic machines, where the ventilator and circle system are linked electronically, various compensatory mechanisms are employed to maintain the set tidal volume despite changes in the FGF (see Chapter 7).

Daily Maintenance of Circle Absorber Systems

During prolonged administration at low FGF rates, water vapour condenses in the expiratory hose and this needs to be emptied from time to time. Condensation also occurs in the expiratory unidirectional valve. Not only may this obscure the glass dome so that the correct operation of the valve cannot be observed, but also a drop of water on the cage retaining the valve disc may cause the latter to adhere to it by surface tension. This holds the valve permanently open, causing the patient to rebreathe repeatedly substantial amounts of exhaled gas from the expiratory pathway in the system. This gas would eventually have a very low oxygen content, which would be catastrophic for the patient. The tendency of the valve discs to stick is a result of their being made of increasingly lightweight materials in order to reduce the resistance to gas flow.

Ideally, to avoid this complication, a low resistance bacterial/hydrophobic filter should be fitted upstream of the expiratory valve V_2. This will protect this valve and absorber system from both bacterial and water contamination. Alternatively, the breathing hoses should be changed between cases.

In locations where the cost of the above exercise would be prohibitive, the tubing should be washed and hung out to dry between cases. Secondly, the expiratory valve should be dismantled and wiped clean with isopropyl alcohol. When, after dismantling, the glass dome of the expiratory valve is screwed back on again, it is important to ensure that the sealing washer is correctly in place, otherwise a serious leak may occur. If a low-resistance bacterial filter is not used, then the circle absorber housing should be autoclaved (where possible) on a regular basis. Some circle absorbers cannot be autoclaved, but may be cleaned by chemical means.

The soda lime should be changed at regular intervals either:

- when the dye indicates that the majority of the granules are exhausted;
- when using an analyser, carbon dioxide appears in the inspiratory mixture; or
- when the absorber is unlikely to be used for some time (e.g. over a weekend).

The soda lime container usually has a mark above which it should not be filled. Overfilling may result in granules of soda lime clogging the threads of canisters that screw into position, or may prevent the correct seating of the sealing washer, thus causing a leak or bypassing of the soda lime. Furthermore, leaving this space at the top reduces the preferential 'channelling' effect of the gas stream along the sides, and ensures a more even flow through the container. Since the canister is held in the vertical position, channelling is less of a problem than in the Waters' canister, although some does occur between the granules and sides of the canister as the air spaces are bigger here than those between granules within the canister.

Gas and Vapour Concentration in a Circle System

Circle systems are unique in that they function effectively (when a steady state of anaesthesia has been reached) using a wide variety of FGF rates. However, the fate of the various gases within the system needs to be understood in order that it may be used safely and effectively. For example, the internal volume of the apparatus (when using a 2 kg absorber), which consists of the intergranular air space in the absorber (1 litre), the breathing hoses (1 litre) and pathways within the absorber (1 litre), totalling 3 litres, along with the functional residual capacity of a patient of 1.25 litres, provides a large reservoir into which the anaesthetic gas is diluted at the beginning of anaesthesia.

In order to minimize this dilution and provide adequate concentrations of anaesthetic agent, high flows of fresh gas and vapour are required initially in order to flush the residual gas out the circle system: the higher the flow, the faster this 'washout' occurs. Lung 'washout' will of course depend on the patient's minute ventilation. The greater this is, the less time the process takes.

Secondly, the alveolar uptake of anaesthetic agent is greatest at the beginning of anaesthesia. Therefore, the higher the initial FGF rate (up to a value equal to the patient's minute ventilation) the greater is the delivery of anaesthetic agent into the system. This in turn minimizes any reduction in concentration of agent caused by uptake by the patient. When near equilibrium of anaesthetic agents has occurred between the alveoli and blood, exhaled agent concentration almost equals that in the inspiratory mixture, and therefore the high initial FGFs may safely be greatly reduced.

In practice the FGF is usually reduced in stages.

First stage The initial flow for patient and breathing system washout, as well as supply of adequate anaesthetic agent to match alveolar uptake, usually takes approximately 5–10 min. (The shorter time is suited to the insoluble anaesthetic agents desflurane and sevoflurane, which reach alveolar equilibrium more quickly.) If this flow rate is at, or greater than, the patient's minute ventilation, then most or all of the exhaled gas will leave the system via the APL (expiratory) valve without passing through the absorber. When used in this mode it may often be referred to as a *high flow system*.

Second stage An intermediate flow rate of 70% of the minute ventilation for a further 5 min will allow purging of the soda lime canister without major changes in anaesthetic concentrations.

Third stage A lower flow may be selected, the value of which will depend on the availability of gas and vapour monitoring within the system, the efficiency of the vaporizer (in or out of circle) and personal preference. Flows of the order of 0.5–2 litres/min are commonly used and when the circle is used in this mode it may often be referred to as a *low flow system*. *A closed flow system* is defined as that which has no gas exit (i.e. APL valve fully closed) and in which the FGF equals the uptake by the patient. In practice, however, few if any commercial anaesthetic circle breathing systems are sufficiently leak proof to be used at such flows.

Oxygen Concentrations in Circle Systems at Low Fresh Gas Flows

As the FGF in a circle is decreased, exhaled gas that is allowed to recirculate exerts an increasing influence on the subsequent inspired gas mixture. The oxygen concentration of this exhaled gas depends on: (a) its original inspired concentration and (b) the alveolar oxygen extraction, which may be unpredictable.

Figure 8.23 (solid line) shows the decrease in alveolar oxygen concentrations of a 50% nitrous oxide and 50% oxygen mixture under controlled conditions. It can be seen that at a fresh gas flow of 1 litre/min the oxygen concentration has dropped to 27% and drops even further at an FGF of 0.5 litre/min. Therefore, in clinical practice the oxygen concentration in a circle at low flows is most unpredictable and monitoring of inspired oxygen with an analyser is essential. In fact, monitoring of all gases and anaesthetic vapours should be considered mandatory for circle systems at low flows.

The Use of Volatile Agents in the Circle System

Volatile inhalational agents can be introduced into the system either by being added to the FGF (vaporizer outside circle/VOC) or by incorporating the vaporizer within the circle (vaporizer in circle/VIC).

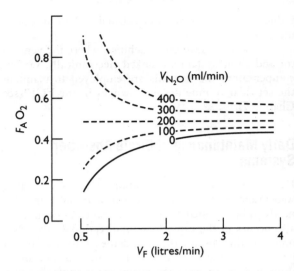

Figure 8.23 Predicted variations in alveolar oxygen concentrations ($F_A O_2$) produced by decreasing fresh gas flow (V_F) and assuming different levels of nitrous oxide uptake in a 50 : 50 mixture of oxygen in nitrous oxide. A constant oxygen consumption of 200 ml/min and a constant ventilation required to produce an alveolar CO_2 concentration of 5% have been assumed. The heavy line shows the fall in alveolar oxygen concentration with decreasing fresh gas flow when the inspired and body levels of nitrous oxide have reached equilibrium (zero uptake). (Reproduced with kind permission from *Scientific Foundations of Anaesthesia*, Butterworth/Heinemann.)

Vaporizer Outside Circle

This is probably the most common method of introducing inhalational agents into the breathing system. At high FGFs, the vapour concentration in the circle is reliably represented by the dial setting of the vaporizer. However, as the FGF is reduced, two phenomena occur:

- Expired gas, which is recycled (and which has a reduced concentration of inhalational agent due to uptake), dilutes the FGF within the system. This reduces the delivered concentration of inhalational agent to below that anticipated by the dial setting on the vaporizer.
- At low FGF, vaporizer efficiency may well be altered, providing a lower or higher than expected concentration of inhalational agent (e.g. TEC 2 vaporizer, see Chapter 5, vaporizers and flow charts of vaporizers).

At low FGFs, therefore, the anaesthetist needs to know:

- the performance of the vaporizer in use at that given FGF;
- the expired concentration of inhalational agent;
- and the degree of dilution of the FGF with expired gas (which in turn depends on the patient's minute ventilation).

The lower the FGF, the more difficult it is to predict the inspired concentration of agent. At flows below 2 litres/min it is highly advisable to incorporate a vapour analyser into the system, especially during controlled ventilation when signs of light anaesthesia may be more difficult to determine, to ensure that adequate amounts of agent reach the patient.

Vaporizer in Circle

If the vaporizer is incorporated into the circle system, it must have a low resistance to gas flow so as to minimize the respiratory work required of a spontaneously breathing patient. High-resistance Plenum vaporizers are unsuitable.

With a vaporizer incorporated in the circle, recirculating gas picks up vapour to add to the vapour already being carried, and therefore the vapour concentration may well be greater than intended. Calibration of vaporizers in this system is therefore impossible. The vapour concentration in this type of system depends on several factors when equilibrium has been reached:

- *The fresh gas flow.* The lower the FGF, the greater will be the recirculation of gas already carrying vapour and the higher will be the concentration of inspired agent.
- *The efficiency of the vaporizer.* The more efficient the vaporizer the higher will be the inspired concentration of agent. This has important implications with potent inhalational agents. At a low FGF and a large assisted or controlled minute ventilation, the anaesthetic gas may well become saturated with agent at that temperature. For halothane, this will represent a concentration of 33% at 21°C (the saturated vapour pressure for halothane).

Therefore, for potent agents, an inefficient vaporizer is preferable. The presence of a wick in a VIC is also unsuitable, since water vapour will condense on the wick, reducing its efficiency and possibly increasing the resistance to gas flow.

Ether, for which much higher concentrations are appropriate, has, however, been widely and safely used with a VIC. Adequate vaporization may be assisted by the use of baffles within the vaporizer that cause the gases to impinge repeatedly on the surface of the ether, or even by bubbling the FGF through the liquid ether. It may also be increased to some extent by the heat from the recirculating expired gases.

MODIFICATIONS OF BREATHING SYSTEMS AND THEIR COMPONENTS

It has long been appreciated that part of the energy required to propel the gases along the passages of a breathing system must be derived from the patient's respiratory effort. The latter, being prejudiced by the depressant effects of narcosis, becomes inefficient, and any form of resistance would further impair respiratory function. On the other hand, any form of assistance to flow or of reduction of resistance would be beneficial. To this end various 'circulators' have been devised and expiratory valves that are not spring-loaded have been advocated. Some of these are described below.

Breathing Systems with Assisted Circulation

These attempt to reduce the problems of resistance to flow, the inertia of gases, and dead space.

Revell's Circulator

Although rarely used nowadays, the device is included as it may be of interest. The design features are of particular benefit in paediatric anaesthesia, and enable a circle system designed for adults to be used for small children. A small fan helps to assist the circulation of gases in a closed system. It will be noted that this is used in conjunction with a 'chimney', which is part of the facemask mount or catheter mount. As is shown in Fig. 8.24, this causes a continuous flow of fresh gases into the facemask, thereby reducing the effects of dead space. The Revell's circulator may be incorporated in a circle system and thereby help to overcome the resistance of the valves and other parts of the system.

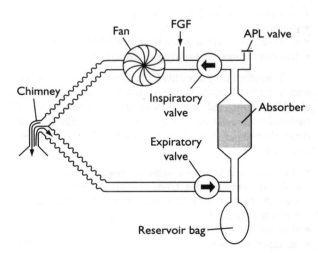

Figure 8.24 Revell's circulator and chimney. Driven by compressed air or other gas, a fan induces the circulation of anaesthetic gases within a circle breathing system. The 'chimney' directs a flow of fresh gases into the facepiece thus minimizing the effective dead space. FGF, fresh gas flow; APL, adjustable pressure-limiting (expiratory) valve.

Neff's Circulator

Again, although rarely used nowadays, the device is also mentioned as it too may be of interest. In 1968 a Venturi circulator was described by Neff, Simpson, Burke and Thompson. It makes use of the power that is latent in the FGF at regulated pressure entering the breathing system from the back bar.

These circulators enabled the exploitation of the advantages of the circle system, such as the economy in FGF and the retention of water vapour and heat, but without the disadvantages of resistance, dead space and the inertia of gases in a large apparatus volume.

Inspiratory Assistance

Some of the more sophisticated anaesthetic machines with integral ventilators and circle systems may have sensors in the breathing system that detect a patient's inspiratory effort and trigger the ventilator to supplement it (a pressure support mode).

PROCEDURES FOR CHECKING BREATHING SYSTEMS

All the breathing systems described above will only function correctly if the components are free of any fault, assembled in the correct order and the connections made gas-tight. A good working knowledge of the apparatus is essential prior to its use by a practitioner. Fatalities have unfortunately occurred where the user:

- was unfamiliar with the equipment;
- included a non-standard item;
- had not noticed that it had been assembled incorrectly;
- had not noticed that it had developed a fault.

Therefore they should be checked prior to each use according to the manufacturer's instructions or against a checklist approved by a hospital department or a national association (e.g. The Association of Anaesthetists of Great Britain and Ireland). A suitable inspection should ensure that:

- the components of the system chosen for use (especially if they are not from the same manufacturer) should always conform to the same national or international standard;
- they are assembled appropriately;
- all tapered connections are secure using a push and twist technique;
- with the APL valve closed, the system is gas-tight when filled;
- when the valve is opened, the gas escapes easily through it.

In addition to this, any co-axial breathing system should have the integrity of the inner limb confirmed. This can be done on a Mapleson D system by occluding the inner limb only (e.g. with a pencil or a 1 ml syringe), observing that the bag remains deflated and that the anaesthetic machine safety valve protecting the back bar gives an alarm signal. With a Mapleson A system (Lack co-axial), occluding the inner limb only should cause the reservoir bag to distend (with the APL valve closed).

THE COMPONENTS OF A BREATHING SYSTEM

Rebreathing and Reservoir Bags

Rebreathing and reservoir bags (Fig. 8.25 are identical, the distinction being solely in the use to which they are put, as explained previously. The commonly used size in adult breathing systems is 2 litres (i.e. that which when fully but not forcibly distended has a capacity of 2 litres; in clinical practice it is seldom filled beyond this capacity). Larger bags are used as reservoir bags in ventilators and smaller ones in paediatric anaesthesia.

In adult breathing systems, the capacity to which the bag may easily be distended must exceed the patient's tidal volume. A larger-capacity bag (2 litres), however, is safer as it more easily absorbs pressure increases. Bags

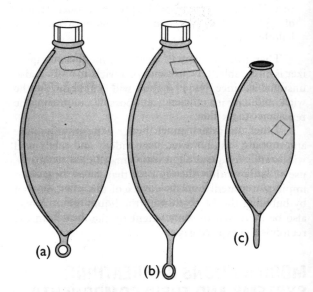

Figure 8.25 Reservoir (and rebreathing) bags. (a) A single-ended 2 litre bag. (b) A 2 litre bag in which the extended tail loop may be removed to convert it into a double-ended bag. (c) A 0.5 litre bag with a small neck, which may be converted into a double-ended bag for paediatric use.

are frequently provided with a loop at the bottom end that makes it possible to double the bag back on itself by hanging the loop from a knob on the top of the bag mount. This manoeuvre can be used when anaesthetizing small children. It does not alter the mechanics of the breathing system, and is justified only in that it makes movements of the bag easier to observe. Certainly it should not be used if it makes the bag 'stiffer'.

The material of which the bag is constructed is important. Where ventilation is spontaneous, the opening pressure of the expiratory valve must exceed that required to prevent the bag from emptying spontaneously owing to its weight or resistance to distension. Therefore, to maintain a low expiratory pressure, the bag must be 'soft'.

A stiffer bag with stronger walls is required for use with minute volume divider ventilators such as the East-Freeman Automatic Vent (see Fig. 12.7), where the back-pressure on the bag may rise to 4 kPa (40 cmH$_2$O) or more, and the elasticity of the bag plays a part in the operation of the valve.

The observed movement of the bag depends on several factors, such as its shape, size, degree of filling, the tension of the expiratory valve and the FGF rate, as well as on the patient's tidal volume. An accurate estimate of the patient's tidal volume cannot be made simply by watching the bag.

When ordering bags, the size of the neck should be specified. Whereas in some bags, including those for the East-Freeman Automatic Vent, the neck is integral with the bag itself and relatively easily stretched, in others the neck includes a stiff moulded rubber fitting that is suitable only for the appropriate size of bag mount.

'Double-ended' bags In the Rees T-piece paediatric attachment, a double-ended bag is added to the expiratory limb (see Fig. 8.15) and the smaller end acts as an expiratory port, the aperture of which can be controlled by the anaesthetist.

Adjustable Pressure Limiting Valves

The purpose of the APL valve is to allow the escape of exhaled (expired) and surplus gases from a breathing system, but without permitting entry of the outside air, even during a negative phase. Usually it is desirable that the pressure required to open the valve should be as low as possible, in order to minimize resistance to expiration. It must, however, present sufficient resistance to prevent the reservoir bag from emptying spontaneously, particularly when a scavenging system is employed that exerts a slight subatmospheric pressure upon it.

A commonly used type of expiratory valve is the Heidbrink (Fig. 8.26). The valve disc is as light as possible, and rests on a 'knife-edge' seating that presents a

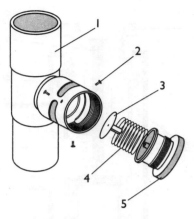

Figure 8.26 The Heidbrink valve: 1, male tapers at both ends; 2, retaining screws; 3, disc; 4, spring; 5, valve top.

small area of contact. This lessens the tendency to adhesion between the disc and seating caused by the surface tension of condensed water from the expired air, or after washing or sterilizing. The disc has a stem that is located in a guide, in order to ensure that it is correctly positioned on the seating, and a coiled spring, of light weight, that promotes closure of the valve.

The spring is a delicate coil and is of such dimensions that when the valve top is screwed fully 'open' there is minimal pressure on the disc when seated. However, during the 'blow-off' phase the disc rises and shortens the spring so that the pressure it exerts on the disc is greater and will close it at the appropriate time. Screwing down the valve top produces progressively increasing tension in the spring. When the top is screwed fully down the valve is completely closed. If, owing to damage or fatigue, the spring is shortened, the top may have to be screwed down a little in order to ensure closure at the start of inspiration. If it has been elongated, the pressure at which it opens may be excessive. Small screws in the body of the valve, and a groove in the skirt of the top, prevent it from being unscrewed so far that it falls apart.

The Humphrey APL Valve

An interesting addition to the standard APL valve is the modification seen on the Humphrey version (Figs 8.13a and 8.27), which is part of the current Humphrey ADE system. Here, the valve disc is attached to a red coloured spindle, which extends through the valve top. When the valve is fully open, the spindle is seen to bob up and down as the disc is lifted up and down during respiration. The valve top is made concave and shiny so that it reflects and magnifies the spindle colour so as to detect even the smallest movement when used in paediatric

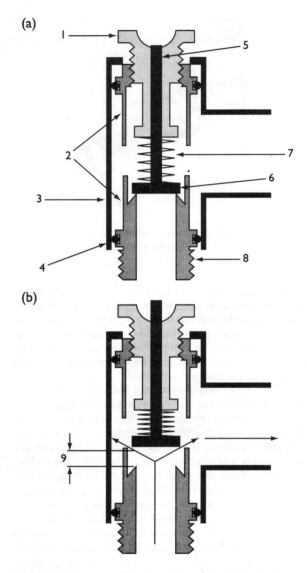

Figure 8.27 'Humphrey' APL valve. (a) Inspiration (with valve disc closed); (b) beginning of exhalation (valve disc just clearing small funnel). 1, Valve top; 2, valve body; 3, exhaled gas scavenging shroud; 4, 'O'-ring seal between the valve body and shroud; 5, valve spindle; 6, valve disc; 7, valve spring; 8, screw thread to secure valve to the breathing system; 9, 5 mm funnel which accentuates movement of the spindle.

anaesthesia. The inside of the valve body has a small funnel through which the disc has to move before significant gas can escape. This initial movement of 5 mm accentuates the bobbing action of the spindle which again is useful when used in paediatric anaesthesia.

When the ADE system is used in the Mapleson A mode, the valve spindle may be held down with a finger if switching from spontaneous to manual ventilation is required. This has several advantages:

- As there is no leak from the valve during inspiration, the patient's lung compliance may be more accurately assessed.
- It becomes as efficient as the Mapleson A mode in spontaneous respiration (i.e. the valve is shut during inspiration and open during expiration).
- The valve top may be kept in the 'open' position at all times and does not require repeated adjustment when switching between spontaneous and manual ventilation.

It was originally thought that the increased respiratory work produced by the expiratory resistance of APL valves was detrimental to anaesthetized patients. This is without doubt true when the valve resistance is high (due to sticky valves, narrow valve apertures) or where the respiratory effort is severely compromised (e.g. in neonates). However, modern valve design (with wider valve apertures, more delicate springs, better screw threads) minimizes this resistance. Furthermore, a small PEEP (positive end-expiratory pressure) effect that these valves may produce is now thought to be positively beneficial, reducing the potential for the functional residual capacity of the lungs to fall below the closing volume in supine anaesthetized patients.

APL Valves with In-built Overpressure Safety Devices

A standard valve, when fully closed, relies on a compliant reservoir bag to absorb any unexpected pressure rise in a breathing system. Should this fail, for instance if the bag were trapped under the wheel of an anaesthetic machine, a dangerously high pressure could develop within the breathing system and be passed on to the patient. Valves are available in which an overpressure safety device has been incorporated.

One example, the Intersurgical APL assembly, is shown in Fig. 8.28. It has two valves:

- the inner (3) which is tensioned with a weak spring (4);
- the outer (5) which is tensioned with a more powerful one (2).

When the valve top (1) is unscrewed fully (Fig. 8.28b), the outer valve is permanently open but the inner one is closed until exhaled gas forces it open. The pressure required to do this is small (0.15 kPa/1.5 cm H_2O). However, when the valve top is screwed down fully, both valves are closed and in this position the outer one is pushed against the inner so that is has no movement of its own (Fig. 8.28c). An excess pressure is now required to move the more powerful spring on the outer valve

(a)

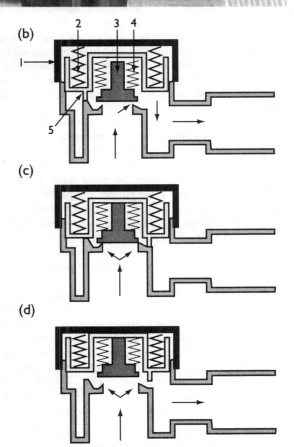

(b)

(c)

(d)

Figure 8.28 (a) The 'Intersurgical' APL valve with an overpressure safety device. 1, Valve control knob; 2, high-pressure spring; 3, valve spindle; 4, light-pressure spring; 5, the part of the asymmetric valve body that rotates during valve closure and occludes the expiratory limb. The figure shows (b) the valve open during exhalation; (c) the valve closed; and (d) the valve closed with the overpressure safety device in action.

which will begin to open at 3 kPa (30 cm H_2O) and be fully open at 6 kPa (60 cm H_2O) when the gas flow is 50 litres/min (Fig. 8.28d).

Breathing Hoses

The hoses connecting the components of a breathing system must be of such a diameter as to present a low resistance to gas flow. Its cross-section must be uniform to promote laminar flow where possible, and although it should be flexible, kinking should not occur. It should drape easily so that a deep loop may hang between the patient and, say, a circle absorber because this tends to trap droplets of moisture that could carry infective organisms back to the apparatus.

The most commonly used type of hosing has for a long time been a corrugated hose of rubber or neoprene (Fig. 8.29). The corrugations allow acute angulations of the hose without kinking. The disadvantages of these materials are that the irregular wall must cause turbulence and may harbour dirt and infection. They are also heavy and, if unsupported, may drag on a facemask or endotracheal tube. The advantage is that the ends are more easily stretched, and will make a good union with other components of different diameters.

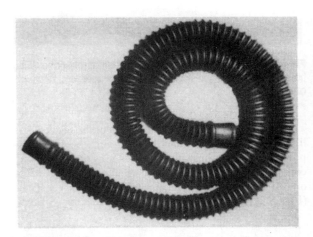

Figure 8.29 A standard length of wide-bore corrugated hose.

Various other materials such as silicone rubber and plastics are in use, both in corrugated and smooth form (Fig. 8.30). Smooth-bore breathing hose produces less turbulence than the corrugated variety at similar gas flows. It can also be produced so that it resists kinking (by the attachment of a reinforcing spiral of a similar material to its external surface). With smooth-bore hosing, a smaller diameter (e.g. 15 mm) may well be acceptable for use with adult breathing systems (see Humphrey ADE breathing system).

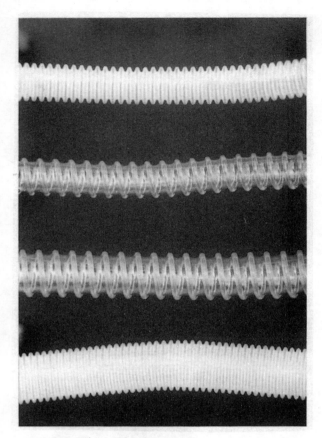

Figure 8.30 From top to bottom: 15 mm corrugated plastic breathing hose; 15 mm smooth-bore hose; 22 mm smooth-bore hose; 22 mm corrugated hose.

Plastic hosing has become very popular because it is lightweight, cheap to manufacture, and therefore disposable. Some of these plastic hoses are supplied in long coils, the appropriate length of which may be cut off at one of the frequent intervals where the corrugations (Fig. 8.31) give way to a shaped connector. Silicone

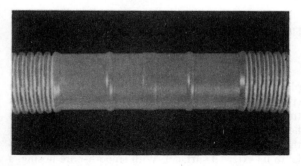

Figure 8.31 Lightweight plastic corrugated hose. At frequent intervals the corrugations give way to a shaped connector, where a long roll of this hose may be cut.

rubber hosing is autoclavable, unlike many plastics, which would melt if so treated. Plastic apparatus is normally sterilized by gamma irradiation as it is intended for single use only.

There are several standard sizes of corrugated hose, both ends of which have smooth walls for about 2–3 cm. These ends are designed to fit either tapered connectors (see below) or tapered components of a breathing system. Breathing hose for adult use is normally 22 mm wide so as to reduce the resistance to breathing to a minimum. Paediatric breathing hose has a narrower bore (15 mm) to reduce its internal volume (*see* Chapter 14) and to make it less cumbersome.

Tapered Connections (Adapters)

Tapered connections (adapters) provide a useful way of joining rigid tubes or other components together in such a manner that the joint will not leak. The joint is described as having a male half and a female half which are *pushed together with a slight twist* to form a gas-tight fit. The joint may be easily dismantled and reassembled, a feature that makes it useful for the interconnection of breathing systems, catheter mounts and endotracheal connectors.

A leak-proof joint relies on its components being completely circular and having the same angle of taper so that the maximum contact between the components of the joint will occur. The standard also requires that male tapers for breathing systems be fitted with a recess behind the taper so that when rubber and plastic hosing is pushed on to a male connector, its leading edge can contract into this recess to provide a more secure fitting. Examples of tapers are shown in Fig. 8.32.

The current ISO and BS recommendations on the sequence of tapers in various breathing systems are set out in Fig. 8.33.

Prior to the introduction of any standards, manufacturers were free to decide the size and angle of tapers used with their equipment. However, there is now an internationally agreed size for tapered connections for use with anaesthetic breathing systems and endotracheal tubes so that there is compatibility between equipment from different manufacturers. The International Standards Organization (ISO.5356, 1987) and the British Standard (BS 3849) specify the use of:

- 30 mm tapered connections for the attachment of scavenging hose to breathing systems;
- 22 mm tapers for connections within a breathing system;
- 15 mm connections for the attachment of a breathing system to an endotracheal tube.

Some 22 mm male breathing hose connections are so manufactured that they incorporate a 15 mm female

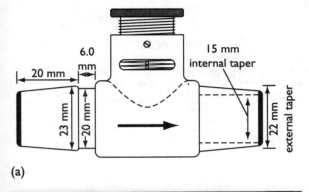

(a)

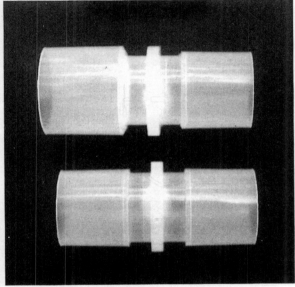

(b)

Figure 8.32 (a) An expiratory valve with the British and International Standard 22 mm taper. Note that the proximal taper may be pushed directly into the end of a corrugated hose and the recessed shoulder will help to secure this joint. The distal 22 mm taper will also accept a 15 mm endotracheal connector. (b) Plastic (disposable) 22 mm tapered adaptors. (Top) Female to male; the male part is normally inserted into each end of a breathing hose. (Bottom) Male to male; this is inserted into the distal end of a piece of corrugated tubing when used as an extension for a reservoir bag (see Fig. 8.33c).

taper for direct connection to an endotracheal tube.

It is worthy of note that the current British Standard requires that a reservoir bag should have a female inlet to fit the male outlet for bag mounts on all breathing systems. However, should a length of breathing hose be required between the bag mount and reservoir bag, a problem arises. The breathing hose has two female ends: one will fit the bag mount (male to female) but the other will not fit the bag (female to female). A

male to male 22 mm tapered adapter is required (see Figs 8.32b and 8.33c).

Problems with Tapered Connections

Many accidents have occurred as a result of the accidental and unobserved disconnection of tapered joints. The material used in the construction may either wear with frequent use (most plastics and rubber), or become distorted by damage (metal connectors). *Disconnection can be minimized by giving the components of the joint a slight twist following their insertion.* Devices designed to prevent accidental disconnection are described below.

Conversely, some metal connectors made from aluminium alloys may stick together by the phenomenon of cold welding produced by the recommended twist above, and may be very difficult to separate.

Anti-disconnect Devices

Accidental disconnection of breathing system components is a common occurrence. Often this is because the recommended procedure of 'push and twist' when connecting tapers is not followed. It may also be due to excessive wear on these tapers (especially when made from plastics) causing them to change shape and become more parallel.

Anti-disconnect devices have been available for some time but sadly have never become popular even though fatalities did occur when unobserved disconnections occurred in patients who were being mechanically ventilated. However, if adequate monitoring (linked to alarms) of both pressure, flow and concentration of exhaled gases (notably carbon dioxide) within a breathing system is maintained, a disconnection will be apparent.

Two anti-disconnect devices are described below.

The Penlon 'Safelock'

In this system (Fig. 8.34a), which is made of plastic, the male taper has a threaded 'cap' which can be screwed onto a matching male thread on the female taper, thus securing the union. The cap is kept on the fitting by an 'O'-ring, but the latter does not contribute to the gastight seal.

The advantage of this kind of system is that items fitted with it can still be joined in the conventional manner with other standard tapers, although the 'safelock' will be ineffectual. The disadvantages are that it is rather bulky, and that its efficacy depends on the anaesthetist taking the trouble to secure the connection. This may be neglected by the same person who fails to give an ordinary tapered connection that important twist as he or she engages it.

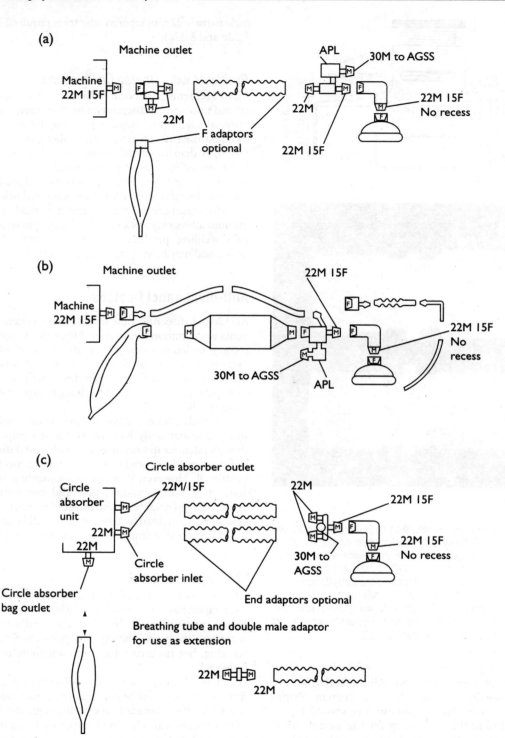

Figure 8.33 Current sequence of tapers in anaesthetic breathing systems as recommended by the ISO and BSI (BS 3849) as from 1988. Typical layout of (a) Mapleson A system; (b) to-and-fro absorption system; and (c) circle absorption system. M, male conical fitting; F, female conical fitting; APL, adjustable pressure-limiting valve.

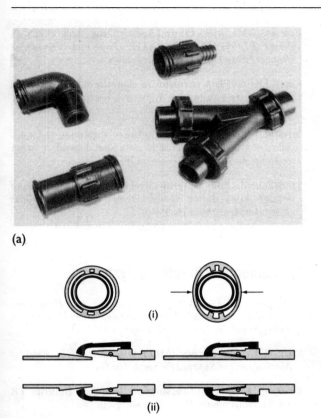

(a)

(b)

Figure 8.34 (a) Penlon 'Safelock' tapered connections showing the nut on the male component and the screw thread on the female connection. (b) Dräger 'Isoclic' safety connection: (i) end-on view showing the distortion required on the female component to retract the claws to enable separation of the connection; (ii) side view showing the components being engaged.

The Dräger 'Isoclic'

This system (Fig. 8.34b) consists of a female taper which is shrouded by a cone that ends in four claws. These engage in the 'groove' ('notch' or 'undercut') on the latest version of the male taper of the ISO connector. A simple push-fit is all that is needed to ensure a secure engagement. Release is achieved by gentle squeezing of the appropriate two sides of the shroud, thus disengaging the claws. The taper is the ISO 22 mm. The gas-tight nature of this joint is completed by an 'O'-ring set within the female taper. The correct seating of this system is therefore assured, provided that the male taper onto which it engages has the appropriate groove (see Fig. 8.34b). In the absence of the latter, which is the case with many parts currently in use, not only is the lock imposs- ible, but the union is far less secure than that with two simple metal tapers. Thus, this system would promote safety only in a department where all appropriate items of

equipment have male tapers with the groove. Otherwise disconnections might become even more common.

Certainly, all hard rubber tapered connectors, which are renowned for jumping apart, should be dis- carded.

Reuse of Breathing System Components

Items that are intended for *reuse* (i.e. to be used on differ- ent patients) are normally made from materials (rubber, neoprene, silicone rubber and metal) that withstand repeated autoclaving.

Some items are designated as *single use* (i.e. to be used on one person only) if they are made from materials such as plastic that are not easily sterilized. Also, if the tapers (see below) are made from materials that are easily distorted with repeated connection they will be desig- nated for single use only.

A third category has been described. Some items that might be designated as single use because they are not easily sterilized may be acceptable for *repeated use*. Provided that these items are protected by a high-quality bacterial filter, some manufacturers will accept product liability if the item is used on several patients provided that the item is thoroughly checked between uses.

FURTHER READING

Mapleson Breathing Systems

Barnes PK, Browne CHW, Conway CM (1977) The work of ventilating in semi-closed rebreathing systems. *British Journal of Anaesthesia* 49: 1173.

Chan AIS, Bruce WE, Soni N (1989) A comparison of anaes- thetic breathing systems during spontaneous ventilation. *Anaesthesia* 44: 194–199.

Cook LB (1996) Mapleson breathing systems. The importance of the expiratory pause. *Anaesthesia* 51: 453–460.

Dorrington KL, Lehane IR (1989) Rebreathing during spon- taneous and controlled ventilation with 'T' piece breathing systems: a general solution. *Anaesthesia* 44: 300–302.

Henville ID, Adams AP (1976) The Bain anaesthetic system. *Anaesthesia* 31: 247–256.

Humphrey D (1983) A new anaesthetic breathing system com- bining Mapleson A, D & E principles. *Anaesthesia* 38: 361–372.

Mapleson WW (1954) The elimination of rebreathing in vari- ous semi-closed anaesthetic systems. *British Journal of Anaesthesia* 26: 323–332.

Miller DM (1988) Breathing systems for use in anaesthesia. *British Journal of Anaesthesia* 60: 555–564.

Nuffield Ventilator Series 200. User's Instruction Manual. Abingdon, UK: Penlon Ltd.

Circle Systems

Bracken A, Cox LA (1968) Apparatus for carbon dioxide absorption. *British Journal of Anaesthesia* **40**: 660–665.

Cossham PS (1992) Obstruction to wet soda lime granules. *Anaesthesia* **47**: 10–11.

Epstein RA (1995) 'Carbon monoxide': what should we do? *Anaesthesia Patient Safety Foundation Newsletter* **9**: 37–41.

Fang ZX, Eger EI (1995) USCF Research shows that CO comes from CO_2 absorbent. *Anaesthesia Patient Safety Foundation Newsletter* **9**: 26–29.

Holmes CMcK, Spears GFS (1977) Very nearly closed circuit anaesthesia: a computer analysis. *Anaesthesia* **32**: 846–851.

Mapleson WW (1960) The concentration of anaesthetics in closed circuits, with special reference to halothane. *British Journal of Anaesthesia* **32**: 298–309.

Morris LE (1974) The circulator concept. *International Anaesthetic Clinics* **12**: 181–198.

Murphy PM, Fitzgeorge RB, Barrett RF (1991) Viability and distribution of bacteria after passage through a circle anaesthetic system. *British Journal of Anaesthesia* **66**: 300–304.

References Medicines Control Agency Drug Alert (1995N 31 May) EL(95) (ALERT) A/17. *Important Precautions Required when Using Halogenated Anaesthetic Agents.*

Revell DG (1959) A circulator to eliminate mechanical dead space in circle absorption systems. *Canadian Anaesthetists' Society Journal* **6**: 98–103.

Strum DP, Eger EI (1994) Degradation, absorption and solubility of volatile anesthetics in soda-lime depend on water content. *Anesthesia and Analgesia* **78**: 340–348.

Versichelen L, Rolly G, Vermeulen H (1996) Accumulation of foreign gases during closed-system anaesthesia. *British Journal of Anaesthesia* **76**: 668–672.

Components of Breathing System

Department of Health (1989) *Anaesthetic and Respiratory Equipment: the Use of 22 mm Breathing System Connections*, Safety Action Bulletin no. 52. London: HMSO.

Medical Devices Agency (MDA DB 9501, 1995) *Reuse of Medical Devices Supplied for Single Use Only.*

Reuse of Equipment, Intersurgical Technical Bulletin TB 5.4.95. Wolzingham, Berks: Intersurgical.

AIRWAY MANAGEMENT DEVICES

Contents

INTRODUCTION

Three of the fundamental principles of modern general anaesthesia are:

- The establishment and maintenance of a patent airway to the patient's lungs (especially as this is almost always obstructed by the collapse of pharyngeal structures as a result of the administration of the anaesthetic). Failure to re-establish patency within a few minutes can result in brain damage or death.
- The provision of a leak-free connection between the patient and the breathing system so as to provide a known and precise concentration of the powerful anaesthetic agents currently used, as well as to apply controlled or assisted ventilation if required.
- The protection of the respiratory system against contamination from refluxed gastric contents or pharyngeal debris.

Crucial to these principles has been the development of the various devices listed below.

ARTIFICIAL AIRWAYS

Terminology To avoid confusion, the term *airway* in this section will be used to describe the air passage in the oropharynx and supraglottis. The term *artificial airway* will be used to describe a device that maintains the patency of the air passage. Also the term *distal* will refer to that part of the device that is inserted the furthest into the patient's airway and the term *proximal* to the part emerging from the mouth or nose.

The maintenance of a clear airway in an anaesthetized patient may be achieved by simple elevation of the jaw, which lifts the tongue, epiglottis and the larynx away from the pharyngeal wall (Fig. 9.1a,b). However, in many instances this is insufficient (usually in those patients in whom this space is already reduced by a large tongue, a small lower jaw, large tonsils or a short fat neck). The relief of the resultant obstruction can be achieved by inserting a device that separates these structures and thus creates an artificial airway. This may be inserted via the mouth (oropharyngeal airway, Fig 9.1c) or nose (nasopharyngeal airway, Fig.9.1d).

Oropharyngeal Airway

These are shaped to emulate and so restore the space in the pharynx, present during consciousness, by pushing the tongue, epiglottis and larynx away from the posterior pharyngeal wall. Artificial airways are usually circular or oval-shaped in cross-section and are produced in varying lengths and diameters to suit different sizes of patient (from neonate to large adult). The proximal end has a

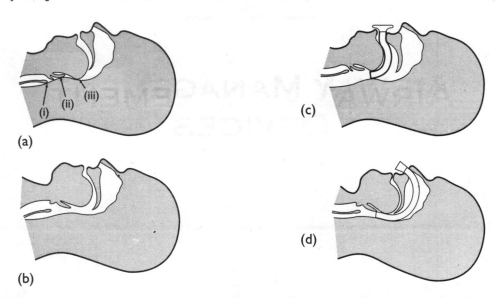

Figure 9.1   (a) The obstructed airway following the administration of a general anaesthetic if the jaw is unsupported. The airway may be obstructed either by the larynx (i), epiglottis (ii) and/or tongue (iii) pressing on the posterior pharyngeal wall. (b) The effect of simple elevation of the jaw in a patient with normal anatomy. (c) An unobstructed air passage produced with an oropharyngeal airway. (d) An unobstructed air passage produced with an nasopharyngeal airway.

flange to limit the depth of insertion and prevent it disappearing into the pharynx. It is also sufficiently rigid or even reinforced to prevent collapse should the patient bite it. When inserted, the distal end should lie just above the epiglottis so as not to irritate the laryngeal inlet. There is a standard colour and number coding for size. The most popular oropharyngeal airway type is the Guedel pattern (Fig. 9.2).

Inserting the Airway

The patient's mouth is opened and the lips and teeth separated. The device, which should be well lubricated,

is inserted so that its curvature follows that of the tongue. If often appears to snag about three quarters of the way in. This is usually overcome by lifting the angles of the lower jaw forward with the middle fingers of both hands and gently pushing on the flange with both thumbs. Alternatively, it can be inserted with its curvature initially facing in the opposite direction and, when halfway in, rotated around to its normal position and fully inserted. However, even correct insertion alone may not be totally sufficient to maintain the airway in a deeply anaesthetized patient. It is often partially pushed out if the patient's jaw is left unsupported and allowed to fall backwards. It may also become dislodged in patients

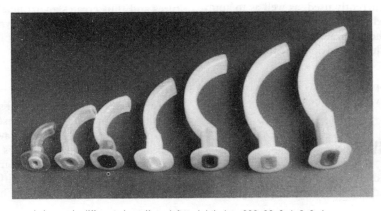

Figure 9.2   Guedel oropharyngeal airways in different sizes: (from left to right) sizes 000, 00, 0, 1, 2, 3, 4.

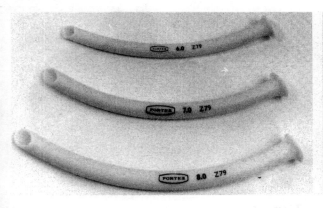

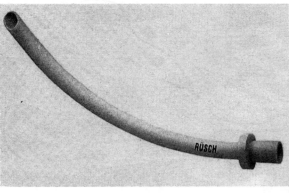

(a)   (b)

Figure 9.3 (a) Nasopharyngeal airways with fixed flanges in different diameters. (b) A nasopharyngeal airway with an adjustable flange.

with marked overbite of the upper teeth. If the lower jaw has to be lifted, both the upper and lower front teeth press on the airway. Because of the overbite, the lower teeth act as a fulcrum so that the downward pressure by the upper teeth on the bite section tends to push the airway out of the mouth causing partial or complete airway obstruction.

Complications

Gagging, retching or laryngospasm will occur if the airway is inserted into a patient whose pharyngeal reflexes have not been sufficiently depressed by topical or general anaesthesia.

The airway may damage the front teeth, especially if there is:

- a porcelain bridge;
- a crowned tooth or teeth;
- excessive pressure on the above due to postoperative masseter spasm;
- overenthusiastic jaw support.

However, the simple expedient of inserting a rubber dental prop between the patient's molar teeth could significantly reduce this problem.

Nasopharyngeal Airway

Where a patient has limited jaw opening, awkward or fragile dentition or where the oral airway is frequently displaced by a marked overlapping bite, an alternative artificial airway may be created via the nose. This is achieved by inserting a soft plastic, polyurethane or latex rubber tube through the nares and passing it along the

floor of the nose and down into the oropharynx to a point just above the epiglottis.

This has either a fixed (Fig 9.3a) or an adjustable flange (Fig. 9.3b) at its proximal end, which limits insertion of an excessive length, so that the device lies in the correct position, i.e. just above the epiglottis. The distal end is bevelled to make its passage through the nose less traumatic. It may also have a hole cut into the wall opposite this so that should the bevel become blocked with mucus during the insertion, airway patency will be maintained. As with oral airways they are produced in a range of lengths and internal diameters (measured in millimetres) for different sizes of patient.

Complications

Complications do occur with the use of nasopharyngal airways. They may traumatize the septal mucosa, nasal polyps or adenoidal tissue producing an epistaxis, which will compromise the airway. Hence they should not be used where there is evidence of a coagulopathy or other causes of epistaxis.

FACEMASKS

Most facemasks are designed to fit over the patient's nose and mouth perfectly, without any leaks, and yet to exert the minimum of pressure, which might either depress the jaw and cause respiratory obstruction or cause pressure sores. The facemask (Fig. 9.4) consists of three parts: the mount, the body, and the edge. A snug fit

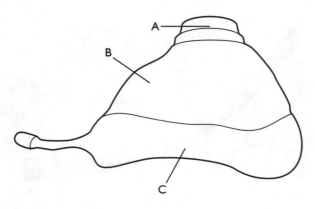

Figure 9.4 The parts of an anaesthetic facemask: A, the mount; B, the body; C, the edge.

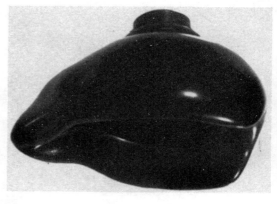

Figure 9.6 The Everseal facemask (M&IE).

is achieved by incorporating one or more of the following features into the design: by anatomically shaping the body, by the use of an air-filled cuff at the edge that has a soft cushioning effect (Fig. 9.5) or by a flap that takes up the contour of the face (Fig. 9.6).

Masks for some dental anaesthetic techniques are designed to fit the nose only so that the dentist has unimpeded access to the mouth (*see* Chapter 15, Fig. 15.3).

The mount normally has a 22 mm female taper if made to ISO (International Standards Organization) or BS (British Standards). It is usually constructed of hard rubber but may be plastic or metal. The former two wear more easily with repeated use and eventually produce a leak or potential for accidental disconnection.

The body may be of rubber, neoprene, plastic or polycarbonate. In some cases a wire stiffener or a wire gauze is incorporated so as to make it malleable in order that its shape may be altered to fit the patient's face. The transparent body of a plastic or polycarbonate facemask is particularly useful as it permits respiration to be

detected by the appearance of condensation during exhalation and also during resuscitation. It allows the early detection of vomit should this unfortunately occur. Also, this type may appear less threatening to anxious adults and small children (Fig. 9.7).

The internal volume (apparatus dead space) within the body of the facemask is relatively insignificant in adults but may assume significance in neonates and infants where it could constitute 30% or more of their tidal volume. Hence, this part of a paediatric mask is filled in to minimize the respirable dead space (Fig. 9.8).

The edge may be anatomically shaped and fitted with a cuff or a flap. A good fit is essential to prevent dilution of inhaled gas by room air during spontaneous respiration and to allow positive pressure ventilation to be administered without leakage. It is advisable to stock a variety of types and sizes of facemask, since none will fit every type of face well. Poor fits occur more frequently in edentulous patients and in those with beards. The cheeks of the former usually sag away from the mask edges producing a leak, which may be solved by selecting a smaller mask or inserting an oral airway. Beards often prevent a good seal around the edge of the mask and a leak-free fit may be achieved with a bigger mask often held on with two hands. Masks with a cuff have a small filling tube fitted with a plug to enable the degree of inflation of the cuff to be regulated. The plug must also be removed and the cuff allowed to deflate if the mask is to be autoclaved.

Whereas some facemasks withstand the high temperatures of autoclaving, others do not. Since these are not easily distinguished, it is advisable to adopt a uniform policy of disinfection. This may be by boiling, pasteurizing or by chemical means, although some chemicals, e.g. chloroxylenol (Dettol), are known to have been absorbed by the material of the facemask and have resulted in injury to the patient's skin.

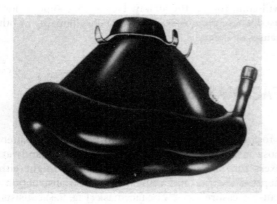

Figure 9.5 The anatomical facemask (Ohmeda).

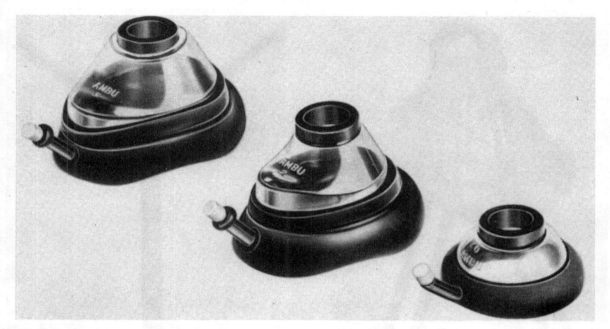

Figure 9.7 Three examples of the Ambu facemask, which has a transparent body that enables the presence of vomitus to be seen.

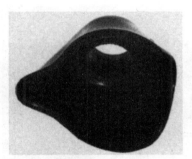

Figure 9.8 The Rendell–Baker paediatric facemask.

Angle Pieces

This is a right-angled connector (Fig. 9.11) which is commonly used to join the facemask more neatly to a breathing system. The downstream end has an external 22 mm male taper that fits the facemask. The upstream end has an internal 22 mm female taper which fits the breathing system.

In some more recent designs, the downstream end has also been fitted with an internal 15 mm *female* taper so that the angle piece may fit an endotracheal tube as well (see below). The upstream (breathing system) end has also been changed. It now has an external 15 mm *male* taper instead of the 22 mm female one. This does not cause any incompatibility problems, however, as the breathing system can accept either taper.

Harnesses

Masks may be held in place by a harness that encircles the head. The mask mount can be fitted with a three, four or five hooked ring, the hooks of which can engage either the holes punched into the arms of the harness or metal clips attached to the latter. The Connell head harness (Fig. 9.9) is fitted with two metal clips for attachment to the mask ring and is popular for securing nasal as well as oral masks. The Clausen harness (Fig. 9.10) has a three-point attachment to the mask and is designed for facemasks.

THE LARYNGEAL MASK AIRWAY

Until recently, maintaining a clear airway in an anaesthetized patient might well involve elevating and protruding the lower jaw, supporting it in this position with a Guedel airway, placing a facemask over the nose and mouth and securing it with a Clausen's harness to provide a gas tight fit. But this can now be accomplished with a single device, *the laryngeal mask airway (LMA)*.

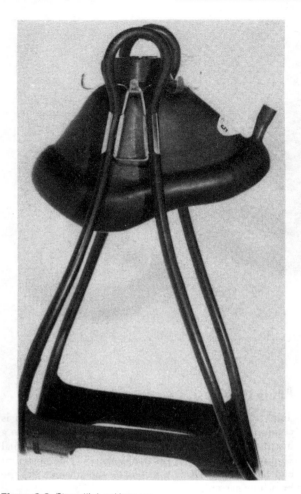

Figure 9.9 Connell's head harness.

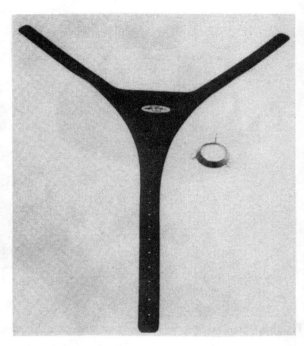

Figure 9.10 Clausen's head harness and ring.

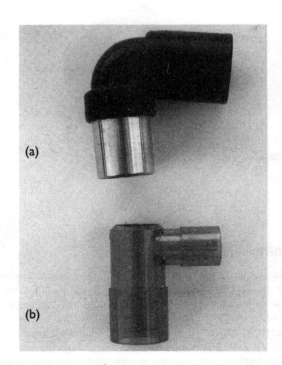

(a)

(b)

Figure 9.11 Angle pieces. (a) Older version with 22 mm tapers; (b) newer version with a proximal 15 mm external taper and a distal dual mode taper (an external 22 mm male and an internal 15 mm female one).

This device is passed through the mouth and into the pharynx so that its distal end lies over the laryngeal inlet.

The distal end consists of a hollow bowl resembling a small facemask which is surrounded by an inflatable tubular cuff. The latter, when inflated, fits around the laryngeal inlet and supports it in a position away from posterior pharyngeal wall. The back of the bowl leads into a tube which passes out of the pharynx and mouth. The proximal end of this tube has a 15 mm ISO male connection so that it can be attached to a breathing system. The tube, at its point of entry into the mask, is fenestrated by two thick silicone rubber strands to prevent the epiglottis falling into it and occluding its lumen. The cuff is supplied by a small tube with a built-in self-sealing valve so that the cuff remains inflated when injected with air.

LMAs are made from silicone rubber so that they

can be autoclaved and reused to the manufacturer's maximum of 40 times and are supplied in five sizes. The manufacturer's recommendations are as follows:

- size 1 should be used for neonates up to 6.5 kg;
- size 2 for patients from 6.5 to 20 kg;
- size 2½ for patients between 20 and 30 kg;
- size 3 for children and small adults;
- size 4 for average-sized adults and size 5 for large adults (Fig. 9.12).

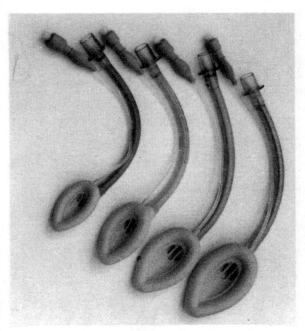

Figure 9.13 The reinforced laryngeal mask airway in sizes 2–4.

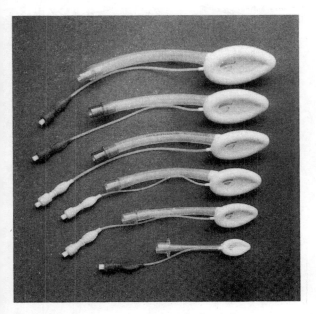

Figure 9.12 The Laryngeal mask airway in sizes 1–5.

An alternative version is available in which the tube is made thinner, narrower and longer and is reinforced with a spiral of steel wire to provide added flexibility without the risk of kinking (Fig. 9.13). This version improves intraoral surgical access for maxillo-facial and ENT surgery as the tube occupies less space and can be positioned away from the operative site.

Discretion should be used in cases where the predicted size does not fit. For example, a large adult may have a smaller than expected pharynx whereas an elderly patient may well have one larger than expected.

Inserting the LMA (Fig. 9.14)

Because the LMA, when correctly placed, would elicit a gag reflex in an awake patient, it should be inserted only in a patient whose pharyngeal reflexes have been sufficiently depressed by adequate general anaesthesia or topical analgesia. As the device is reusable, it is subject to wear and tear and should be checked for damage as well as for leaks or a hernia in the inflatable cuff. The latter two, if present, will be identified by filling the cuff to 50% more than the recommended volume.

The manufacturer's recommended insertion technique requires that the cuff, having been checked (see above), is deflated fully with the concave part of the mask pressed against a hard surface. This causes the cuff to fold backwards behind the bowl. The back of the mask is lubricated with a water-based gel and the tubular section is grasped like a pen, with the tip of the operator's gloved index finger placed at the junction of the tube and mask. The operator's other hand extends the patient's neck by cradling the occiput so that the patient's mouth falls open. The mask is then pushed with one firm movement through the mouth and down the posterior pharyngeal wall as far as possible (Fig. 9.14b). The fingers are withdrawn and the tube pushed further in until a resistance is felt (Fig. 9.14c). This is usually the point of full insertion. Without holding the tube, the cuff is then inflated with the recommended volume:

- 4 ml for size 1;
- 10 ml for size 2;
- 14 ml for size 2½;
- 20 ml for size 3;
- 30 ml for size 4;
- 40 ml for size 5.

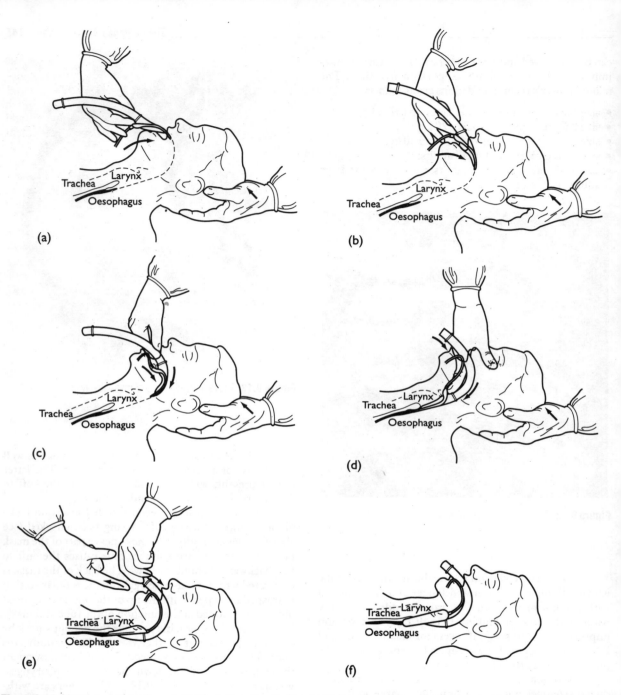

Figure 9.14 Manufacturer's recommended method of insertion. Position the head and neck as for normal intubation. (a) Keep the neck flexed and the head extended by pushing on the occiput with one hand while inserting the mask into the mouth with the other hand. When inserting the mask, hold it like a pen, with the index finger placed anteriorly at the junction of the cuff and tube. (b) Using the index finger, keep pressing upwards as you advance the mask into the pharynx to ensure the tip remains flattened and avoids the tongue. (c) Keeping the neck flexed and head extended, press the mask into the posterior pharyngeal wall using the index finger. Note that the index finger must be directly in line with the mask aperture. (d) Continue pushing with the tip of the index finger guiding the mask downward into position. By withdrawing the other fingers and slight pronation of the forearm, it is usually possible to push the mask fully into position in one fluid movement. (e) Now grasp the tube firmly with the other hand and withdraw the index finger from the pharynx. Press gently downward with this other hand to ensure that the mask remains fully inserted. In the event insertion to the correct depth has not been achieved using the index finger, this action will ensure full insertion. (f) Inflate the mask with the recommended volume of air. Do not over inflate. Do not hold the tube of the LMA while inflating unless the position is obviously unstable. Normally the mask should rise slightly out of the hypopharynx as the cuff is inflated, and the mask finds its correct position.

This frequently causes the tube to ride upwards as it settles into the correct position. Overinflation of the cuff may distort its shape and interfere with the correct anatomical fit, therefore only the recommended amount of air should be used to fill it.

Alternative Methods of Insertion

Other methods of insertion have been described. For those with short fingers, the tube may be grasped like a dart close to its connector although this will not work for the reinforced version of the LMA because it is too flexible to transmit the force required to push it down the pharynx. For this version, stiffening it by inserting a malleable introducer or smaller endotracheal tube into its lumen may aid placement. Elevating and protruding the jaw by placing a thumb into the mouth and pulling on the jaw from behind the lower front teeth (instead of cradling the occiput) also aids insertion and lessens the chance of the mask colliding with the epiglottis.

A longitudinal black line is marked along the full extent of the dorsal surface of the tube. This should lie in the midline when the tube is in situ. If not, it will indicate a degree of rotation or misplacement.

Confirmation of Correct Placement

Remarkably, for a device that is inserted blindly, the mask almost always adopts the correct position and provides a patent airway. In a spontaneously breathing patient, the sound of breathing should be non-stridorous and the reservoir bag of the breathing system should show a normal excursion. In an apnoeic patient, squeezing the reservoir bag should produce normal chest movements with an applied pressure no greater than 2 kPa (20 cmH$_2$O). A small leak is permissible; a large leak or an inflation pressure higher than expected will usually indicate the possibility of either a misplacement or of breath holding by the patient.

Indications for Using the LMA

- It may replace the use of a facemask and pharyngeal airway in a spontaneously breathing patient, with the added benefit of:

  (a) releasing the anaesthetist's hands to deal with other matters; and

  (b) providing a more reliable airway in patients placed in positions other than supine (such as on their side).

- It may replace an endotracheal tube:

  (a) in elective procedures where this would have been used to facilitate surgical access to the head, neck

and pharynx, dispensing with the need to use muscle relaxant drugs usually required for endotracheal intubation;

(b) where a difficult intubation is predicted in which conventional laryngoscopy could be traumatic and damage dentition, or where neck movement should be minimized;

(c) as an alternative airway especially in an emergency following failed intubation, or as used by para-medical staff who are not regularly trained in endotracheal intubation, or ventilating a patient with a facemask;

(d) in balanced anaesthesia using controlled ventilation where intubation may elicit undesirable cardiovascular or respiratory responses. Although the device was originally designed to maintain the airway in spontaneously breathing patients, leak-free positive pressure ventilation is possible in most instances where the peak inflation pressure required is less than 2.5 kPa (25cm H$_2$O). However, it is more easily dislodged than an endotracheal tube and it is therefore inadvisable to use it in situations where access to the airway is difficult in case its position requires readjustment or it requires replacement by an endotracheal tube during the procedure.

- It may be used to aid a difficult intubation. For example, a suitably sized, uncut, cuffed endotracheal tube may be inserted through the LMA so that its tip projects just beyond the protective bars of the mask. The LMA is then inserted in the normal manner and when in situ, the endotracheal tube can often be advanced into the larynx, the cuff inflated and the connector attached to a breathing system.

  Occasionally, the epiglottis may become folded over inside the bowl of the mask and can prevent successful insertion. A flexible fibreoptic laryngoscope can be used to bypass the obstruction and confirm correct placement.

- Where a patient needs resuscitation in a position in which a laryngoscope cannot easily be employed.

Contraindications

In its present form the LMA does not necessarily protect the larynx from aspiration of refluxed gastric contents. Its use should therefore be avoided where regurgitation is potentially possible as in a patient with a full stomach or untreated hiatus hernia.

ENDOTRACHEAL TUBES

There are various situations in which it is not feasible to administer anaesthetic gases via a facemask, laryngeal mask or nasal mask. Where positive pressure ventilation is contemplated, or where the trachea and lungs require protection from refluxed gastric contents or pharyngeal debris, it is necessary to secure a leak-free passage between the trachea and the anaesthetic apparatus. In these cases an endotracheal tube is the most appropriate device to use. Most commonly this is inserted through the mouth and through the larynx into the trachea. It should be of sufficient diameter that it either fits snugly into the larynx with only a minimal leak (in neonates, infants and small children) or the tracheal portion may be surrounded by an inflatable cuff which is filled to seal the space between the tube and tracheal wall. It may also be inserted through the nose, passed down the nasopharynx and through the larynx when surgical access to the oropharynx is required. Here, the size of tube required is limited by the size of the nares, and reduced accordingly.

Design

An orotracheal tube (Fig. 9.15) usually has a preformed curve that vaguely conforms to the anatomical shape of the pharynx. This aids insertion and ensures that, when the tube is further flexed when in situ, it is unlikely to kink. The distal end is cut obliquely (bevelled) so that the aperture faces to the left when held in the operator's right hand. When inserted into the larynx, the bevel allows the tip of the tube to be seen passing between the vocal cords. There may be a hole in the wall (a Murphy eye) opposite the bevel. This is designed to provide a secondary port for gas movement in and out of the tube should the bevel become blocked or wedged against the tracheal wall. Part of the distal end of the tube may be surrounded by an inflatable cuff which, when inflated, fills to seal the space between the tube and the tracheal wall. The tube carries several markings, one of which is a longitudinal line of radio-opaque material so that correct placement can be verified from an X-ray if required. The distance from the tip of the bevel is also marked (in centimetres) on the wall, along with the internal diameter.

Construction Materials

Traditionally, endotracheal tubes have been made of red rubber or latex, which can be cleaned and sterilized for reuse. However, these materials are opaque and inadequate cleaning is not always apparent from a superficial examination. Occlusion of the lumen occurs occasionally with foreign objects and dried mucus. Perishing may cause the wall of the tube to weaken, increasing the possibility of kinking. The material itself (red rubber) is potentially an irritant when used for long periods and has been blamed for producing laryngeal granulomata.

Currently, plastics (polyvinyl chloride (PVC) and more recently polyurethane) and, to a lesser degree, silicone rubber have replaced red rubber and latex as primary materials for the following reasons:

- they are non-irritant and are now cheap to produce to allow single patient use;
- they can be sterilized more reliably during manufacture;

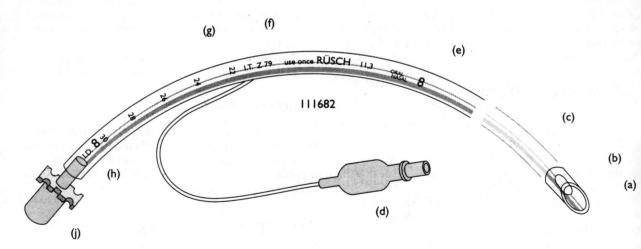

Figure 9.15 An uncut orotracheal tube. (a), Bevel; (b), Murphy eye; (c), tracheal cuff; (d), self-sealing valve which keeps gas in the cuff; (e), marking to show the internal diameter of the tube in millimetres; (f), marking (I.T.Z 79) to show that the plastic has been tested for tissue toxicity; (g), the length of the tube in millimetres, (h), longitudinal line of radio-opaque material; (j), 15 mm connector.

- blockages may be visible as the material is usually clear;
- the manufacturing tolerances are much closer with plastics, so that there is much less variation in the size of the lumen (important in neonatal endotracheal tubes).

However, plastic tubes do not have the 'springiness' of rubber and may be more difficult to insert in difficult situations. Also, the relative rigidity of plastic (PVC) tubes at room temperature appears to cause more trauma when they are inserted via the nasal route compared with rubber ones. However prewarming, by immersing them in warm water, does make the plastic softer. Polyurethane is softer and more 'springy' and may be less traumatic for nasal intubation. Silicone rubber is both soft and has the advantage in that it will withstand autoclaving and so can be reused.

The type of plastic used in the construction of endotracheal tubes is tested to make sure that it is non-irritant. Each endotracheal tube is marked with a test number, which can be seen on the body of the tube labelled 'I.T.' (implant tested) Z.79. This refers to the Z79 Toxicity Subcommittee of the ANSI (American National Standards Institute) set up in 1968 in the USA, which established the current test method. The test consists of implanting four samples of the plastic, under sterile conditions, into the paravertebral muscle of anaesthetized rabbits along with two samples of Reference Standard Negative Control plastic, for 70–144 h. The implant sites are then examined both micro- and macroscopically for signs of inflammation.

Size

Conventional wisdom dictates that the widest diameter tube that will pass *easily* through the narrowest part of the airway should always be used in order to minimize the resistance to gas flow within it, and so reduce the work of breathing. In children, the narrowest part of the airway is the cricoid ring, which being conveniently circular can accept a snug fit from a tube (see below). In adults, the narrowest part is the larynx, which is oblong in shape and would not accept a snug fit from a round tube without inflicting mucosal damage. Hence, in adults, a leak is more likely to occur unless the tube is fitted with an inflatable cuff. Again, conventionally, the tube should be as short as possible so as to further reduce the work of breathing and to prevent the tube from entering a main bronchus (usually the right main bronchus) and ventilating one lung only. Both statements are uncontested in paediatric anaesthesia. However, in adults, selection of the largest tube was also a consequence of early cuff design (see below).

Endotracheal Cuffs

Originally cuffs were made of relatively thick rubber, which could withstand cleaning and autoclaving so that the endotracheal tubes could be reused. If a small tube was repeatedly used in a large trachea, the cuff would become stretched and baggy and develop a weak spot, which could herniate over the tip of the tube and occlude it. Hence, large tubes were used preferentially because these would not require the same degree of cuff distension to effect a tracheal seal, so that the likelihood of herniation was less likely to occur.

This type of cuff nevertheless requires high pressure to distend it (*high pressure cuff*) (Fig. 9.16a). It inflates into a circular shape (Fig. 9.16b) and when a seal is just achieved, only the widest circumference touches the tracheal wall, with little transmission of cuff pressure. Overdistension increases the area of contact but causes the high pressure within the cuff to be transmitted to the tracheal wall. This cuts off the blood flow to the underlying mucosa, which then suffers ischaemic damage.

The cuff on a modern disposable tube can be made so that it does not require the same high pressures for inflation. For example, it can be made from a much thinner elastic material such as latex rubber, which fits snugly to the tube in the deflated state without appearing bulky (Fig. 9.17a). The cuff is referred to as a *medium pressure cuff* because it requires some degree of pressure for inflation, although a seal can be achieved with a pressure below that in the capillaries supplying the underlying mucosa. However, being compliant, overinflation of the cuff causes less pressure rise than the *high pressure* variety. Unfortunately, it may be more easily damaged if

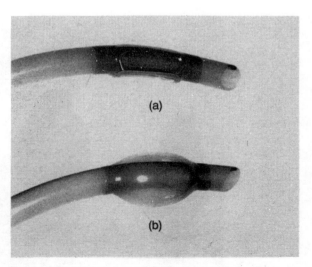

Figure 9.16 A high-pressure tracheal cuff: (a) deflated, and (b) inflated.

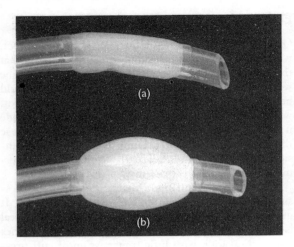

Figure 9.17 A medium-pressure tracheal cuff: (a) deflated, and (b) inflated.

snagged against teeth, instruments, intubation guides or bony spurs in the nasopharynx.

Alternatively, the cuff may be made from a thin inelastic material (PVC) which when inflated would have a larger than required volume to effect a seal (Fig. 9.18 a,b). In situ, there is a large area of contact between the cuff and tracheal wall before the material is fully stretched. The pressure can therefore be kept low enough (*low pressure cuff*) so as not to occlude mucosal blood flow. However, the cuff should be inflated only to a pressure (around 2.5 kPa/25cm H_2O, see Fig. 9.18c) that would normally:

- prevent a gas leak during assisted ventilation and
- prevent pharyngeal contents being leaked past the cuff into the lungs.

If overfilled, the material will be stretched to the limit of its compliance, at which point the pressure will rise dramatically to levels well above that of the blood flow to the underlying mucosa.

Modern cuff design allows narrower bore tubes to be used. This reduces the potential for another complication, that of vocal cord damage. The larger the tube, the greater is the area of contact between it and the vocal cords and the greater the likelihood of damage. The limiting factor governing tube size now becomes that resistance to gas flow within the tube and connectors which is acceptable in a particular situation. For example, a 5 mm internal diameter tube is acceptable in an average adult male undergoing microlaryngoscopy provided that both assisted ventilation and sufficient time to exhale is allowed. However, the same tube would be too small to allow the same patient to breath spontaneously for all but the shortest of periods. In adult male breathing spontaneously, a 7–8 mm tube would be acceptable.

Tubes for orotracheal use are usually cuffed (sizes 6–11 mm internal diameter). Below 6.0 mm internal diameter, the cuff, added to the size of the tube wall, increases the relative bulkiness of the tube so that a smaller size is required in order to pass as easily into the larynx and trachea. This causes a reduction in the internal diameter of the resultant air passage and produces a sharp rise in resistance to gas flow (see Chapter 1, Poiseuille's law), so that below this value (6 mm) the use of a plain tube is preferable. Also, the narrowest part of

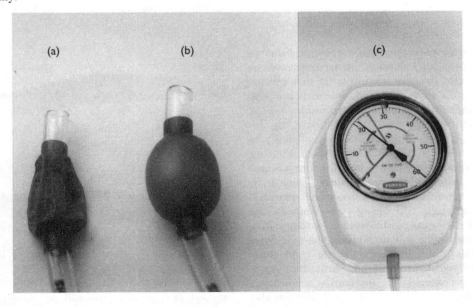

Figure 9.18 A low-pressure tracheal cuff: (a) deflated, and (b) inflated; (c) shows a pressure manometer.

the airway of a child or infant (the cricoid cartilage) is almost circular and a more snug fit is possible, therefore reducing the need for a cuff on a tube. There are a few exceptions to this rule, however (see the section on Special Tubes and also Chapter 14).

Cuffs are inflated via a small-bore inflation tube, which is either welded *onto* the outside of the endotracheal tube or *built into* its wall. The inflation tube is connected, at its proximal end, to a small pilot balloon which is designed to give an indication of the distension of the cuff. The cuff (and pilot balloon) are inflated, usually with air, via a syringe. The proximal end of the inflation tube is often fitted with a self-sealing valve, which prevents air escaping when the syringe is removed. Cuffs on tubes should be inflated with just sufficient air or gas to prevent leaks. This limits the pressure on the ciliated columinar epithelium of the trachea, so as to prevent damage or even necrosis. Also, if there were overpressure in the breathing system it would permit leakage around the cuff thereby:

- allowing excess gas under pressure to escape and
- giving a warning by the gurgling noise produced.

Nitrous oxide diffuses into a cuff filled with air. The rate at which this occurs depends on:

- the permeability of the material from which the cuff is constructed (rubber being more permeable than plastic);
- the surface area of cuff exposed to the nitrous oxide;
- the partial pressure of nitrous oxide.

The rise in pressure caused by this diffusion into the cuff depends on the compliance of the cuff. Low-volume, high-pressure cuffs suffer the greatest pressure rise and may well transmit this rise in pressure to the tracheal mucosa. High-volume, low-pressure cuffs, constructed of plastic, expand with only a slight increase in pressure until all the slack in the cuff is taken up. At this point, owing to the inelasticity of plastic, the pressure rise increases rapidly (up to 12 kPa/90 mmHg) to that which can damage the tracheal mucosa.

Methods of Preventing the Pressure Increase

This phenomenon can be avoided if the cuff is filled with either sterile water or a gas mixture identical to that of the inspired gas.

Alternatively, there are several devices that limit the pressure rise. For example, the Mallinckrodt Brandt device has a pilot balloon made from a material that allows the nitrous oxide, which has diffused into the cuff, to escape (Fig. 9.19).

The Mallinckrodt Lanz device consists of a secondary balloon made of thin latex which is placed inside the plastic pilot balloon on the tube. When air is intro-

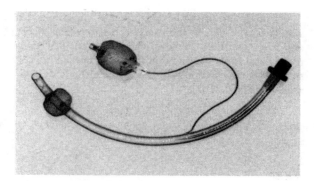

Figure 9.19 The Mallinckrodt Brandt device.

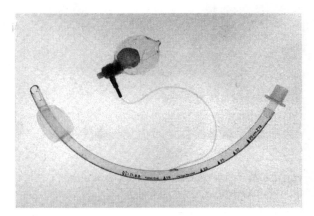

Figure 9.20 The Mallinckrodt Lanz device.

duced into the system, the tube cuff and this latex balloon are both inflated. As the cuff pressure starts to rise due to the diffusion of nitrous oxide, the latex balloon absorbs this pressure by expanding (Fig. 9.20). More recently, materials that are impervious to the diffusion of nitrous oxide have been used in the construction of cuffs.

Nasotracheal Intubation

The size of tube that can be passed via the nasal route is limited by the size of the nares and the potential obstruction caused by the nasal turbinates or a deviated nasal septum. Tubes made from standard plastic (which is relatively hard), as well as those with cuffs, may well be more difficult to insert and may increase the likelihood for epistaxis. Most manufacturers use softer plastics, latex or silicone rubber for specialist nasal tubes, which are less traumatic.

The design of the bevel tip is also important. The standard type has, in the past, been sharp (Fig. 9.21a) and may tear the turbinates when inserted. Currently, many nasal tubes have a bevel tip that is curved inwards so that any obstruction is pushed aside rather than traumatized (Fig. 9.21b).

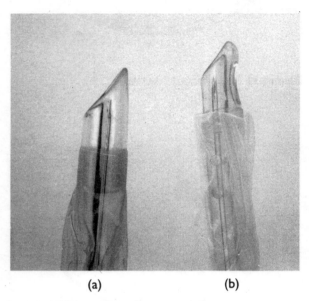

(a)   (b)

Figure 9.21 (a) Standard nasotracheal tube bevel (sharp); (b) cupped nasotracheal tube bevel (blunt).

Plain (uncuffed) tubes made from a softer material and with a cupped bevel tip still seem to be the least traumatic and are appropriate where spontaneous respiration is planned, regurgitation of gastric contents is not anticipated and where the pharynx is securely packed in case of surgical bleeding. If a cuffed tube has to be used, then one with the softest and smoothest exterior surface is best. This will include one that incorporates the inflation tube within its walls, and one that has a close fitting streamline cuff of fine latex. Plastic tubes may be preheated to body temperature by immersion in warm water to soften them prior to insertion.

Maintenance of Reusable Endotracheal Tubes

Endotracheal tubes that are designed for reuse should be autoclavable. Connectors should be removed and cuffs deflated before treatment. The self-sealing valves should be kept open with an autoclavable syringe (with the plunger removed) so as to release any residual gas or water vapour, which might expand during the autoclaving process. Tubes may be wrapped separately, in which case a transparent packet should be used so that they may be inspected before opening. The cuff should be inflated before reuse and if it shows any weakness or herniation, it should be rendered unusable and discarded. Tubes should also be tested for resistance to kinking, and any that show signs of ageing or perishing should also be discarded.

Endotracheal Tube Lengths

Endotracheal tubes are supplied from the manufacturer longer than normally required. Many anaesthetists cut their tubes to a shorter length so that when inserted they are less likely to enter a main bronchus (Table 9.1).

Common Problems with the Use of Endotracheal Tubes

These are as follows:

- A tube may be passed too far down the trachea and may enter the right main bronchus. This occurs because the tube selected is too long and it needs shortening.
- There may be a leak between the cuff and the trachea. This may be either because the cuff has not been sufficiently inflated in the first place, or because it has leaked. The latter may be due to a fault in manufacture, or to overinflation. (The presence of a leak may be demonstrated by immersing the whole tube in water, inflating the cuff and watching for bubbles.) It is possible to kink the pilot tube accidentally and prevent inflation of the cuff even though the pilot balloon is blown up.
- The tube may be obstructed in one or more of several ways. The opening may be occluded if the larynx or trachea is deviated to one side as seen in Fig. 9.22. This may happen particularly during thyroidectomy, when the gland is being pulled to one side by the surgeon. The 'Murphy eye' (Fig. 9.23) will prevent this hazard.
- During nasal intubation the tube may be blocked as it harvests a polyp or adenoidal tissue. It may also kink when bent into too small a radius, particularly if soft. If it must be acutely bent when in situ, an armoured tube or one that is specially shaped should be used (see Tubes for Special Purposes below). A tube may be compressed by a throat pack that has been inserted too firmly, and it may also be obstructed if the patient is lightly anaesthetized and bites it. This may be prevented either by inserting an airway alongside the tube or by using a rubber dental prop to keep the jaws apart. In tubes with high pressure cuffs, sufficient pressure can develop to cause inward herniation of the tube wall underneath the cuff and obstruct gas flow.

Table 9.1 Lengths of endotracheal tubes

Internal diameter (mm)		Age (years)	Length (cm)	
Oral	Nasal		Oral	Nasal
2.5	2.5	PREMATURE	10.5	13.0
3.0	3.0		10.5	13.0
3.5	3.5	0-1	11.0	14.0
4.0	4.0		12.0	14.5
4.5	4.5	1-2	13.5	15.0
5.0	5.0		14.0	16.6
5.5	5.5	2-4	14.5	17.0
6.0	6.0		15.0	17.5
6.5	6.5	5-12	16.0	18.5
7.0	7.0	13-16	17.5	19.0
8.0	8.0		18.5	19.5
—	6.0	Small women	—	24.0
—	6.5		—	24.0
7.0	7.0	ADULTS	—	24.0
7.5	7.5		—	25.0
8.0	8.0		23.0	26.0
8.5	—		24.0	—
9.0	—		25.0	—
9.5	—		25.0	—
10.0	—	Large men	26.0	—
11.0	—		26.0	—

A widely used formula for selecting the diameter of an endotracheal tube suitable for children over the age of 1 year is:

$$\frac{\text{Age in years}}{4} + 4.5\ \text{mm}$$

The exact length to which a new tube should be shortened cannot be categorically specified. In some operations it is necessary to pass the tube further down the trachea than in others. Cuffed tubes are generally trimmed to a centimetre or so longer than plain ones.

Endotracheal tubes may become kinked in the mouth (Fig. 9.24) or nasopharynx when the patient's neck is flexed, and this is particularly likely when procedures such as oesophagoscopy are being performed, or during operations when extreme flexion of the head or the neck is required, as in some neurosurgical procedures.

With any endotracheal tube it is important that it is cut to the correct length so that the connector is as close as possible to the patient's mouth. If there is an excess of tube sticking out of the mouth, kinking may easily occur at that point. A tube may also be obstructed by being twisted in its long axis if the position of the catheter mount is altered (Fig. 9.25). This is especially true with PVC tubes, which soften in situ as they warm up.

All sorts of foreign bodies, including the tops of ampoules, have been found within reusable endotracheal tubes, blocking them. This emphasizes the fact that tubes, airways, etc. that are to be reused should not be placed in the same 'dirty dish' as discarded syringes, needles, ampoules, etc. A diaphragm of dried mucus or K-Y Jelly has been found blocking a tube, and even if the tube is straightened so that one can look through it to confirm patency, it is almost invisible.

ISO Connectors

The endotracheal tube is attached to the other components of a breathing system via a male to female 15 mm International Organization for Standards (ISO) tapered connection. The male connector is fitted with a tapered cone, which is pushed into the lumen of the endotracheal tube (see Fig 9.15j). It is slightly bigger than the tube so that the tube material has to be stretched to fit. This produces a secure connection, which can often only be broken by cutting the tube. This principle is important where manufacturers supply the tube and connector separately as too small a connector may become loose and separate from the tube, probably at the most inopportune moment.

Either the breathing system or 'catheter mount' houses the female part of the connector (see below).

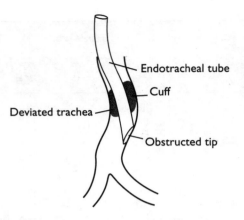

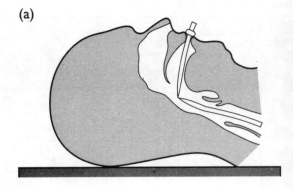

(a)

Figure 9.22 If there is marked deviation of the trachea, the end of the tube may be obstructed.

(b)

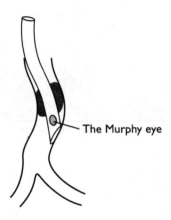

Figure 9.23 The distal end of an endotracheal tube with a 'Murphy eye'

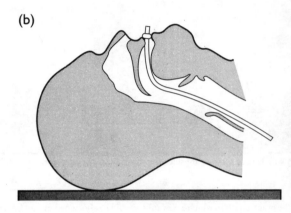

Figure 9.24 (a) Kinking of an endotracheal tube inside the mouth due to excessive neck flexion and softening of the tube owing to its becoming warmer during anaesthesia, all having seemed well at induction. (b) Head in correct position.

This two part design permits a rapid disconnection and reconnection. However, the connection should be made secure with a 'push and twist' movement if possible to prevent accidental separation under normal working conditions. Tapers made from soft plastic are prone to wear if the connection is repeatedly disrupted and so this material is normally found only on single use items. High density nylon and, better still, metal can be used repeatedly but should be discarded as soon as signs of wear become apparent.

Other Connectors

The early pioneers in anaesthesia produced connections in a variety of shapes and sizes designed mostly to streamline the fit and to improve surgical access to the head and neck of a patient, or to minimize resistance to gas flow and so reduce the work of breathing. This func-

tion has largely been incorporated into the design of the various specialist endotracheal tubes (see below), allowing a single size of connection (15 mm ISO) to be developed. However, a smaller size of 8.5 mm is becoming popular for use in neonates as this reduces the weight of the components (see Fig. 14.7, p. 237).

An endotracheal tube that has been cut to size (see Table 9.1) and fitted with a 15 mm male ISO connector can be connected directly to a breathing system which has at its outlet a dual mode ISO connector, i.e. its inner diameter being a 15 mm ISO female connector for this purpose (whereas its outer diameter is a 22 mm male ISO connector for use with other breathing system components). The direct coupling of a standard endotracheal tube to the breathing system may increase the relative bulkiness of the system in such close proximity to the face and may interfere with surgical access, the preparation of the operating field, or it may drag on the

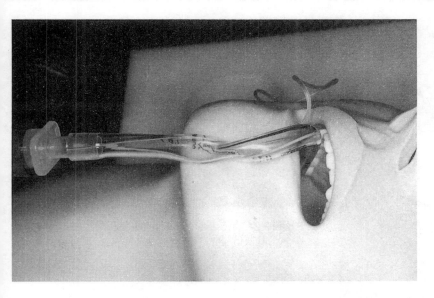

Figure 9.25 Obstruction of the lumen of an endotracheal tube due to a twisting force from a breathing system.

tube causing it to change position within the larynx. There are two possible solutions to this:

- design elongated tubes with individual shapes (see Tubes for Special Purposes below);
- include a short adapter or 'catheter mount' between the two pieces of apparatus in question.

Catheter Mounts

The term 'catheter mount' does not appear in BS 6015 (ISO 4135), which is the official glossary of terms used in anaesthesiology. Its modern equivalent, 'tracheal tube adaptor', will probably be slow to replace the older and more familiar term, as will the term 'tracheal tube' rather than the older 'endotracheal tube'. Some explanation of these terms would perhaps be apt.

Before the introduction of the Boyle's machine with the Magill breathing attachment, the mixed gases, with added vapour of volatile agents, were fed via a narrow-bore tube (*catheter mount*) to the patient, with no reservoir bag or expiratory valve in the positions in which we now know them. The end of the tube could be attached to a Boyle-Davis gag or to a catheter that was passed through the larynx into the trachea. In the latter case, the gases and/or vapours were blown constantly down the catheter and were exhausted to the atmosphere by passing out through the trachea but outside the catheter.

Currently, a catheter mount usually consists of a short piece of flexible, kink-resistant 15 mm tubing with a 15 mm female tapered connector for attachment to the endotracheal tube (Fig. 9.26 a–c). The connector may be either straight or angled and often incorporates swivels to reduce any torsion caused by the breathing system. The angled version may also have a port with a detach-able cap so that suction catheters or a bronchoscope may be passed into the trachea.

The other end may have either a 15 mm male taper that fits inside the end of the breathing system or a 22 mm female taper that fits on the outside of it. Although the device increases the apparatus dead space of the breathing system, this is probably insignificant in adults but may be important in the very young.

ENDOTRACHEAL TUBES FOR SPECIAL PURPOSES

Many 'special' tubes have been devised but they are too numerous for all to be described here. A few examples are shown below.

RAE Preformed Tubes (Fig. 9.27)

There are two separate versions of these tubes (named after their inventors: Ring, Adair and Elwin). The tube for orotracheal intubation (Fig. 9.27a) has a preformed bend on that part of the tube where it exits the mouth, so that the part housing the ISO connector passes down the chin and away from the face thus improving surgical access to the mouth, nose and head of the patient. The nasotracheal version (Fig. 9.27b) is bent where it exits the nose so that the part housing the ISO connector passes upwards to the forehead. It is used to improve surgical access in intraoral procedures.

The main disadvantage of both designs is in the fixed length of the intraoral section. This is rarely too short but is occasionally too long and can enter a main bronchus

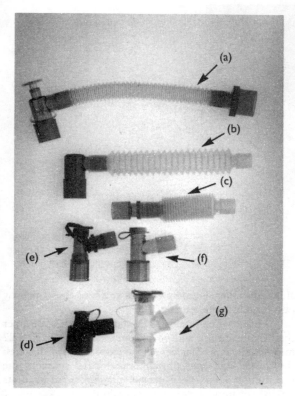

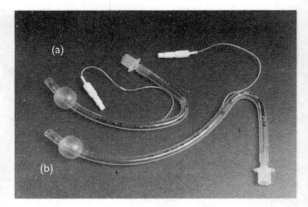

Figure 9.27 (a) Oral version of the RAE preformed tube; (b) nasal version of the RAE preformed tube.

Figure 9.26 (a) A catheter mount with right-angled connector fitted with a suction port; (b) a similar version but without a suction port; (c) a straight catheter mount, (d) an angled swivelled connector with a suction port; (e), (f) and (g) similar versions but with optional gas-tight seals in their suction ports through which a fibreoptic scope may be passed during ventilation.

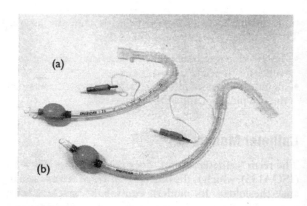

Figure 9.28 Sheridan 'Flexibend': (a) orotracheal version; (b) nasotracheal version.

causing unilateral ventilation. If this happens, the tube may be withdrawn back into the trachea, but then the preformed curve no longer fits the face snugly and securing the tube becomes difficult. Furthermore, the acute curvature impedes the passage of fibrescopes and suction catheters. A version is available with a flexible bend, which overcomes some of these problems. The 'flexi-bend' resembles a catheter mount and can be supplied separately so that the endotracheal tube portion may be cut to suitable lengths for individual patients (Fig. 9.28).

Reinforced Tubes

Most endotracheal tubes will kink when bent into an acute angle or when compressed by an external force such as from a surgical instrument. There are situations where either or both can occur during the course of certain surgical operations. Tubes may be made kink-resistant by embedding a reinforcing spiral of either steel or nylon into

the wall, which can then be made of a more elastic material than usual (i.e. silicone rubber or latex rubber, Fig. 9.29). This makes the tube very flexible with little preformed shape so that it is more difficult to insert into the trachea. It may be introduced over a bougie which has first been passed into the trachea. Alternatively, a malleable stylette can be inserted into its lumen to shape it.

The reinforcing spiral will not stretch to accommodate a connector so the tubes cannot be cut to be a shorter length than supplied. The ISO connectors are therefore usually bonded to a small non-reinforced part of the tube at the factory. Some that are supplied for both oral and nasal use are long and if inserted too far will result in endobronchial intubation. Reusable tubes may be prone to kinking at the 'soft spot' between the end of the connector and the start of the spiral reinforcement (Fig. 9.30) if the connector is not inserted fully.

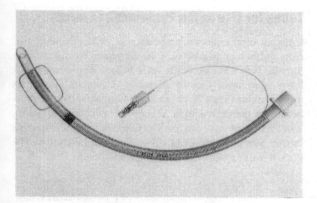

Figure 9.29 A reinforced endotracheal tube for oral or nasal insertion.

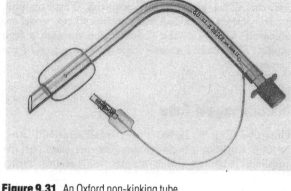

Figure 9.31 An Oxford non-kinking tube.

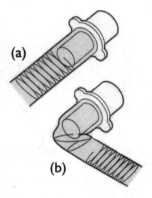

Figure 9.30 Obstruction at the 'soft spot' between the connector and the spiral of an armoured tube. (a) With the connector placed correctly; (b) with incorrect placement leaving an unarmoured segment of tube.

The Carden Tube

This was developed to facilitate microsurgery of the larynx. The body resembles a shortened cuffed endotracheal tube and is served by a long pilot tube for the cuff and a catheter for insufflation of gas (Fig. 9.32). It is inserted into the upper trachea so that only the pilot tube and insufflation catheter occupy the larynx during surgery, and being slender, these can be kept out of the way of the surgeon's manipulations.

The tube may be inserted either by grasping it with the Magill's endotracheal forceps, or as follows. The Carden tube and an uncut plain tube, just wide enough to fit inside it, are threaded in series onto a stylet. This assembly is then introduced through the larynx so that the Carden tube and a centimetre or so of the plain tube pass into the trachea. The cuff on the Carden tube is inflated, the stylet is then withdrawn, and until all is ready for the laryngoscopy, the anaesthetic is maintained

Oxford Tube

For situations that require a patient's neck to be flexed (as in neurosurgical anaesthesia), an alternative to the reinforced tube is an anatomically shaped tube such as the Oxford non-kinking tube (Fig. 9.31), which may be either cuffed or plain. In the older red rubber version, the pharyngeal section is made thicker to resist kinking and the tracheal part is tapered to maximize the internal diameter (especially in the paediatric version). There is a special stylet or 'director' available to straighten the curvature and assist with the insertion of these tubes.

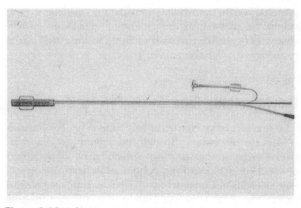

Figure 9.32 A Carden tube for microlaryngeal surgery.

through the plain tube. When the laryngoscopy is to be performed, the plain tube is removed. The breathing system is then discarded and the anaesthetic gases are delivered directly to the Carden tube through a feed mount. The expired gases escape via the lumen of the Carden tube.

Microlaryngeal Tube

This tube (Fig. 9.33), has a very small internal diameter (5–6 mm) but a high-volume, low-pressure cuff. As supplied, it is not cut to length for insertion either

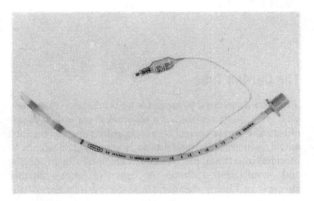

Figure 9.33 A tube for microlaryngeal surgery.

nasally or orally. Its small external diameter takes up little space in the laryngeal inlet so that endoscopy and surgical procedures on the larynx may be performed relatively unhindered. The high volume cuff provides a tracheal seal to enable controlled ventilation to be performed during anaesthesia. (The high resistance to gas flow in these tubes is probably too great for spontaneous respiration for anything but the shortest of periods. With controlled ventilation, sufficient time should be allowed for the prolonged exhalation, otherwise a progressive increase in lung volume will occur resulting in a Valsalva effect.)

Laryngectomy Tube

The preformed curvature of this tube (Fig. 9.34) makes it ideal for placement through tracheotomies. The relatively long, straight portion conveniently allows direct connection to a breathing system away from the operation site without producing an excessive apparatus dead space. The tip may be cut close to the cuff to minimize the risk of endobronchial intubation.

Tubes for Use in the Presence of Lasers

Conventional endotracheal tubes of either rubber, silicone rubber or plastic may be damaged by the carbon dioxide Nd-YAG or KTP laser beam. These materials burn more fiercely in the presence of oxygen (as well as nitrous oxide) than in air, and can be ignited by the temperatures generated by a 'direct hit' with a laser beam. The resultant fire can produce serious upper airways burns. Some examples of tubes that can be used in the presence of a laser beam are described below.

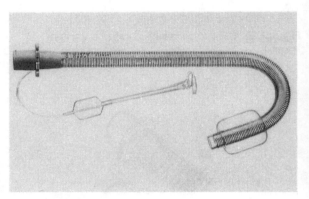

Figure 9.34 A laryngectomy tube.

Bivona 'Fome Cuf' (Fig. 9.35) **and Mallinckrodt 'Laserflex' endotracheal tubes** (Fig. 9.36). These tubes are constructed in a similar fashion. However, the metal links are incorporated into the wall of the tube, which is made

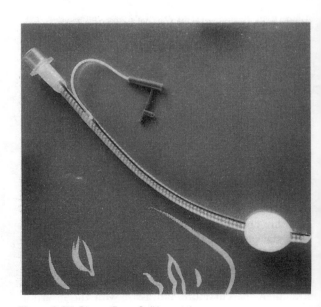

Figure 9.35 Bivona 'Fome Cuf' Laser tube.

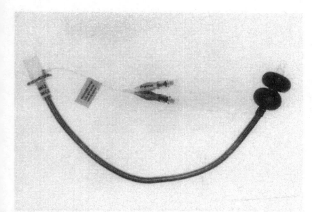

Figure 9.36 Mallinckrodt 'Laser-flex' tube.

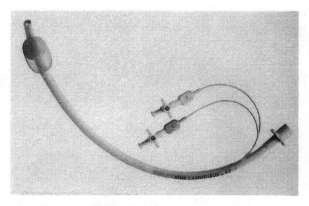

Figure 9.38 The Rusch 'Lasertubus'.

of silicone rubber. The cuff of the former is packed with a sponge, which can be filled with either air or water, so that if the cuff were to burst, the sponge would prevent the cuff from deflation. The cuff can be forcibly deflated by extracting the air or water from within so that a traumatic insertion and removal of the tube from the larynx is possible. The tube, however, is intended for single use only. The 'Laser-flex' has a double cuff so that should the first be punctured the second can then be inflated to provide a seal so obviating the need to change the tube.

Foil wrapped tubes An alternative approach used by some manufacturers is to wrap a suitably small tube spirally with a narrow strip of good quality aluminium or copper foil (which may be stippled to disperse the beam), ensuring that the ends are well secured and the edges are smoothed down. The *Sheridan Laser Trach* (Fig. 9.37) is coated in such a fashion. The foil is then overwrapped with Teflon to provide an outer, smooth coat.

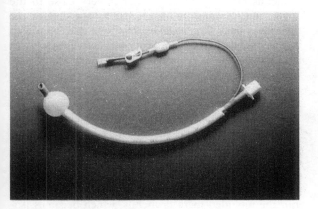

Figure 9.37 The Sheridan Laser Trach.

The pilot balloon may contain methylene blue crystals, which dissolve in saline, which is recommended for inflation of the endotracheal cuff. Should this cuff puncture, the leak of dye would then cause this hazard to be detected easily at operation. The *Rusch 'Lasertubus'* (Fig. 9.38) has a porous sponge coating, which is soaked in water to help absorb the laser energy, and a double cuff (one inside the other).

Disadvantages of 'Laser' Tubes

All the tubes described have thick walls and because they must not be so bulky as to obscure surgical access, a suitably sized tube will have a smaller than usual internal diameter. This may provide too great a resistance for spontaneous respiration and assisted ventilation is often required.

If surgical access is going to be significantly impaired by a laser-resistant tube, a rigid straight-bladed operating laryngoscope (Fig. 9.39) may be substituted so that its tip lies within the glottis but just above the cords. An injector needle is attached to its inside wall and connected to a manually operated gas gun (see Fig. 9.71), which can supply intermittent pulses of high-pressure oxygen. The device has an adjustable regulator to alter the driving pressure of the oxygen. The injector needle acts as a venturi and entrains ambient air to supplement ventilation. Unfortunately, the position of the needle, being adjacent to the wall of the laryngoscope, reduces its ability to entrain air and so it may deliver inadequate ventilation if higher than normal lung inflation pressures are required (as in obese patients). In these cases, ventilation may be supplemented from an anaesthetic breathing system using a cuffed endotracheal tube, which is passed intermittently down the operating laryngoscope and the cuff inflated to provide a seal.

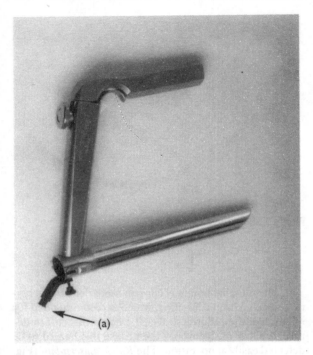

Figure 9.39 A rigid, straight-bladed operating laryngoscope with (a) an injector needle attached.

Tracheostomy Tubes

The distance between a tracheal stoma and the carina in a patient is both variable and often short. Tubes placed in the trachea via a tracheostomy are therefore designed to be non-bevelled, short in length and with the cuff bonded closer to the tip of the tube to prevent accidental endobronchial intubation (Fig. 9.40). Some may have a variable flange to control the depth of insertion (Fig. 9.41). They are also usually preformed into a right angle to prevent kinking during neck flexion.

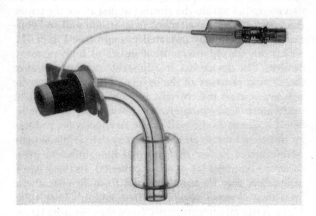

Figure 9.40 A tracheostomy tube.

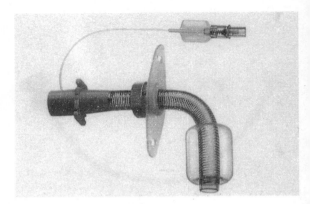

Figure 9.41 A tracheostomy tube with an adjustable flange to control the depth of insertion.

Paediatric Tubes

These are discussed in Chapter 14.

Tubes for Use in Thoracic Surgery

Operations within the thoracic cavity may require the collapse of a lung to improve access to other organs or to isolate that lung for its removal or repair or to prevent contamination from a diseased lung spreading to the other side. This may be achieved in one of three ways.

Endobronchial Tubes

Firstly, a long tube may be passed, often under endoscopic control, beyond the carina and into the unaffected lung so that the cuff can be inflated within a main bronchus. The other lung is not ventilated and collapses, especially when the pleura on that side is opened. This technique is normally applicable only to the left lung. This is because the right upper lobe bronchus enters its main bronchus very close to the carina and it would be obstructed by the cuff of the tube described. The *endobronchial* tube may be placed in the trachea initially so as to use both lungs for as long as possible and then advanced when required to isolate the appropriate lung.

Tubes with Endobronchial Blockers

The second method of isolating a lung is to use a special endotracheal tube through which a fine balloon catheter can be passed either through the lumen of the tube or through a channel in the wall. The balloon tip is then passed, usually with the aid of a fibreoptic endoscope, into the intended main bronchus, which becomes isolated when the balloon is inflated (Fig. 9.42).

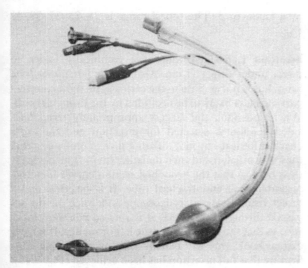

Figure 9.42 An endotracheal tube with endobronchial blocker.

Double-Lumen Tubes

The third and most popular method is to use a combination (or double lumen) tube. These are made by bonding together two tubes of similar diameters but different lengths. The shorter tube fits and seals the trachea with its own cuff whilst the longer one is designed to fit a main bronchus and seal it with a separate cuff. The cuffs are supplied by separate inflation tubes and balloons which are colour coded and labelled to aid identification between the two. The devices are produced in two different preformed shapes to fit either the anatomy of the left (Fig. 9.43) or right (Fig. 9.44) main bronchus. A small soft hook (carinal hook, Fig. 9.45) is fitted below the tracheal lumen on some designs, which wedges at the carina to ensure correct insertion. The right bronchial versions also have a side hole to accommodate the right upper lobe bronchus and the bronchial cuff is also designed so that it does not occlude it (Fig. 9.45b).

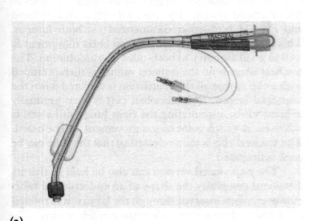

(a)

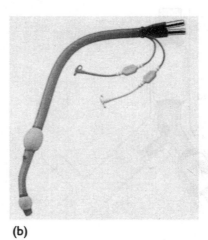

(b)

Figure 9.43 (a) A plastic and (b) a rubber double-lumen tube for left endobronchial intubation.

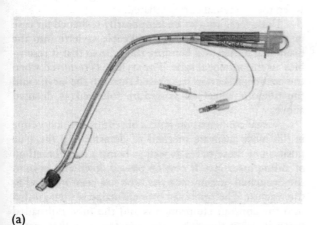

(a)

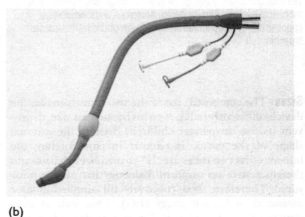

(b)

Figure 9.44 (a) A plastic and (b) a rubber double-lumen tube for right endobronchial intubation.

(a)

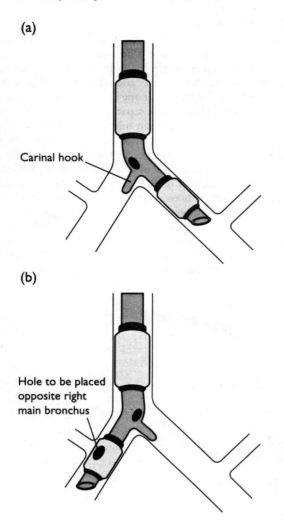

Carinal hook

(b)

Hole to be placed
opposite right
main bronchus

Figure 9.45 (a) The endobronchial section of the tube in the left main bronchus with the carinal hook limiting the depth of insertion. (b) The endobronchial section of the tube in the right main bronchus with the carinal hook limiting the depth of insertion and the side hole opposite the right upper lobe bronchus surrounded by the adapted bronchial cuff.

Sizes The combined size of the two lumens makes the device sufficiently bulky, even in the smallest size, to prevent its use in younger children. Because the external shape of the device is circular in construction, the lumens of its two tubes are 'D'-shaped back to back and therefore have no uniform diameter that can be measured. Therefore, these tubes are still supplied in sizes measured in French gauge (FG). This scale is constructed from the external diameter of the widest portion of the device, measured in millimetres, multiplied

by a factor of 3. The tubes' range is 28–35–37–39–41 FG.

Insertion Left-sided tubes are technically easier to insert under direct vision. Also, as the left upper lobe bronchus is not as close to the carina as its right counterpart, it is less likely to be occluded by the bronchial cuff. Where possible, the largest appropriately sized left-sided version is selected for insertion and the cuffs checked for leaks by first inflating them, confirming that they stay inflated and then deflating them. The device is then held so that the bronchial section curves forwards resembling an endotracheal tube. It is inserted under direct vision using a laryngoscope and, once the tip has passed through the larynx, it is rotated counter-clockwise so that the tip will enter the left bronchus. If it has a carinal hook, this will usually snag on the carina confirming that full insertion has been achieved (Fig. 9.45). The two connectors are then joined to those on a twin tube adapter (catheter mount), which links the tubes to the breathing system. The tracheal cuff is then inflated and manual ventilation commenced via both lumens. This should produce visible bilateral chest movement as well as good air entry to both sides on auscultation. The tracheal adaptor on the catheter mount is then occluded with a clip so that all the ventilation is directed down the bronchial lumen. The bronchial cuff is then gradually inflated whilst auscultating the right lung until a seal is achieved, at which point no gas movement will be heard. The tracheal clip is then released so that the tube can be used as intended.

The right-sided version can also be held so that its distal end resembles the shape of an endotracheal tube. However, when inserted through the larynx, it is rotated clockwise and then pushed in until it is felt to snag. The procedure for confirming correct placement is similar to its left-sided counterpart with the added proviso that gas entry should also be heard over the right upper zone when the bronchial cuff is inflated.

Both versions may be temporarily reshaped for ease of placement by inserting a malleable stylette into the bronchial lumen and bending the tube so that it resembles an endotracheal tube. The stylette is removed when the bronchial section has passed through the larynx and the relevant insertion procedure followed as detailed above.

Visual confirmation with a fibreoptic bronchoscope is the most accurate method of determining the true position of these tubes as well as being a useful method of aiding insertion. It may be passed down and beyond the bronchial lumen once the tube has been inserted in the trachea. The tip of the bronchoscope is then guided into the appropriate bronchus and the tube railroaded down it. With the right-sided version, it is then withdrawn as far as the lateral hole in the lumen to confirm that this is opposite the opening of the right upper lobe bronchus. Prior to using this instrument, one should confirm that, when well lubricated, it will pass easily through the appropriate lumen. For the smaller-size tubes a paediatric fibrescope may be required.

Confirmation of Correct Placement of Endotracheal Tubes

Scrupulous attention should be paid to the insertion of endotracheal tubes and confirmation of their correct placement. Vigilance should be maintained throughout the anaesthetic as movement of the tube down, up or out of the larynx is well documented. The consequences to the patient of inadvertent oesophageal placement are disastrous if unrecognized. The following tests should be employed where appropriate:

- Visual confirmation of the tube passing through the larynx. However, the tube may be subsequently dislodged by insertion of throat packs or surgical instrumentation of the pharynx, or by traction from a breathing system when the tube has been inadequately secured.
- Visible equal and bilateral expansion of the thorax using a low inflation pressure with assisted ventilation.
- Confirmation by auscultation of the apices and bases of both lungs. Even this may be masked in an obese patient or one with bronchospasm or where the tube is marginally in one main bronchus.
- Testing carbon dioxide in the exhalate, although this is unreliable in a patient with little or no blood flow to the lungs for whatever reason. (Carbon dioxide can also be retrieved from an oesophageal intubation if there has been undue pressure in providing ventilation before intubation as expired gases can be forced into the stomach.)
- The use of pulse oximetry. Although the device samples blood that had been previously in the lungs some 30–60 s earlier and so is an indicator of prior events (it is NOT an early warning system!), it can be useful in determining the position of the tube. A normal steady reading of above 95% is reassuring whereas one that continually displays a steady value between 90 and 92% despite an increase in inspired oxygen concentration is almost certainly a result of endobronchial intubation. A continuously falling oxygen saturation should indicate oesophageal intubation until proven otherwise!
- Confirmation of tracheal placement using a modified Wee's detector. This consists of an angle piece attached at one end to a 50 ml rubber bulb. The other end connects to the endotracheal tube. The rubber bulb is evacuated first, then attached to the tube and then released. If the tube is in the trachea, the bulb will

reinflate from the gas therein. If there is oesophageal placement, the bulb does not reinflate as the oesophagus acts as a flap valve over the end of the tube.
- A recent but novel method of identifying tracheal intubation using a portable, battery powered microphone (Penlon 'Scoti', Fig. 9.46). This, when connected to the endotracheal tube, emits a continuous sound wave to excite the gas just beyond its tip (*sonomatic confirmation of tracheal intubation, 'Scoti'*). It analyses and differentiates between those acoustic properties of gas in the trachea (which is an open tube) with those in the oesophagus (which is a closed tube). Both audible and visual confirmation of placement are displayed on the device.

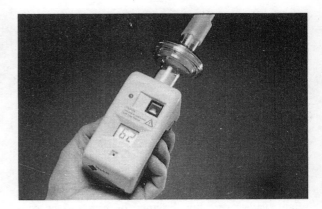

Figure 9.46 Penlon 'Scoti' device.

LARYNGOSCOPES

Visualization of the vocal cords for intubation was popularized by Sir Robert Macintosh and Sir Ivan Magill in the early 1940s. It was during the insertion of a Boyle-Davis gag that Sir Robert conceived the idea of his laryngoscope, which is still the most popular design in use today and has spawned a wide variety of modifications. It consists of a blade that elevates the lower jaw and tongue, a light source near the tip of this blade to illuminate the larynx and a handle to apply suitable leverage to the blade. The handle also contains the power supply (battery) for the light source. This blade is so hinged on the handle that, when opened to the right angle position, the light comes on automatically.

Blades

Macintosh designed a slightly curved blade (Fig. 9.47) with a small bulbous tip that was to be inserted anterior

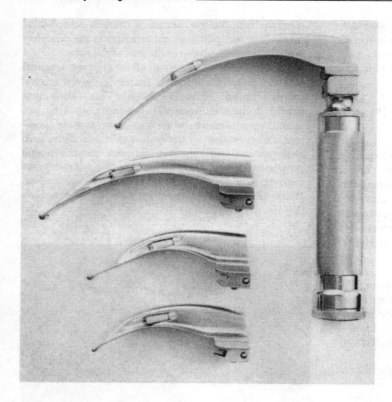

Figure 9.47 The Macintosh laryngoscope with four sizes of hook-on blade.

to the base of the epiglottis in an adult. The child and infant blades were not designed by him and he condemned them as being anatomically wrong and unnecessary. Most blades for infants and children and some of those for adults tend to be either straight or with a shallow curve at the tip only. These are designed to be inserted deeper into the pharynx as well as posterior to the epiglottis and hence the blades are correspondingly longer.

Figure 9.48 shows the wide variety of blades currently available and the choice of blade for routine use is probably largely a matter of personal preference. Most blades are detachable from the handle for ease of cleaning and change of blade size where appropriate. The 'hook on' connection, which allows easy detachment, is very convenient and was developed by Welch Alleyn Ltd in the early 1950s. Although this has become the standard with most manufacturers, there is no agreement to the dimensions of the connection and so blades will rarely fit another manufacturer's handles.

Illumination

The illumination system of the laryngoscope has been greatly improved in recent years, but some points are still worthy of note:

- The bulb may be fitted with a screw thread connection close to the tip of the blade (as in Fig. 9.47), so that when fully inserted into the 'light carrier' (a discrete channel attached to the blade), an electrical contact is made. The light carrier terminates at the base of the blade as a single insulated contact. When the blade is pushed into the handle, the latter connects with the central contact on the handle. This in turn is pushed inwards to make contact with the battery. The handle and blade complete the circuit back to the bulb, which then lights up. The bulbs often appear to 'unscrew' when brushed during cleaning so that when next used they fail. This type should always be checked prior to each use to confirm that the bulb is firmly screwed in.
- The light carriers, if detachable, are not interchangeable with different blades and should be removed and cold sterilized when the blade is autoclaved. The electrical contacts between the handle and the blade mount may need cleaning from time to time with some fine abrasive material or a smooth file.
- When replacing the batteries in the handle, it should be ensured that the spiral spring is still in the base of the battery compartment; leak-proof batteries should be used. (It is most aggravating to find, in an emergency, that not only are the batteries exhausted but they have also corroded within the handle, making replacement impossible.)

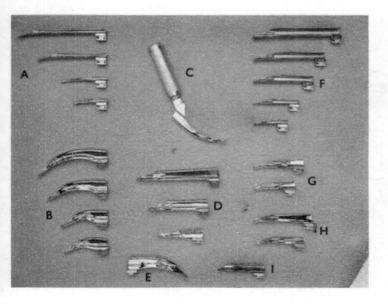

Figure 9.48 Laryngoscope blades. A, Miller pattern: 3, large; 2, adult; 1, infant; 0, premature. B, Macintosh pattern: 4, large; 3, adult; 2, child; 1, baby. C, Macintosh polio blade. D, Soper pattern: adult; child; baby. E, Macintosh pattern left-handed version. F, Wisconsin: large, adult, child, baby, infant. G, Robertshaw's: infant and neonatal. H, Seward: child and baby. I, Oxford: infant.

Recent Advances in Laryngoscope Design

Light Source

Many laryngoscopes are currently produced with the light source sited within the handle and with the light projected to the tip of the blade via a fibreoptic bundle (see below). This bundle may be manufactured as an integral part of the blade (Fig. 9.49), making the blade very easy to clean and sterilize. Alternatively, the fibreoptic bundle may be detachable so that should it become damaged and opaque it may be replaced without having to buy a new blade.

The siting of the light source within the handle increases the reliability of this design over traditional light sources sited on the blade. Rechargeable nickel-cadmium batteries are gaining popularity as the power source for these laryngoscopes.

A brighter light is now possible with the use of xenon gas filled bulbs rather than the conventional tungsten type. However, they require the power from alkaline batteries to work efficiently.

The laryngoscope blade may be cleaned between cases with soap and water, applied using a scrubbing brush, followed by spirit or chlorhexidine swabbing to disinfect it, and should be autoclaved, without the light carrier, as often as circumstances permit.

Laryngoscopy

The larynx, tongue and palate normally form a 'V' shape anatomically, the base of which is the tongue, which hides the larynx from direct view (Fig. 9.50a). Laryngoscope blades are designed to pass behind the tongue and bring it forwards so making the 'V' shape more shallow. Optimal jaw protrusion is achieved with

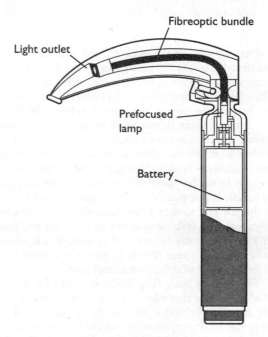

Figure 9.49 The Heine fibreoptic laryngoscope. Note that the lamp is within the handle, thus avoiding unreliable electrical contacts between the handle and the blade.

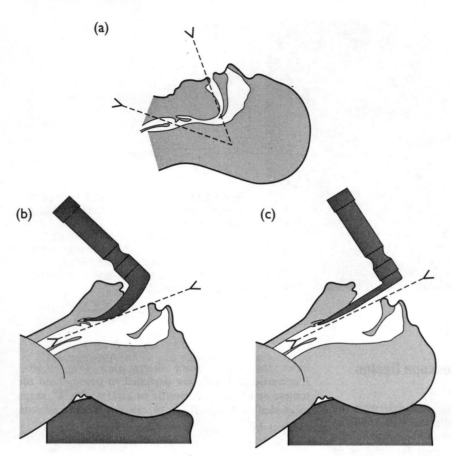

Figure 9.50 (a) The 'V' shape of the normal upper airway. The larynx cannot be seen from outside the mouth. (b) With the neck extended at the upper cervical spine and the jaw protruded forward by the laryngoscope blade, the 'V' extends into a straight line bringing the larynx into view. The curved blade fits between the base of the tongue and the epiglottis. (c) The straight blade passes behind the epiglottis.

the strap muscles of the neck relaxed and the cervical spine flexed. Moving the palate away from the larynx, by extending the upper cervical spine, extends the now shallow 'V' into a straight line and brings the larynx into view. In practice, this is achieved as follows. With the lower cervical spine flexed by suitable support behind the neck and the jaw rotated upwards, the curved blade (Fig. 9.50b) is inserted through the mouth and passed conventionally behind and to the right of the tongue displacing it to the left until the tip reaches the vallecula. The handle is gripped firmly in the operator's left hand and the jaw and tongue lifted away from the posterior pharyngeal wall (taking care not to lever on the front teeth) to expose the larynx and epiglottis. This manoeuvre creates a space that is larger on the right-hand side for insertion of the endotracheal tube.

The straight blade (Fig. 9.50c) is inserted in a similar fashion except that when the epiglottis is exposed the blade is passed behind it so that the tip lies just at the laryngeal inlet. It is particularly useful in an adult with a long and floppy epiglottis. However, it may also be used in a manner similar to the curved blade. Straight blades may also provide a better view in the very young.

Difficult Laryngoscopy and Intubation

Although standard blades for laryngoscopes perform satisfactorily for the majority of cases, there are times when alternative devices may be better. For example, as the extended blade normally forms a right angle with the handle, this may prove difficult to insert in patients with abnormal anatomy, e.g. limited neck extension or large breasts, or who are in unusual situations (e.g. in a cabinet ventilator). Various alternative angles for blades have been produced by modifying the 'hook on' angle (e.g. the polio blade, Fig. 9.51) or by producing a handle with multiple locking positions (the Patil-Syracuse handle, Fig. 9.52).

Left-handed Blades

At least one company (Penlon Ltd) manufactures a Macintosh laryngoscope the blade of which is the mirror image of that to which we are accustomed. The left-handed laryngoscope is not, as sometimes imagined, for use by an anaesthetist who is left-handed, but for patients in whom the nature of the teeth or maxilla make

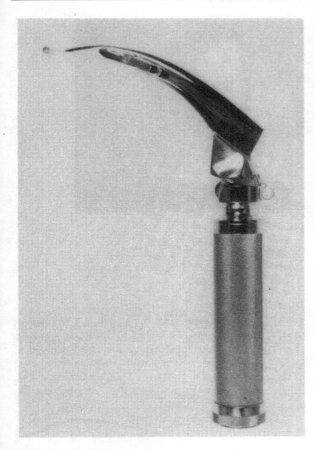

Figure 9.51 The Polio laryngoscope.

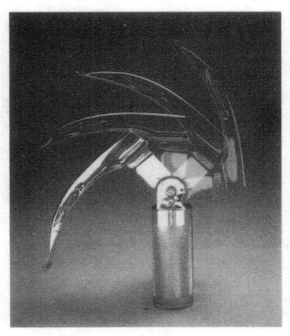

Figure 9.52 Patil-Syracuse handle, which allows multiple locking positions of the attached laryngoscope blade.

it undesirable to exert pressure that might damage a particular area. This may be due to:

- complicated dental restorations;
- loose or ill-positioned teeth;
- the presence of cysts or tumours of the maxilla.

A left-handed laryngoscope should be carefully marked and kept in an appropriate place. Those with no experience will be amazed to find how difficult it is to use it to begin with. It would be wise to obtain some practice with it so that when a difficult case does arise the user will be familiar with it.

McCoy Blade

This is based on a standard Macintosh blade with the addition of an adjustable tip that is operated by a lever on the handle (Fig. 9.53). The blade is inserted in the normal way, and if the view of the larynx is obscured, the tip can be flexed so that it elevates the epiglottis. It allows a

decrease in the force required to bring the larynx into view and moves that point on the blade which acts as a fulcrum further into the pharynx so that inadvertent contact with the upper teeth should be eliminated.

Bullard Laryngoscope

The blades described above are designed to bring part or all of the larynx into direct view by requiring varying degrees of jaw protrusion and upper neck extension. The Bullard laryngoscope has a curved blade (Fig. 9.54a), which is designed to pass behind the tongue and lift it away from the posterior pharyngeal wall but without neck extension. Although this manoeuvre does not make the larynx visible directly, a fibreoptic viewing channel and light source built into the blade allow indirect laryngoscopy to be achieved.

The blade may be passed anterior to the epiglottis as with a Macintosh-type blade or posterior to it as with a straight blade. A wire guide is fitted to the side of the device (which runs parallel to the blade), which is preloaded with a suitable endotracheal tube (Fig. 9.54b). The tip of the guide has a slight bend that can be seen via the fibreoptics if the guide is pressed against the laryngoscope. Following successful laryngoscopy, the tube is passed down the guide and can be seen, via the

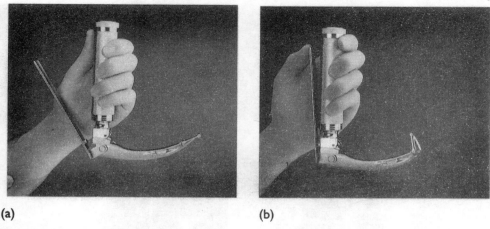

(a)   (b)

Figure 9.53 (a) The McCoy modification of the Macintosh blade; (b) the blade with the tip flexed.

fibreoptics, to enter the larynx. A reinforced tube is ideal for this as it passes more easily down the guide and can be readily rotated if necessary to make intubation easier.

The device is very useful in patients with limited neck movement and/or limited jaw opening. It is important that the fibreoptics at the distal end are pretreated with an anti-fogging solution prior to use so as to obtain the best view.

There is an adult version that may be supplied with an attachable extension for patients with long necks, or a smaller version for paediatric use.

Upsherscope

This has a curved blade (Fig. 9.55a) which is 'C' shaped in cross-section in order to cradle the endotracheal tube (Fig. 9.55b). It also has built in fibreoptic viewing and light carrying channels. As with the Bullard blade, it is designed to elevate the jaw only without extending the neck. The tip has a spatulate shape designed to pass behind the epiglottis in the same manner as a straight blade.

The blade is inserted along the floor of the oropharynx with the head in the neutral position. The depth of insertion is then adjusted so that the tip lies behind the

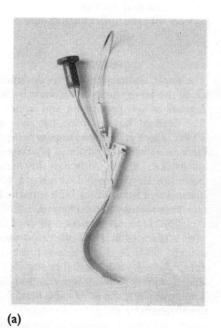

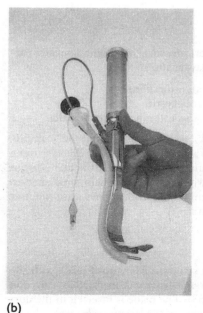

(a)   (b)

Figure 9.54 (a) The Bullard laryngoscope; (b) preloaded with a suitable endotracheal tube.

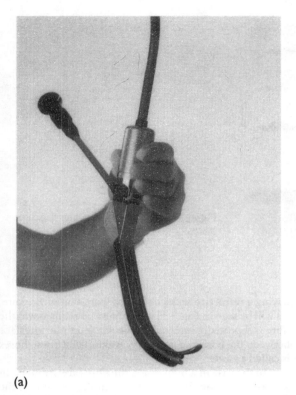 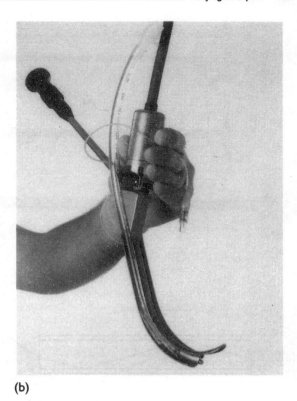

(a)   (b)

Figure 9.55 (a) The Upsherscope; (b) preloaded with a suitable endotracheal tube.

epiglottis and at the glottic opening. The jaw is elevated by lifting the blade forwards and indirect laryngoscopy performed through the eyepiece. The tube may then be advanced under fibreoptic control into the larynx. Reinforced tubes are again the easiest to pass. The blade has the standard 'hook on' attachment and can accept either a handle with a xenon bulb powered by batteries, or one that can be attached to an external light source.

Bronchoscopes

There are simple emergency bronchoscopes that work on the same principles as laryngoscopes. The dimensions are different, however, and a smaller bulb is employed.

It is an advantage to obtain blades that fit the same universal handle as the laryngoscope. They are made in various sizes, a set of three diameters, viz. 11 mm, 8.5 mm and 3.5 mm, being convenient.

Figure 9.56 shows three blades for the Magill emergency bronchoscope, which incorporates a side tube through which oxygen may be blown. By occluding the open end with the finger, the patient's lungs may be inflated with what becomes a type of T-piece system.

Although this may be less convenient for the operator than a jetting device (see Fig. 9.40 above) it should be pointed out that this is an emergency bronchoscope, to be used at times when the latter may not be available. Metal suction tubes or plastic suction catheters may be used for aspiration.

Flexible Fibreoptics

The object of the flexible fibreoptic system is to transmit light from a powerful external light source through an instrument that, being flexible, can be passed through a series of curvatures, and return an image of the area being illuminated to an eyepiece or camera. It may be used for endoscopy by various routes, for example:

- laryngoscopy;
- bronchoscopy;
- oesophagoscopy.

The pathways through which the illumination and the image pass consist of bundles of thousands of very fine glass fibres. Typically these fibres have a diameter of the order of 20 μm. Each consists of a central glass core surrounded by a thin cladding of another type of glass

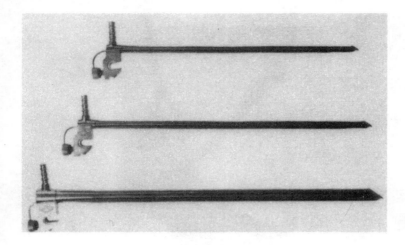

Figure 9.56 Magill emergency bronchoscope blades.

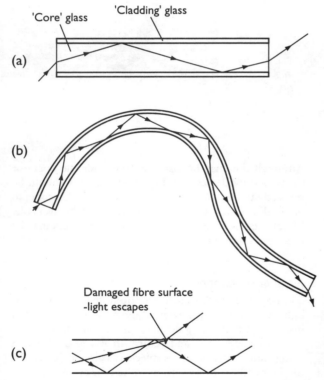

'Core' glass   'Cladding' glass

(a)

(b)

Damaged fibre surface
-light escapes

(c)

Figure 9.57 (a) A single optical fibre. Note that the light ray is repeatedly internally reflected from the interface between the core and cladding glass. (b) If the fibre is curved, the ray is still internally reflected within it. (c) If the surface of the fibre is damaged, the light ray may not be totally internally reflected and some light may escape from the bundle.

having a refractive index different from that of the core. As will be seen in Fig. 9.57 the light ray passing down the fibre is repeatedly internally reflected from the interface between the core and cladding. A bundle of these fibres is called a guide.

In the case of a light guide the fibres are arranged in a random fashion. With the image guide, the ends of the fibres at each end of the bundle are precisely located relative to each other so that each fibre carries the light from one small portion of the image in the same way that many small dots make up the printed representation in a book or newspaper of an original photograph. The fibres are so fine that they are easily flexible and they are lubricated so that they can move relative to each other. The whole bundle may therefore be flexed.

The light source of a fibrescope (Fig. 9.58) is usually powered by the mains electricity supply and uses a lamp very much brighter than that seen at the distal end of a

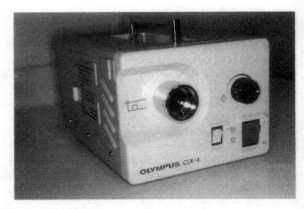

Figure 9.58 A light source for a fibrescope.

laryngoscope. It provides sufficient illumination not only for visualization, but also for the taking of colour photographs with a suitably adapted camera. The trunk of the instrument may carry all of the following:

- an optical bundle (image guide);
- one or two light guides;
- a channel for suction or air insufflation;
- another channel for the passage of instruments such as biopsy forceps.

At the distal end of the optical bundle there is a lens to focus the image from the ends of the fibres; at the proximal end there is an eyepiece with an adjustable focus. The eyepiece mount also carries:

- a connection for the vacuum/insufflation channel;
- a valve to make a seal for the instrument channel.

A fibreoptic laryngoscope is shown in Fig. 9.59.

Care of the Fibrescope

The care of the fibrescope and of its light cables in general is of great importance. The optical bundles, in particular, are extremely expensive to manufacture and are easily damaged. Although they can be flexed into acute angles of relatively small radii, they are easily damaged if they are pinched or knocked, as for example by a towel forceps on the operating table, or by being shut in the lid of the case in which they are transported. The covering over the distal 6 cm or so of the instrument is very delicate, and it is at this point that the greatest flexion takes place. It may well have to be replaced at about yearly intervals, the whole instrument being serviced every 6 months, according to the maker's instructions.

After use, the instrument may be cleaned by wiping it with a solution of aqueous chlorhexidine and then rinsed in water. It can be disinfected between cases with gluteraldehyde (Cidex) or per-acetic acid (Nu-Cidex) based solutions, but it is essential that in older models the eyepiece and head of the instrument are not immersed in the solution, otherwise water may track down between the fibres and damage the lubricant between them. If the trunk is immersed in the sterilizing solution, it should not be hung vertically, since gravity may be sufficient to drive water inside the cable and damage the lubricant as mentioned above. There are specially designed dishes into which the instrument is laid horizontally, with the head supported well above water level. Currently marketed models are now totally immersible and these restrictions do not apply. Although the instrument may be better protected by returning it to its carrying case after sterilization, it is, in fact, better to hang it vertically in a cupboard with the eyepiece at the top, so that any moisture contained may evaporate.

Fibreoptic Laryngoscopes

These instruments are invaluable as an aid to difficult intubation either by the oral or nasotracheal route. There are two versions: the adult version has an external diameter of 4 mm whereas the paediatric one is 2.2 mm. Several techniques involving their use have been advocated, but all of them require regular practice on routine cases before they can be of benefit in an emergency or difficult situation.

Fibreoptic laryngoscopy may be performed on both an awake or asleep patient. Following suitable topical anaesthesia or nerve block, the fibrescope may be inserted through the mouth or nose of an awake patient and advanced behind the tongue and into the larynx. The patient should be encouraged to protrude his or her

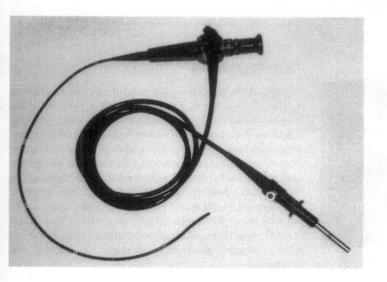

Figure 9.59 A fibreoptic intubating laryngoscope.

lower jaw to create a space in the pharynx, which is almost essential for this technique to succeed. Failure to do this requires that the scope be pushed past the tongue, contact with which often causes misting of the optics. Once in the larynx, the endotracheal tube, which should have been preloaded onto the fibrescope, may then be slid down it and into the larynx.

In an anaesthetized patient, the jaw protrusion can be maintained manually by an assistant or by the insertion of a suitable airway such as the Berman (Fig. 9.60) or alternatively the Ovassapian airway (Fig. 9.61). The large internal bore of the former holds the pharyngeal structures out of the way and also protects the fibrescope tip from pharyngeal secretions. Both have splits in their walls so that the endotracheal tube and fibrescope can be peeled off and the airways removed without disturbing the position of the tube. Where anaesthesia is maintained with an inhalational anaesthetic, endoscopy may be carried out through a mask and angle piece (Fig.

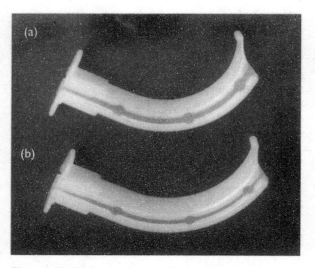

Figure 9.60 The Berman airway in different sizes: (a), 9 mm; (b), 10 mm.

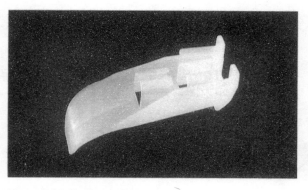

Figure 9.61 The Ovassapian airway.

9.62), which separate to release the fibrescope and endotracheal tube when required.

AIDS TO INTUBATION

Bougies and Stylets

Occasionally at direct laryngoscopy, the larynx may be only partially visualized or hidden behind the epiglottis and beyond reach with the normal curvature of an endotracheal tube. Intubation may then possibly be accomplished by either:

- altering the curvature of the endotracheal tube using a malleable plastic coated metal stylet; or
- initially inserting a long, thin gum-elastic bougie and using this as a guide over which the tube may be passed ('rail-roaded') into the trachea (Fig. 9.63). A bougie and stylet are illustrated in Fig. 9.64. Malleable metal stylets should be plastic-coated so that, in the event of a metal fracture (from repeated bending), part of the stylet will not detach and disappear into the bronchial tree. Most are designated for single use only to prevent such a fracture occurring.

Adjustable and Flexible Guides

Malleable stylets are bent to shape prior to insertion into the pharynx, the curvature being carefully adjusted since it cannot be changed in situ. Also, once in the larynx the curvature, if acute, may not allow easy passage of the tube over it. Guides are available that have an adjustable tip operated by a plunger mechanism (Fig. 9.65). This bends the tube to the correct curve at laryngoscopy and then straightens it at insertion.

Tube Exchangers

Should an endotracheal tube require changing following a difficult intubation, a suitable length of hollow tubing (the exchanger) may be passed down the tube, which is then removed leaving the former in situ. (The exchanger should be long enough to be held at all times during the procedure so that it cannot slip further into the larynx and out of view.) A new endotracheal tube can then be 'railroaded' over it and guided into the trachea. Commercial versions of this are available, such as the Cook Airway Exchanger (Fig. 9.66a), which have adaptors (15 mm ISO and luer connections) (Fig. 9.66b) to allow oxygen insufflation through it during the exchange.

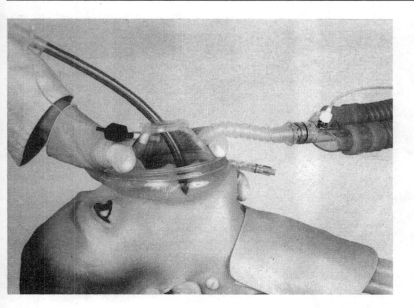

Figure 9.62 A mask and angle piece which separate to release the fibrescope and endotracheal tube when required.

Retrograde Intubation

The larynx may be intubated using the following technique. A cannula is introduced diagonally through the cricothyroid membrane with its tip pointing cephalad. A steel 'J'-tipped guide wire is then passed through the cannula, through the larynx and into the pharynx where it is retrieved and brought out through the mouth. A thick Teflon catheter is passed over the 'J' tip and back along the guide wire and into the larynx. The guide wire is then removed and an endotracheal tube 'railroaded' over the catheter into the larynx. A kit (Fig. 9.67), which includes all the above components, is available.

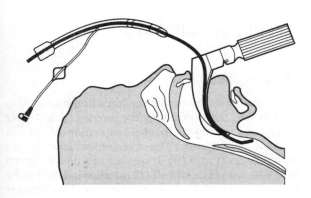

Figure 9.63 The Eschmann endotracheal introducer.

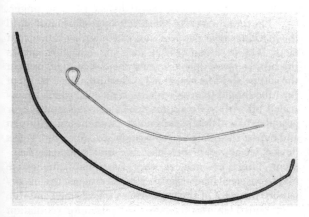

Figure 9.64 A bougie and stylet.

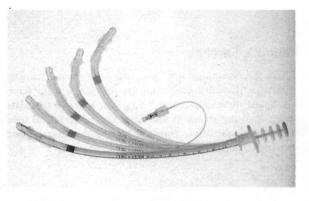

Figure 9.65 A guide with an adjustable tip operated by a plunger mechanism fitted to an endotracheal tube (Rusch).

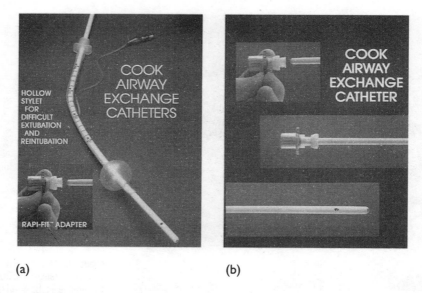

Figure 9.66 (a) The Cook airway exchanger; (b) 15 mm ISO connector.

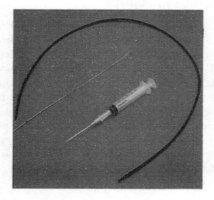

Figure 9.67 The Cook retrograde intubation kit.

Magill's Forceps

These are ergonomically designed forceps, the handles of which fit comfortably into an operator's right hand like a pair of scissors (Fig. 9.68). The tips are spatulate and ridged for gripping the tip of an endotracheal tube so that it can be lifted from the back of the pharynx and into the larynx.

EMERGENCY AIRWAYS

The Combitube

There may be occasions when endotracheal intubation is not possible, but maintaining the patency of the upper airway and preventing tracheal aspiration of foreign material is required. The Combitube meets these requirements (Fig. 9.69). It consists of a double-lumen tube with a small distal cuff (15 ml when inflated) and a large proximal cuff (100 ml when inflated). One lumen is patent throughout whilst the other lumen is sealed at its distal end and has large perforations in that part of its wall between the two cuffs. The two halves are identified by having separate proximal mounts (each fitted with a connector), the one to the sealed distal end being longer.

The tube is inserted blindly through the mouth until the markings near the proximal end align with the front teeth. The proximal cuff is then inflated. This causes the tube to move upwards until the cuff wedges against the soft palate. The lower cuff is then inflated. The tip of the tube should then be in the oesophagus, which is now sealed off. Any refluxed material from the stomach or oesophagus will thus pass through the open-ended lumen and bypass the pharynx. An oesophageal detector (Wee's device, see above) is then used to confirm correct placement. This is essential as, very occasionally, the device may be inserted inadvertently into the trachea. In this situation, the roles of the two lumens are reversed and the open-ended (shorter) lumen will be used for ventilation (functioning as an endotracheal tube).

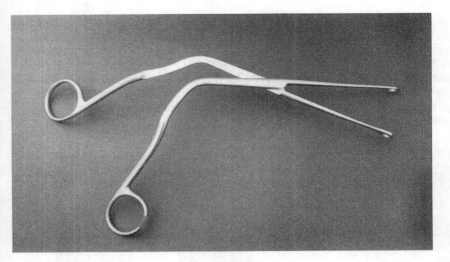

Figure 9.68 Magill's introducing forceps for endotracheal tubes.

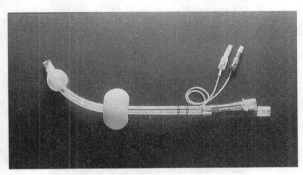

Figure 9.69 The Combitube.

When inserted correctly, the longer lumen may be connected to a breathing system for spontaneous or manual ventilation. Gases pass down this and escape through the perforations between the two cuffs into the pharynx and into the larynx. The seal between the two cuffs is usually so secure that airway pressures up to 4 kPa (40 cm H_2O) can be achieved.

If endotracheal intubation is attempted at any time after insertion, the proximal cuff is deflated, the tube pushed to the left hand side of the mouth and conventional laryngoscopy performed. The oesophageal seal effected by the distal cuff prevents soiling of the pharynx by gastric contents during the procedure.

Cricothyrotomy Devices

Oxygen may be delivered to the trachea by puncturing the cricothyroid membrane either as an emergency procedure, in a 'can't ventilate can't intubate' scenario, or as a planned procedure if this is anticipated.

Some of the devices are similar to intravenous cannulae in that they have a metal cannula sheathed by a plastic catheter. They are inserted through the cricothyroid membrane with a syringe attached. This is aspirated to confirm correct placement in the trachea, the metal cannula withdrawn and the plastic catheter inserted fully. The proximal end of the latter often has a luer lock for connection to a high-pressure gas supply (especially with the narrower gauge ones) as well as a 15 mm ISO

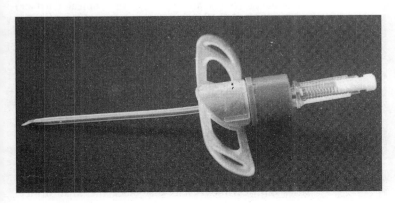

Figure 9.70 A 13-gauge internal diameter cricothyroid cannula.

male connector for attachment to a breathing system. The distal end of the narrow gauge (13 or 14 G) cannula (Fig. 9.70) has small lateral holes in its walls so that when high-pressure gas is used (transtracheal ventilation, Fig. 9.71), some of this escapes via these to produce stabilizing jets which prevent the cannula from 'whipping' inside the trachea. Larger devices are available with an internal diameter of 2 mm for paediatric and 4 mm for adult use (Fig. 9.72).

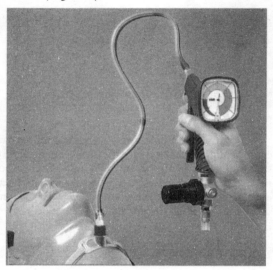

Figure 9.71 Transtracheal ventilation through using high-pressure gas from a manual gas gun (VBM Manujet III).

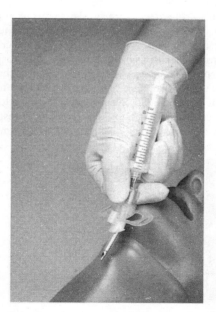

Figure 9.72 A 4 mm internal diameter cricothyrotomy device for adult use (VBM).

Even larger devices (6 mm internal diameter, Fig. 9.73) are available although the method of insertion is different. This type is inserted by firstly establishing correct placement with a small cannula through which a Seldinger wire is passed. The cannula is then removed and a dilator used to widen the aperture so that the airway can be passed easily into the trachea.

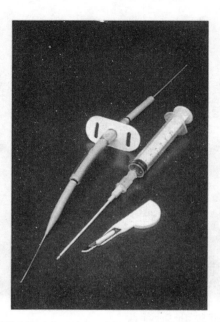

Figure 9.73 A Cook 6 mm internal diameter cricothyrotomy device.

DRUG DELIVERY SYSTEMS

Sprays

Nebulizing sprays are used for the topical (surface) application of local analgesic solutions, such as 4% lignocaine, to the larynx and trachea, and sometimes of vasoconstrictors to the nose. The general principle is the same in all of them: when the air reservoir bulb is compressed, a part of this is blown into the chamber containing the solution of the agent to be used. This forces the latter up and along a narrow-bore delivery tube to the tip of the apparatus. The rest of the air from the bulb is directed to the tip where it mixes with and nebulizes the solution. Figures 9.74 and 9.75 show two popular types.

They tend to block up if they are not cleaned shortly after use, because the solution remaining at the nozzle dries out, leaving crystals that block the small orifice.

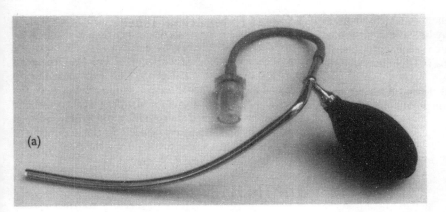

(a)

Figure 9.74 (a) The Forrester spray. (b) Working principles. Note that the diameters of the tubes leading to the nozzles are very small and if analgesic solution is allowed to collect and crystallize out in this area the spray will be blocked. (c) The air inlet valve.

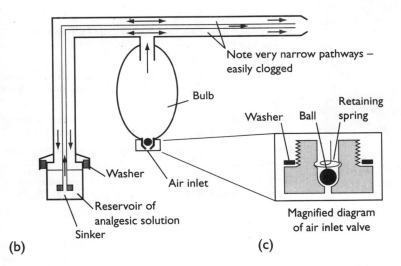

Note very narrow pathways — easily clogged

Bulb

Washer

Air inlet

Washer

Reservoir of analgesic solution

Sinker

Washer Ball Retaining spring

Magnified diagram of air inlet valve

(b)

(c)

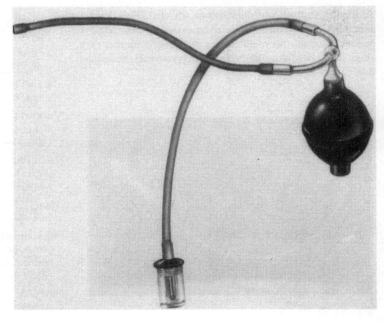

Figure 9.75 The Macintosh spray.

This may be avoided by rinsing them out with distilled water or spirit after use. They may be cleaned after use by any cold sterilizing solution, but a scrub with a brush and soapy water followed by soaking in 70% alcohol for 3 min is considered adequate.

Versions dispensing metered doses of anaesthetic from multi-use bottles but with disposable nozzles are also available (Fig. 9.76).

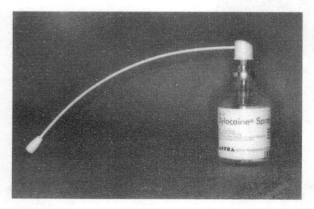

Figure 9.76 A commercial spray (Astra).

Jets

Local anaesthetic solutions may be injected through a preformed, stiff plastic, blind-ended narrow-bore cannula with multiple side holes near the tip. The device, attached to a syringe of local anaesthetic solution, is passed between the vocal cords and into the upper trachea, both of which can then be sprayed with the solution (Fig 9.77).

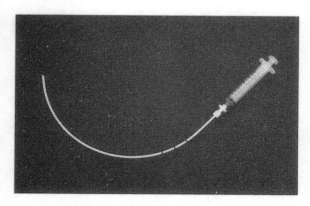

Figure 9.77 The Tracho jet.

Adapted Endotracheal Tubes

An endotracheal tube may have an extra narrow-bore tube fitted to its wall (Local Instillation of Tracheal Analgesia (LITA tube), Sheridan Corp.). This exits near the tip either through the outer wall or within the lumen of the tube. The former is useful for instilling local anaesthetic into the trachea to reduce coughing and hypertension at extubation. The latter may be used for the deposition of drugs such as adrenaline further down the trachea.

FURTHER READING

Bolder PM, Healy TEJ, Bolder AR, Beatty PCW, Kay B (1986) The extra work of breathing through adult endotracheal tubes. *Anesthesia and Analgesia* **65**: 853–859.

Borland L, Casselbrandt M (1990) The Bullard laryngoscope: a new indirect oral laryngoscope. *Anesthesia and Analgesia* **70**: 105–108.

Brain AIJ (1983) The laryngeal mask: a new concept in airway management. *British Journal of Anaesthesia* **55**: 801–804.

Chandler M (1986) Pressure changes in tracheal tube cuffs. *Anaesthesia* **41**: 287–293.

Clark AD (1958) Potential dead space in an anaesthetic mask and connectors. *British Journal of Anaesthesia* **30**: 176–181.

Editorial (1991) The Laryngeal mask airway. *Lancet* **338**: 1046–1047.

Fujiwara M et al. (1995) A new endotracheal tube with a cuff impervious to nitreous oxide: constancy of cuff pressure and volume. *Anesthesia and Analgesia* **81**: 1084–1086.

Jephcott A (1984) The Macintosh laryngoscope. *Anaesthesia* **39**: 474–479.

Leach AB, Alexander CA (1991) The Laryngeal mask – an overview. *European Journal of Anaesthesia* **4**:(suppl) 19–31.

McCoy EP, Mirakhur RK, (1993) The levering laryngoscope. *Anaesthesia* **48**: 516–519.

Murray D, Ward ME, Sear JW (1995) Scoti: a new device for identification of tracheal intubation. *Anaesthesia* **50**: 1062–1064.

Nandi PR, Charlesworth CH, Taylor SJ, Nunn JF, Dore CJ. (1991) Effect of general anaesthesia on the pharynx. *British Journal of Anaesthesia* **66**: 157–162.

Nunn JF (1988) The oesophageal detector device. *Anaesthesia* **43**: 804.

Seegobin RD, van Hasselt GL (1984) Endotracheal cuff pressure and tracheal mucosal blood flow: endoscopic study of effects of four large volume cuffs. *British Medical Journal* **288**: 965.

Sosis M (1990) Hazards of laser surgery. *Seminars in Anaesthesiology* **9**: 90–97.

EQUIPMENT FOR THE INHALATION OF OXYGEN AND OF ENTONOX

Contents

INTRODUCTION

This chapter describes equipment used for two classes of patient who are conscious and breathing, but require assistance by the administration of:

(a) extra oxygen; and
(b) analgesia on a self-administered, and often intermittent, basis the agent being Entonox.

There are two categories of patients who require oxygen therapy:

- The first includes those in whom the oxygen-carrying capacity of their haemoglobin is normal but are hypoxaemic because they have an underventilation or ventilation/perfusion abnormality of the lungs (as most commonly seen in the immediate postoperative period). Depending on the cause and severity, supplemental oxygen from a range of devices delivers oxygen therapy at or just above atmospheric pressure to correct it (*normobaric oxygen therapy*).
- The second includes those in whom either the oxygen-carrying capacity of their haemoglobin is compromised (e.g. carbon monoxide poisoning) or if extra tissue oxygen is required (in severe burns and tissue infections). Here, supplemental oxygen may be delivered by dissolving it, under pressure, in plasma (*hyperbaric oxygen therapy*).

Entonox, a 50:50 mixture of oxygen and nitrous oxide is used in a variety of situations, the commonest being obstetrics and the transportation, usually in an ambulance, of patients in pain.

NORMOBARIC OXYGEN THERAPY

If the hypoxaemia is responsive to supplemental oxygen alone, then a *low dependency system* may be adequate. However, if a patient requires both supplemental oxygen and a continuous positive airway pressure (CPAP) to correct the hypoxaemia, a *medium dependency system* may be selected. If a patient is clearly unable to breathe spontaneously and mechanical ventilation with supplemental oxygen is required, then a *high dependency system* is necessary.

Low Dependency Systems

When supplemental oxygen alone is required to correct hypoxia, it may be delivered by a miscellany of devices. These can be divided into two groups by convention.

Variable Performance Devices

Oxygen is delivered at a predetermined flow (usually between 2 and 12 litres/min) through the device to the patient. As the patient inhales, the oxygen is diluted by ambient air that is entrained in order to match the inspiratory flow. As the flow of the latter varies during the inspiratory cycle and from cycle to cycle, the final inhaled oxygen concentration is both variable and unpredictable. The degree to which this occurs also depends on the design of the device and the flow rate chosen for the oxygen. The different types are described below.

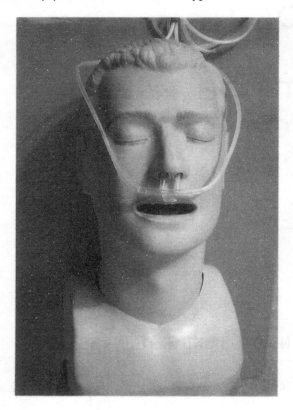

Figure 10.1 A variable performance, no capacity device (nasal prongs).

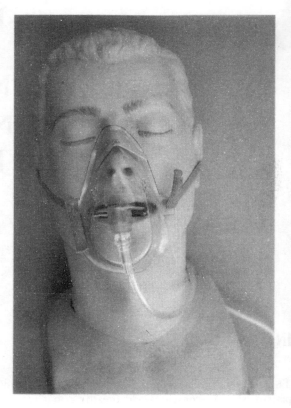

Figure 10.2 A variable performance, small capacity device (facemask).

No capacity systems (Fig.10.1). Here, the oxygen is delivered directly, via a catheter or nasal cannulae (nasal prongs), to the patient's nose or mouth. The oxygen is diluted by inhaled air in the manner described above. Although oxygen enrichment is low, these devices appear to be better tolerated by patients at low flows (up to 2 litres/min) than other devices described below.

Small capacity systems (Fig.10.2). If the flow of oxygen in the above system is increased above 2–3 litres/min, it will displace air in the oro- and nasopharynx (especially if there is an expiratory pause), which creates a reservoir of oxygen that supplements the next breath. This effect is very small. However, the increased flow rate of oxygen can reduce the amount of air subsequently entrained and so enhance the final oxygen concentration inhaled. In addition, the flow (by a flushing effect) can reduce functional dead space by a small amount, but these higher flows are uncomfortable for patients.

More commonly, oxygen can be fed into a small lightweight facemask that is attached loosely to the patient's face. The apparatus dead space collects a small amount of oxygen at the end of expiration that is inhaled

at the beginning of the next breath. The inhaled oxygen concentration drops when the inspiratory rate increases and causes more air to be entrained. The amount of oxygen inhaled will depend on its delivered flow rate and the inspiratory effort of the patient. With the advent of continuous pulse oximetry, the average patient may be managed satisfactorily in the recovery room with this system. The flow of oxygen may be titrated against pulse oximeter readings until adequate oxygenation occurs. It may then be reduced gradually as the patient recovers. The facemask actually increases the functional dead space although this has little effect in the average patient when adequate flows are used.

Large capacity systems (Fig. 10.3). Neither of the systems above stores the oxygen flowing towards the patient during exhalation. It is blown away by the exhaled gases and is wasted. In large capacity systems, this wasted oxygen can be preserved in several ways.

(a) A reservoir bag can be attached to the facemask and the oxygen fed directly into it. The patient inhales oxygen preferentially from the reservoir until it empties and then ambient air from vents in each side of the mask

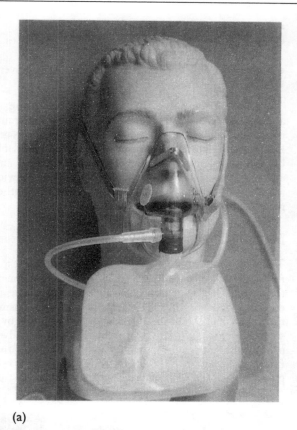 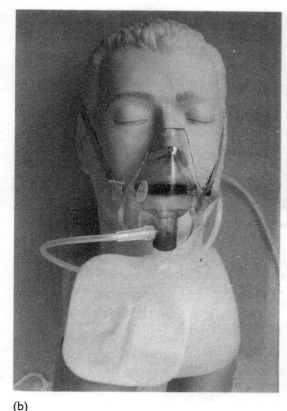

(a)   (b)

Figure 10.3 A variable performance, high capacity device. Facemask and oxygen reservoir (a) fitted with a non-rebreathing valve and (b) without a non-rebreathing valve.

body if necessary. The vents can be fitted with flap valves (on the outside of the mask) that prevent air entrainment and so increase the inspired oxygen. (The flap valves, being on the outside, do not impede exhalation.) The final delivered oxygen concentration of the latter depends upon the ratio of air to oxygen that is finally inhaled. High inspired oxygen concentrations can be achieved with:

- high fresh gas flows of oxygen;
- large reservoir bags;
- the inclusion of flap valves;
- slower respiratory rates (to allow the reservoir to fill);
- smaller tidal volumes.

(b) A one-way valve can be fitted between the reservoir bag and mask to prevent rebreathing. This is important in situations where carbon dioxide accumulation is undesirable (e.g. in patients with head injury). The device may also be valveless, in which case there is some rebreathing. In the latter situation, the exhalate that enters the bag has an oxygen concentration that is only slightly lower than the inspired mixture and may be used to supplement subsequent breaths. This allows some

reduction in the fresh gas flow (in situations where conservation of oxygen may be important).

These types of mask can be used in situations where a high concentration of oxygen is required for a spontaneously breathing patient. It is the recommended mask in the ATLS (Advanced Trauma and Life Support) manual. Where some rebreathing is acceptable and the oxygen supply may be limited, the valveless type may be used, for example, on commercial aircraft for the supply of emergency oxygen in the event of sudden loss of cabin pressure. Table 10.1 shows a range of oxygen concentrations that can be achieved at different oxygen flow rates.

Table 10.1 Approximate values of inspired oxygen concentration (%) delivered by high capacity oxygen masks

Oxygen flow (litres)	No valve	One-way valve
3	50–65	45–60
6	60–75	60–75
9	65–80	65–80
12	70–85	70–85
15	75–90	75–90

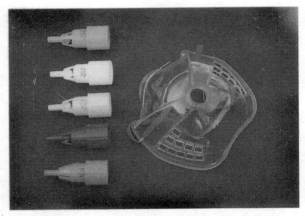

Figure 10.4 A fixed performance device (high volume facemask and venturi injectors for oxygen used to entrain supplemental air). From top to bottom, the injectors supply 60 litres/min of 24% oxygen (at an oxygen flow of 2 litres/min), 28% oxygen (at an oxygen flow of 4 litres/min), 35% oxygen (at an oxygen flow of 8 litres/min), 40% oxygen (at an oxygen flow of 10 litres/min) and 60% oxygen (at an oxygen flow of 15 litres/min).

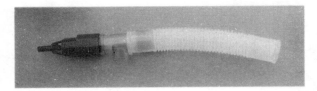

Figure 10.5 A fixed performance device. 'T'-piece fitted with a venturi injector for oxygen used to entrain supplemental air. The injector that is fitted supplies 60 litres/min of 40% oxygen (at an oxygen flow of 10 litres/min).

(c) The oxygen supply may be fed into a tent or incubator. The inspired concentration will depend on the volume of the tent, the flow of oxygen and any leak.

Fixed Performance Devices

Either a special facemask (Fig. 10.4) or a 'T'-piece attachment (Fig. 10.5) that fits a laryngeal mask, endotracheal tube or tracheostomy tube may be fitted with a venturi that is driven by a set flow of oxygen and which entrains a known amount of air into the device. The latter must have an apparatus dead space large enough to ensure even mixing of the air and oxygen so that the concentration of inspired oxygen remains constant. The combined gas flow is also sufficient to match or surpass the peak inspiratory flow of the patient. It is also sufficient to flush away the exhaled gases so that none is subsequently rebreathed. The venturi is available in a range of jets that can supply 24, 28, 35, 40 or 60% inspired oxygen at a total flow of 60 litres/min.

A fixed performance device should be used to deliver supplemental oxygen where the patient:

- is less well supervised (as on a ward);
- has a chronic respiratory pathology that causes a dependency on a hypoxic drive for ventilation;
- requires an objective assessment of his/her recovery (as in an Intensive Care Unit).

It should be noted that a venturi is sensitive to any resistance downstream. This reduces the entrainment and must be accounted for in the design. Furthermore, sufficient space must be made available beyond the venturi to allow mixing of driving and entrained gas. Therefore, a venturi from one device may not function as expected if fitted to another manufacturer's product.

Medium Dependency Systems

There are times when a patient may have a normal respiratory drive but nevertheless requires both supplemental oxygen and a degree of respiratory assistance to correct a hypoxaemic state. In many instances, raising the pressure of the inspired gas above atmospheric by a small amount is sufficient to prevent the collapse of alveoli, in the lung periphery, that may be the main causative factor. The pressure is usually raised throughout the respiratory cycle (CPAP) and is best achieved by a leak-free

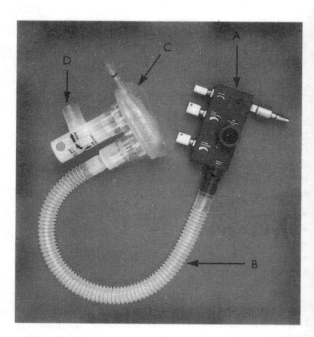

Figure 10.6 A CPAP device. The flow generator (A) plugs into a terminal outlet for oxygen. It has an ON switch, a flow adjustment and an oxygen concentration adjustment. A section of wide-bore tubing (B) connects it to a close-fitting facemask (C) that has two one-way valves in the body of the mask. One is an inlet valve and the other, fitted with a disposable PEEP valve (D), is the outlet valve.

connection between the patient and the device delivering the respirable gases. This may be in the form of a tight-fitting facemask, nasal mask, head box (for infants) or connection to an endotracheal tube or other similar device.

The CPAP delivery system (Fig. 10.6) must be capable of delivering the gases to the patient at, or greater than, the inspiratory flow if the raised pressure is to be maintained. These can be delivered via:

- A ventilator with a patient trigger that responds to respiratory efforts and provides sufficient flow at a preset pressure above atmospheric. The oxygen concentration in the inspired gases can be set at a predetermined level by using *a blender (see below)* to supply the ventilator.
- A breathing system incorporating both a venturi to deliver the high gas flow and a spring-loaded expiratory valve that maintains the raised airways pressure. The size of the venturi and the flow of oxygen can be changed to alter the delivered oxygen concentration.

High Dependency Systems

If a patient is clearly unable to breathe spontaneously, mechanical ventilation using a suitable concentration of inspired oxygen is required. Mechanical ventilators are described in Chapter 12. However, methods of providing them with the ability to vary the inspired oxygen concentration will be discussed here.

Metered Sources of Oxygen and Air

In most hospital environments, oxygen and medical air are provided under pressure to terminal outlets in a treatment area. The supplies can be tapped in two ways.

1. *Flowmeters* may be inserted into the supply terminals for the different gases and their outlets linked with a 'Y'-shaped connection to form a single supply to a ventilator. The concentration of oxygen delivered depends on the ratio of the flows chosen. Nomograms (Fig. 10.7) are available that compute this for different flows (taking into account that air itself contains 21% oxygen). This method is most suitable for minute volume divider ventilators and 'mechanical thumbs'.
2. The terminal outlets for air and oxygen may be connected to *a blender*. This device (Fig. 10.8), proportions the flows of the two gases via a special valve that can be adjusted to deliver a known oxygen concentration. The valve contains two variable restrictors (one for each gas) that are linked so that when the aperture of one is reduced the other increases (Fig. 10.9a). The outputs of the restrictors form a single exit. The two restrictors are operated by a single control knob that is calibrated for delivered oxygen concentration.

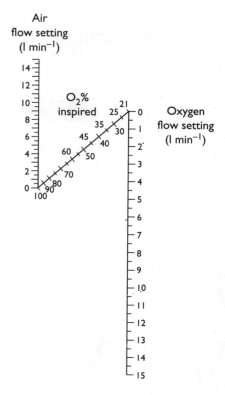

Figure 10.7 A nomogram for air and oxygen mixtures.

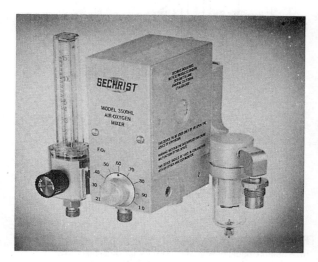

Figure 10.8 An air and oxygen blender.

However, the accuracy of the device depends upon the two gases having the same driving pressure. To ensure this, both gases pass first through a nulling regulator (Fig. 10.9b). This device works by allowing each gas to pass through identical needle valves that are arranged

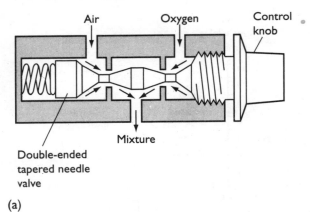

(a)

Air — Oxygen — Control knob

Double-ended tapered needle valve

Mixture

Air 350 kPa (50 psi) — Oxygen 420 kPa (60 psi)

Inlet

Filter

Check valve

Needle valve/ seat

Central diaphragm

Air 330 kPa (49 psi) — Oxygen 330 kPa (49 psi)

(b)

Figure 10.9 (a) The proportioning valve that is part of a gas blender. (b) A nulling regulator which ensures that the different gases, supplying the proportioning valve in a blender, are at the same pressures.

on opposite sides of a central diaphragm. The gas entering at the higher pressure passes through its valve and pushes the diaphragm towards the opposite gas supply. The valve spindle, being attached to the

diaphragm, is pulled through the valve seat and occludes its gas supply, causing the pressure on the diaphragm to drop until it reaches the counter balancing pressure of the other gas. The regulator is able to use the pressure of one gas to control the other, but either gas may be the controlling gas. It will, therefore, reduce whichever gas pressure is the higher to a value equal to the lower gas pressure.

There are two types of blender:

• One type is designed to provide continuous low flows (up to 15 litres/min). Here, the cross-sectional areas of the variable restrictors are suitably graduated for these flows so as to increase the accuracy of the blender.
• The second type has restrictors with greater cross-sectional areas that are designed to work at higher flows (up to 60 litres/min). These can be used where there is a demand for high, but intermittent flow. This design is most suited to supply sophisticated ventilators that may require additional gas if the patient is allowed to breathe in between controlled breaths.

Metered Sources of Oxygen Only

There may be occasions where there is access to a pressurized oxygen source only. In order to deliver air/oxygen mixtures the ventilator or resuscitator must have the facility to entrain supplemental air. There are two methods commonly employed:

1. The oxygen may be passed through a venturi injector that is built into the ventilator. Depending on the driving pressure of the oxygen and the design of the injector, the entrained air plus the oxygen can develop sufficient force that it may be used by the ventilator to ventilate a patient's lungs. The entrainment ratio of the venturi is usually fixed by its design to deliver a predictable oxygen concentration at or around 45–50% across a wide range of tidal volumes. Also, the dilution with air will prolong the duration of ventilation available from a portable cylinder source. This can be an important consideration when transporting a ventilated patient.
2. If the bellows of a ventilator or resuscitator is either mechanically expanded in the expiratory phase or self-filling (a manual resuscitator), it is capable of entraining air. The entrained air can be supplemented by oxygen supplied from a metered source. The oxygen pathway may contain a reservoir which stores that part of the flow that cannot enter the bellows during the inspiratory phase. The final concentration of oxygen in the ventilator bellows is difficult to predict as it depends on:

• the flow rate of the oxygen supply;
• the size of the oxygen reservoir (if present);
• the speed at which the bellows sucks in gas;

- the resistances of the air and oxygen pathways into the bellows.

An oxygen analyser must therefore be placed in the inspiratory pathway of the breathing system to measure the inspired oxygen concentration.

HYPERBARIC OXYGEN THERAPY

If the oxygen-carrying capacity of haemoglobin is compromised (e.g. in carbon monoxide poisoning) or if extra tissue oxygen is required (in severe burns and tissue infections), hyperbaric oxygen therapy may be indicated. This uses the ability of plasma and tissue fluid to accept an increased amount of oxygen that is dissolved under pressure. Normally, 100 ml of plasma in a patient breathing 100% oxygen at atmospheric pressure carries 2 ml of dissolved oxygen. If the inspired pressure of oxygen is raised to 3 atm (absolute pressure), this amount increases to 6 ml. The extra 4 ml per 100 ml in the plasma equates to 40 ml/litre, which, if the cardiac output is 5 litres/min (in an adult), results in an extra 200 ml/min of oxygen delivered to the tissues. This is close to the amount of oxygen used by the tissues per minute at rest.

A single patient chamber for hospital use is shown in Fig. 10.10. A few features of interest to anaesthetists are described below.

- The chamber has multiple antistatic points to prevent any build-up of electrical charge. A spark within the chamber containing 100% oxygen at 300 kPa (absolute pressure) would ignite any combustible material within the chamber and cause an explosion that would certainly kill the patient.

- The chamber temperature and humidity must be closely controlled. Compressing gas to 300 kPa causes its temperature to rise.
- The gas flow through the chamber is sufficient to prevent accumulation of carbon dioxide.
- Some chambers are pressurized with air at 300 kPa (absolute pressure) but allow the patient to breathe 100% oxygen at the same pressure from a breathing system with a close-fitting facemask. This reduces the risk of an explosion.

ENTONOX

The properties of this 50:50 mixture of nitrous oxide and oxygen are described in Chapter 1 (pp. 5–6) and the storing and handling of cylinders in Chapter 3 (pp. 26–27). It is administered with a patient-demand valve and facemask.

'Demand' Valves

Demand valves may be used by the patient for self-administration. Suitable instruction and only general supervision, which may be by a nurse or ambulanceman, is required. Two valves for the delivery of Entonox – a 50:50 mixture of nitrous oxide and oxygen, supplied in cylinders by BOC – will be described.

The BOC Entonox valve

The valve (shown in Fig. 10.11) clamps directly onto a pin-index cylinder. It contains a first-stage regulator and a second-stage demand valve. A sensitive diaphragm,

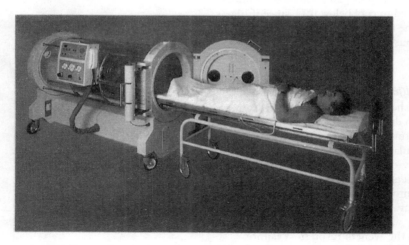

Figure 10.10 A single patient hyperbaric chamber. (Reproduced with permission of HYOX Systems Ltd, Aberdeen, Scotland.)

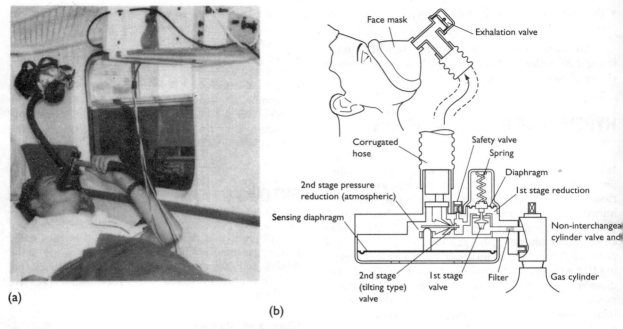

(a)

(b)

Figure 10.11 (a) The Entonox valve, (b) Working principles.

which is deflected by the patient's inspiratory effort, operates a push rod which tilts the valve lever, opening the valve and letting the gases flow. Very little inspiratory effort is required to achieve a high gas flow rate, making this a most efficient demand valve.

Since the nitrous oxide is in the gaseous state in the cylinder of premixed gases, the pressure gauge gives a direct indication of the cylinder contents. When small cylinders are used they may be placed in any position, but large ones should be maintained upright.

As mentioned on page 26, Entonox cylinders should not be allowed to cool below 0°C, since if it gets very much colder the nitrous oxide and oxygen may separate out, with serious consequences.

The Pneupac Analgesia Valve

Although the valve shown in Fig 10.12 also uses Entonox and may be used on demand by the patient, it embraces some additional features to those mentioned above.

A pressure regulator is attached to the cylinder yoke and clamps directly onto the cylinder. A narrow-bore delivery tube connects this to the demand valve which is mounted directly onto the facepiece. Two versions of the demand valve are available, one having a push-button manual override by which the attendant can inflate the lungs of a patient in the event of respiratory failure.

The delivery tube between the regulator and demand valve may be several metres long, and this may facilitate its use in the roadside treatment of accident cases and also allows the cylinder to be kept inside the ambulance so that during cold weather it will not become too cold. The joints at either end of the tube are secure, and this makes disconnection less likely.

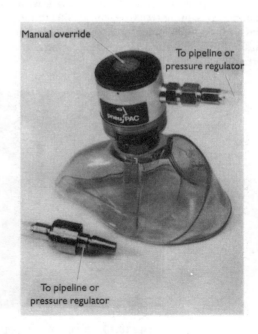

Figure 10.12 The Pneupac analgesia valve.

– 11 –

MANUAL RESUSCITATORS

Contents

INTRODUCTION

There are occasions both in and out of hospital when a patient needs emergency ventilatory support requiring a device that is easily portable and does not rely on a source of pressurized gas or of electricity for its operation. A manual resuscitator fulfils these requirements. The number of different designs available bears testimony to their usefulness. However, they all have three similar components:

- a self-inflating bag;
- a fresh gas input with or without a reservoir;
- a non-rebreathing valve.

COMPONENTS

The Self-inflating Bag

The bag is strengthened either by making its wall thicker, or incorporating circular 'ribs' of identical material during manufacture (Fig. 11.1), or by lining it with thick foam (Fig. 11.2) so that in the resting state it is expanded. The respirable gas inlet mechanism is housed at one end and the non-rebreathing valve at the other.

The Respirable Gas Inlet

The respirable gas inlet (Fig. 11.3) has several components:

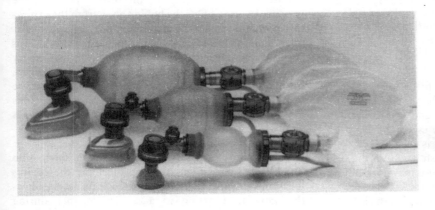

Figure 11.1 The Laerdal system (back to front): adult, child and infant sizes. The versions shown all have oxygen reservoir bags attached. The child and infant versions show the overpressure safety valves fitted.

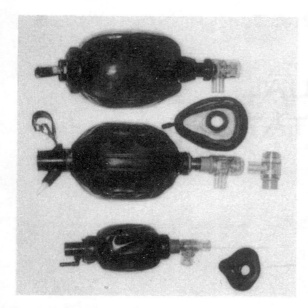

Figure 11.2 The Ambu system (top to bottom): Mark III, Mark II,

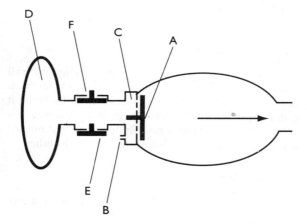

Figure 11.3 The respirable gas inlet of a self-inflating bag showing the wide-bore gas inlet (C), oxygen inlet (B), one-way flap valve (A) and the reservoir (D) with its overpressure valve (E) and entrainment valve (F).

- *A one-way flap valve* (A). This is fitted to the inlet of the self-inflating bag. When the bag is squeezed, the gas pressure inside the bag rises and causes the flap valve to close. This prevents the escape of gas back through the inlet. When the bag is released, its self-inflating characteristic causes fresh gas from the respirable gas inlet to be entrained. This may normally be either air, oxygen or a mixture of both.
- *A small bore nipple* (B). This is mounted on the inlet, to allow the oxygen supply to be attached.

- *A wide-bore gas inlet* (C). This supplies the bulk of the gas entering the bag and is usually air, unless oxygen above is added. In the latter situation the final concentration of oxygen delivered is a function of the added oxygen and its dilution with entrained air.
- *A reservoir system* (D). This inlet may be fitted with a reservoir system that is now widely used in almost all manual resuscitators. Its purpose is to store the oxygen supply that cannot enter the bag whilst it is being compressed but which can supplement the next filling cycle to provide a greater concentration (up to 100%). The reservoir may take the form of an elongated wide-bore hose (popular in paediatric and infant resuscitators) or it may be a large-capacity bag (see Fig. 11.1). The latter must be fitted with an overflow valve (E) to prevent overfilling from too high a flow of oxygen and an entrainment valve (F) to allow ingress of air should the bag collapse as a result of under filling. Tables 11.1 and 11.2 show typical oxygen concentrations that are delivered under a variety of conditions with two popular makes of resuscitator. The differences reflect the size of the relevant reservoirs used.

The Non-rebreathing Valve

This is housed at the opposite end of the bag to the gas entrainment system described above. It has several components which ensure that during the inspiratory phase gas flows out of the bag and only into the patient port. When the patient exhales, the valve also ensures that this exhaled gas escapes through the expiratory port without mixing with the fresh gas stored in the bag. Functionally, most non-rebreathing valves are similar, although there are some differences in their efficiency and their tendency to jam (see below).

The Ruben Valve

The Ruben valve (Fig. 11.4) has a spring-loaded bobbin within the valve housing. In the resting position, the very weak spring holds the bobbin away from the expiratory port and against the inspiratory port, allowing relatively unhindered exhalation via the patient port. This prevents any exhaled gases from mixing with inspiratory gas in the self-inflating bag. When the bag is squeezed, the bobbin is forced across the valve housing, so that the inspiratory port is connected to the patient port. This movement also occludes the expiratory port and allows inspiratory gas to enter the patient's lungs without leaking out through the expiratory pathway.

The differential resistance of the inspiratory limb (0.7 kPa/0.8 cmH$_2$O at 25 litres/min) and the expiratory limb (0.98 kPa/1 cmH$_2$O at 25 litres/min) allows the valve to function in a similar manner during spontaneous ventilation. In this situation the patient

Table 11.1 Oxygen concentrations (%) in a Laerdal resuscitator (with and without the reservoir bag)

Adult: Ventilation bag volume 1600 ml; reservoir bag volume 2600 ml

O_2 flow (litres/min)	Tidal vol. (ml) × bag cycling rate per min					
	500 × 12	**500 × 24**	**750 × 12**	**750 × 24**	**1000 × 12**	**1000 × 24**
3	56 (37)*	39 (32)	47 (33)	34 (29)	41 (32)	30 (28)
5	81 (52)	52 (38)	62 (41)	42 (33)	52 (39)	38 (31)
10	100 (73)	84 (48)	100 (56)	65 (42)	84 (55)	53 (39)
12	100 (84)	97 (53)	100 (61)	74 (45)	94 (60)	59 (42)
15	100 (89)	100 (59)	100 (69)	86 (48)	100 (69)	66 (44)

* Data are O_2 concentrations using reservoir (without reservoir).

Child: Ventilation bag volume 500 ml; reservoir bag volume 2600 ml

O_2 flow (litres/min)	Tidal vol. (ml) × bag cycling rate per min			
	250 × 20		**100 × 30**	
	w/reservoir	wo/reservoir	w/reservoir	wo/reservoir
10	100	75	100	90

Infant: Ventilation bag volume 240 ml; reservoir bag volume 600 ml

O_2 flow (litres/min)	Tidal vol. (ml) × bag cycling rate per min			
	40 × 30		**20 × 40**	
	w/reservoir	wo/reservoir	w/reservoir	wo/reservoir
4	98	89	98	98

Table 11.2 Oxygen concentrations (%) in the Ambu system with reservoir

O_2 flow (litres/min)	Ventilation volume (ml) × frequency			
	250 × 12	**600 × 12**	**750 × 12**	**1000 × 12**
2	74	43	38	34
5	100	76	65	54
10	100	100	100	87
15	100	100	100	100

preferentially draws gas from the inspiratory limb, thus forcing the bobbin to move and occlude the expiratory port. This valve has a tendency to jam in the inspiratory position if high upstream gas pressures are allowed to develop and can result in lung overinflation. For example, if the valve is used to replace the APL valve in a Mapleson A system during spontaneous ventilation, and the reservoir bag is allowed to overdistend, the valve will jam. In this situation an open APL valve upstream of the Ruben valve should always be fitted so as to provide a pressure relief facility if required.

Ambu Series of Valves

The Ambu 'E' valve (Fig. 11.5). In this system, the unidirectional flow of gas is controlled by two labial flap valves:

- The upstream valve 'A', in the resting position, seals the inspiratory port but leaves the pathway into the expiratory port 'B' open, so that relatively unimpeded expiration can occur. During controlled ventilation the valve 'A' is forced open and seals port 'B' so that inspiratory gas enters only the patient port.
- The labial valve 'D' is included to prevent the inhalation of downstream gas should the Ambu valve be used during spontaneous ventilation. This downstream gas may be air when the valve is used as a resuscitator but it

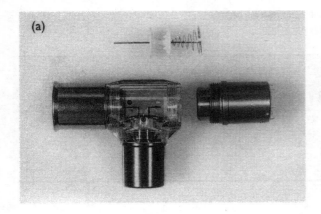

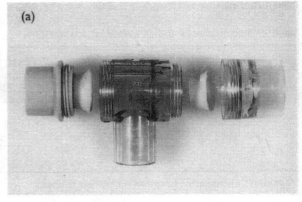

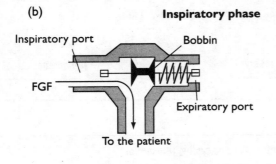

Inspiratory phase

Inspiratory port

Bobbin

FGF

Expiratory port

To the patient

Expiratory phase

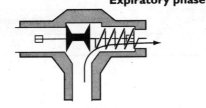

Figure 11.4 (a) The Ruben valve. (b) Working principles: (top) in the inspiratory phase the bobbin occludes the expiratory port; (bottom) during exhalation the spring causes the bobbin to occlude the inspiratory port.

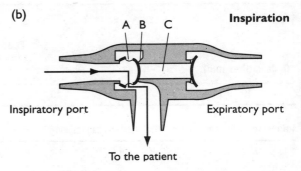

Inspiration

A B C

Inspiratory port

Expiratory port

To the patient

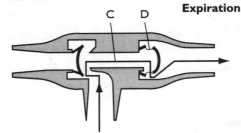

Expiration

C D

To the patient

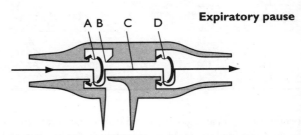

Expiratory pause

A B C D

could be exhaled gas if used in a circle breathing system.

When this Ambu E valve is used for controlled ventilation, a high initial surge of gas is required to produce sufficient movement in valve 'A' to effect a complete expiratory seal. This model is relatively inefficient at lower inspiratory gas flow rates, and in this situation the seal may be incomplete allowing some of the inspiratory gas to pass straight across the valve. This results in lower than expected tidal volumes. In fact, it is possible to occlude totally the patient port and gently squeeze the contents of the self-inflating bag out through the valve!

Figure 11.5 (a) The Ambu E valve. (b) Working principles. (Top) During assisted inspiration. Note that the port B is closed by the pressure of the head of the 'mushroom' valve A. (Centre) During expiration. (Bottom) During the expiratory pause, excess gases may pass straight through the valve, so preventing excessive build-up of pressure. A, upstream (inspiratory) valve; B, expiratory port; C, expiratory pathway; D; downstream (expiratory) valve.

This relative inefficiency greatly decreases the potential for valve jamming. For instance, if any high gas pressures were to begin to develop upstream, excess gas would be dumped across the valve. Because of this the Ambu E valve *should not be used* with automatic resuscitators that do not produce the initial high surge of gas required to produce an effective seal.

The Ambu E2 valve (Fig. 11.6). This model contains only the main labial valve (A) seen in the E valve. Hence it functions in a similar fashion when used with controlled ventilation, but behaves differently if used with spontaneous respiration. In this situation the absence of the downstream valve allows the patient to breathe ambient air via the expiratory port and not the gas mixture from the self-inflating bag.

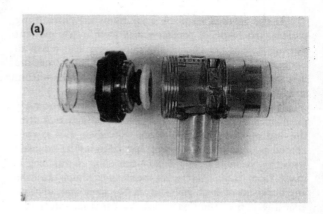

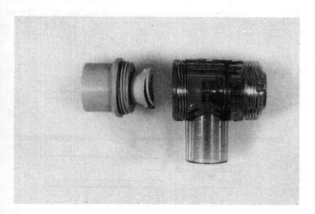

Figure 11.6 The Ambu E2 valve.

The Ambu Mark III valve (Fig. 11.7). This valve overcomes the potential problem of leakage across the E valve at low flow rates. The valve mechanism has three components: an inspiratory leaf valve, an expiratory leaf valve and a mushroom valve.

When this valve is used for controlled ventilation, a very small increase in pressure within the self-inflating bag, due to manual compression, expands the elastic mushroom valve, which then totally occludes the expiratory port, providing a complete seal. Further compression of the bag opens the inspiratory leaf valve, forcing gas from the bag into the inspiratory port, thus providing an inspiratory flow.

At the beginning of the exhalation phase, the self-inflating bag starts to re-expand. The reduced pressure within causes the mushroom valve to collapse and the inspiratory leaf valve to close, sealing the bag off from the main valve. The exhaled patient gas then leaves the system through the expiratory port via the expiratory leaf valve.

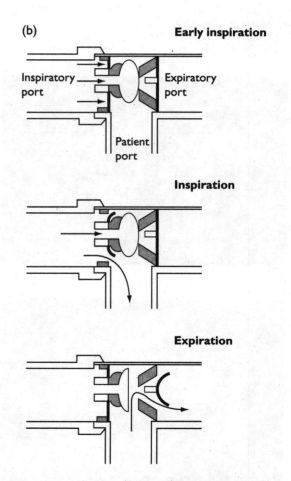

Figure 11.7 (a) Ambu Mark III valve. (b) Working principles. (Top) Very early in inspiration, inspiratory gas causes the mushroom valve to balloon out and occlude the expiratory port. (Centre) Shortly afterwards, the inspiratory valve opens to allow inspiratory gas to enter the patient port. (Bottom) Expiratory phase, the mushroom valve retracts to its resting position and allows exhalation to occur.

If the valve is used on a spontaneously breathing patient, the negative pressure produced by the patient during inspiration causes the expiratory leaf valve to close, sealing the expiratory port. This ensures that the inspired gas is drawn from the bag contents and not from ambient air through the expiratory port.

This type of valve could jam in the inspiratory position if high upstream gas pressures persisted after the end of an inspiratory phase. However, this is prevented by a new self-inflating bag designed to be used with this valve. The gas-tight outer skin of this bag is made from thin, distensible neoprene, which absorbs any build-up of high pressure in the same way that an anaesthetic breathing bag does. As a further safety feature, the diameter of the inspiratory port of this valve (24 mm) prevents this valve being used with other breathing systems. It also prevents misassembly with other self-inflating bags.

The Ambu single shutter valve (Fig. 11.8). This valve has been simplified by ingenious design to incorporate a single, multifunction shutter. When this valve is used for controlled ventilation, manual compression of the new self-inflating bag pushes gas against the concave aspect of the shutter causing it to move and occlude the expiratory port. The same movement opens the patient port to allow ingress of the gas. At the beginning of the exhalation phase, exhaled gas impinges on the convex aspect of the shutter causing it to move in the opposite direction, so that it opens the expiratory pathway as well as occluding the inspiratory port.

With spontaneous respiration, because inspiratory resistance (0.7 mbar at 10 litres/min) through the valve is less than expiratory resistance (0.8 mbar at 10 litres/min), gas is drawn preferentially from the bag. Initial movement of gas also causes the shutter valve to

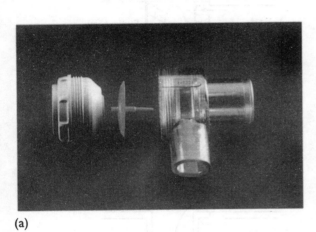

(a)

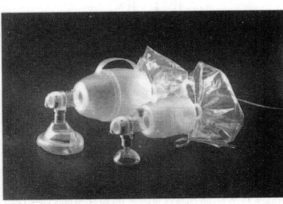

(b)

Inspiration

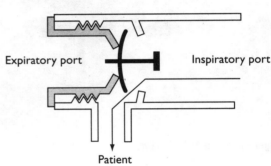

Expiratory port   Inspiratory port

Patient

Expiration

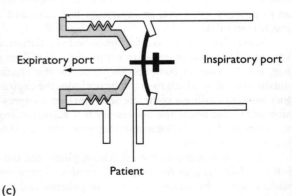

Expiratory port   Inspiratory port

Patient

(c)

Figure 11.8 (a) Ambu single-shutter valve. (b) A SPUR system (Single Patient Use Resuscitator) based on the valve. (c) Working principles. (Top) The valve is pushed onto the expiratory port and occludes it so that gas can enter only the patient port. (Bottom) Exhaled gas pushes the valve against the inspiratory port, occluding it so that the gas can escape only through the expiratory port.

occlude the expiratory path so that the valve behaves in a similar manner to controlled ventilation.

The guide stem of the shutter is clearly visible through the transparent valve body and its 'to and fro' movement is an indicator of correct function.

The self-inflating bag supplied with this valve is made from silicone rubber and the gas inlet is fitted with the two pressure relief valves described above.

The Laerdal valve (Fig. 11.9). This high efficiency non-rebreathing valve is made in three sizes (adult, child, infant). The valve itself has three components: a duck-billed inspiratory/expiratory valve, a valve body housing inspiratory and expiratory ports, and a non-return flap valve sited in the expiratory port. It operates as follows:

- *Inspiratory phase.* The central duck-billed portion of the main valve opens when the attached self-inflating bag is squeezed, or when a patient inhales through it. Almost simultaneously the outer disc-shaped portion of the valve is pushed against the apertures in the valve body, thus sealing the expiratory pathway.
- *Expiratory phase.* Positive expiratory pressure from the elastic recoil of the patient's lungs causes the duck-billed section of the valve to close thus preventing rebreathing into the bag. It also lifts the outer disc-shaped portion off the expiratory apertures, allowing exhaled gas to escape. Escaping gas also lifts the flaps on the non-return valve in the expiratory port. This is a supplementary valve that prevents air from being aspirated into the expiratory port during spontaneous respiration. The valve is constructed of autoclavable materials and is made in three sizes. All the sizes have a 23 mm external diameter expiratory port and a 22 mm external diameter/15 mm internal diameter inspiratory port so as to minimize the possibility of misconnection. The child and infant models have overpressure safety valves built into the inspiratory port of the valve and which are set to blow off at a pressure of 45 cmH$_2$O. If these pressures ever need to be exceeded, the safety valve can be overridden by finger pressure or a lock clip over the valve.

The self-inflating bag supplied with Laerdal resuscitators has thickened ribs of silicone rubber that provide the rigidity for the self-inflating action. These bags can be supplied with a supplementary reservoir bag (larger than that for the Ambu) for the supply of high oxygen concentrations to patients (see Table 11.1). The reservoir bags are fitted with a double valve (for air entrainment and relief of high pressure) to ensure adequate but not excessive gas pressures in the system.

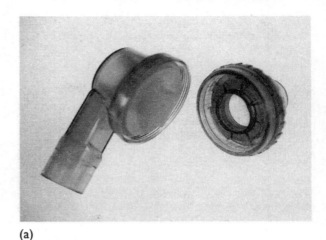

(a)

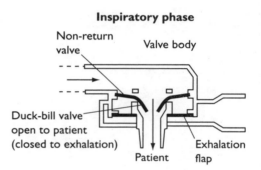

Inspiratory phase

Non-return valve

Valve body

Duck-bill valve open to patient (closed to exhalation)

Patient

Exhalation flap

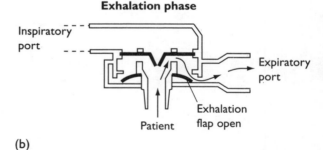

Exhalation phase

Inspiratory port

Expiratory port

Exhalation flap open

Patient

(b)

Figure 11.9 (a) The Laerdal valve; (b) working principles.

OTHER USES FOR MANUAL RESUSCITATORS

Most of the devices described above can be used with draw-over anaesthetic equipment to provide controlled ventilation when required. An example of such a system is described more fully in Chapter 30.

AUTOMATIC VENTILATORS

Contents

INTRODUCTION

In order to inflate a patient's lungs adequately with a mechanical ventilator, sufficient pressure must be generated in the respirable gas within a ventilator or resuscitator (*positive pressure ventilation*) to overcome the elastic properties of the lungs (their compliance) and the resistive properties of the airways (their resistance). Compliance and resistance may be normal in healthy patients, requiring the generation of modest (low) pressures for inflation, or may be grossly abnormal in disease, requiring the generation of much higher pressures to overcome them in order to provide the same degree of ventilation. Furthermore, some surgical procedures may make it more difficult to inflate the lungs, e.g. by restricting the movement of the diaphragm, due to posture or internal intervention. An additional factor during anaesthesia is the resistance of the artificial part of the airway, which may increase accidentally, e.g. by mucus accumulation or kinking of the endotracheal tube.

A patient's lungs may also be inflated by using 'negative pressure'. The patient's body (from the neck downwards), or thorax only, is encased in a gas-tight container to which an intermittent subatmospheric pressure is applied. The thorax is 'sucked outwards' causing air/respirable gas to enter the lungs (*negative pressure ventilation*). Exhalation is achieved passively as a result of the elastic recoil of the latter.

POSITIVE PRESSURE VENTILATORS

Methods of Pressure Generation

Respirable gas may develop sufficient pressure either:

- by being compressed in a ventilator bellows or bag. The bellows may be compressed *mechanically* by attaching it to a spring, a weight, a gas-powered piston, or via a cam or gear chain to an electric motor. It may also be compressed *pneumatically* by placing the bellows in a gas-tight canister into which a separate pressurized gas source is fed or;
- by the adaptation of a suitable source of gas that is already pressurized (cylinder or pipeline supply). If the source is able to supply the high flows required for ventilation, it may be fed directly into a ventilator to be divided up into suitable tidal volumes. If not, lower flows can be used to distend a reinforced rubber reservoir bag with the gas and allowing the elastic recoil properties of the bag to provide the suitable driving pressure and gas flow.

The pressure created within the bellows may be constant, as produced by a weight placed on top of it, or variable when produced by some of the other methods. Distensible bags, and bellows attached to springs, produce pressures that steadily decline as the contents are released, whereas those attached to, say, an electric motor that progressively compresses the bellows produce pressures that gradually increase as the bellows is compressed.

Ventilator designs fall into two categories: those developing modest pressures suitable only for relatively normal lungs (*low-powered ventilators*) and those developing higher pressures that can cope with both normal and abnormal lungs (*high-powered ventilators*).

Classification of Ventilators According to their Power

Low-Powered Ventilators

Low-powered ventilators (Fig. 12.1a) generate only the modest gas pressures required to deliver reasonable tidal volumes to lungs with normal and near-normal compliances and resistances. These pressures are often insufficient to overcome the increase in airways resistance and reduction in lung compliance that are seen in diseased lungs. As a result of this, the tidal volume delivered may well be less than the volume anticipated. Their use is therefore limited. When these ventilators are used, the need to monitor lung ventilation must be emphasized. Either expired minute volume or capnometry can be used to check that ventilation remains satisfactory throughout a procedure. However, these ventilators are simpler and more cheaply constructed and are also less likely to cause lung damage than those generating high pressures.

High-Powered Ventilators

In order to prevent a reduction in ventilator performance in the presence of deteriorating lung conditions, a ventilator needs to be powerful enough to develop a sufficiently high gas pressure in order to overcome most of the increases in airways resistance and reduction in compliance with little alteration in desired gas flow, but without producing lung damage. These ventilators are more costly to produce and require the addition of certain safety features to protect patients with both normal and abnormal lungs from excessive pressures. For example, a safety valve is always included in the gas pathway to the patient to release any build-up of potentially dangerous pressures that might damage the lungs. Figure 12.1b shows an example of a typical high-powered ventilator. The pressure-relief valve can either be preset (usually at 4.4 kPa/ 45 cmH$_2$O) or, in more sophisticated machines, can be adjustable (up to 7.8 kPa/80 cmH$_2$O) to cope with severe conditions such as asthma and adult respiratory distress syndrome. The higher the preset safety limit, the narrower becomes the safety margin between safe ventilation and barotrauma.

Those high-powered ventilators that always generate high gas pressure in the ventilator system prior to its delivery (by using powerful springs, heavy weights or a

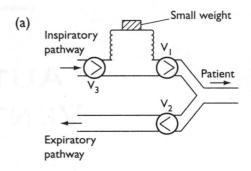

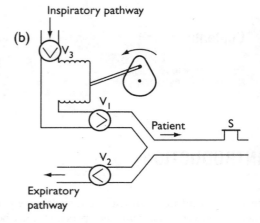

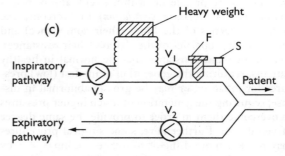

Figure 12.1 (a) Low-powered ventilator generating constant low pressure. (b) High-powered ventilator generating an increasing pressure. (c) High-powered ventilator generating a constant high pressure, V$_1$, inspiratory valve; V$_2$, expiratory valve; V$_3$, non-return valve; F, flow restrictor; S, overpressure relief valve.

pipeline gas source) (Fig. 12.1c) require the fitment of a further safety device, a flow restrictor, in the inspiratory pathway. This reduces the flow to the patient and prevents too rapid a build-up of pressure in the lung.

Alternative Classifications

A popular classification with British anaesthetists has been described by Mushin. Those ventilators that by their design produce only a sufficient pressure to ventilate normal or mildly abnormal lungs are classified as *pressure generators*, i.e. the tidal volume delivered to the patient is limited by the pressure generation. Those ventilators that develop sufficiently high pressures to deliver a desired flow even to grossly abnormal lungs are deemed *flow generators*.

However, as most other electromechanical devices in common usage are described in terms of *power*, the authors prefer the first classification.

Efficiency of Ventilators

This may be defined as the ratio of the intended tidal volume (as determined by the settings on the ventilator) over the actual delivered tidal volume. For example, when a ventilator acts on a bellows containing patient gas at atmospheric pressure, the gas undergoes a degree of compression in order to raise the pressure sufficiently to provide an inspiratory flow. Part of the bellows travel is taken up in compressing the gas. If the bellows travel is calibrated for delivered tidal volume, it becomes apparent that the amount actually delivered is less than that indicated on the calibration scale. The greater the pressure required to ventilate a patient's lungs, the greater will be the amount of gas lost in compression. This type of ventilator is regarded as relatively inefficient, as the discrepancy between anticipated and delivered tidal volumes may be as great as 25% in patients with significant pathological lung conditions. Furthermore, the effective inspiratory time is shortened as, initially, time is wasted in compressing the gas to the required pressure.

More efficient ventilators store respiratory gas under a pressure greater than that required to ventilate a patient's lungs, so that the gas is already compressed prior to being released and, therefore, none is lost in a 'compression volume'. This concept is important to grasp, as there may be a marked difference in the anticipated performance of ventilators. Inefficient ventilators (which include most anaesthetic ventilators that supply circle systems) may well require validation of the delivered tidal volume, using a spirometer or capnograph. However, once recognized, any reduction in delivered tidal volume can be anticipated and corrected, provided that these ventilators are still of the high-powered variety.

Some more sophisticated ventilators are designed to receive information from a spirometer in the breathing system and automatically compensate for any discrepancy between the intended and delivered volumes.

Inspiratory Characteristics of Ventilators

Ventilators may produce a variety of pressure waveforms and inspiratory flow characteristics, depending on the method of generation of gas pressure and the resistance to flow that the gas meets during delivery of the intended tidal volume.

Low-Powered Ventilators

Low-powered ventilators (Fig. 12.2) normally generate their power from gas stored under modest pressure in a bellows or distensible bag. Those ventilators exerting a constant gas pressure (weighted bellows) on the patient airway will have an inspiratory flow rate of gas that is greatest in early inspiration, when the pressure differential between the ventilator and the lung is wide, but that slows during expansion of the lung as the pressures approximate (Fig. 12.2(a)). Similar flow patterns will be seen with those ventilators exerting a gradually declining pressure (by storing gas in a distensible bag and the bellows attached to a weak spring) (Fig. 12.2 (b)).

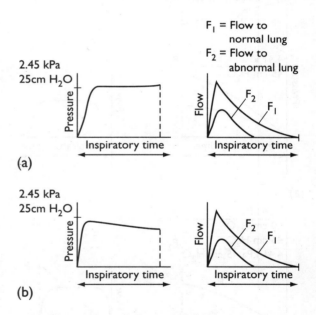

Figure 12.2 Inspiratory characteristics of low-powered ventilators. (a) Constant pressure (weighted bellows); (b) variable (declining) pressure (i.e. bellows attached to a weak spring).

High-Powered Ventilators

High-powered ventilators (Fig. 12.3) that function by creating a constant high pressure of gas (e.g. bellows compressed by a heavy weight), or by using a high pressure gas source, do not directly exert these pressures at the patient airway, as this would be potentially very dangerous. The presence of an obligatory flow restrictor proximal to the patient (see above) determines both the pressure waveform, and the flow waveform of gas leaving the ventilator. A fixed performance flow restrictor produces a constant flow of gas through its orifice, resulting in a gradual pressure rise downstream of the device sufficient to deliver the preset tidal volume. As the lungs expand, the pressure rise that occurs within them is insufficient to alter the flow from the ventilator, which remains virtually constant (Fig. 12.3(a)).

Some high-powered ventilators generating a constant high pressure have flow restrictor apertures that can be varied electronically (Servo ventilators, see below) and so are able to respond to user-programmed inspiratory flow patterns (constant or increasing flows) (Fig. 12.3(b)).

Ventilators can be designed to allow their bellows to be gradually compressed either mechanically, via a linkage from a power source (Fig. 12.3(c)), or pneumatically,

by placing the bellows in a gas-tight container into which a pressurized gas source is fed (bag-in-bottle arrangement, Fig. 12.3(d)). The bellows in this type of ventilator normally fills with gas at near atmospheric pressures, so that when it is compressed, the pressure developed rises as it overcomes the resistive properties of the lungs. The resultant pressure waveforms can be sine wave (from a crank driven electric motor) or ramp shaped (from any linear power source, e.g. gas piston). In either type the delivery of the intended tidal volume is assured owing to the power developed by the ventilator (unless the pressure relief valve opens). More sophisticated ventilators provide an alarm signal if this occurs. The flow waveform produced depends in turn on the method of pressure generation.

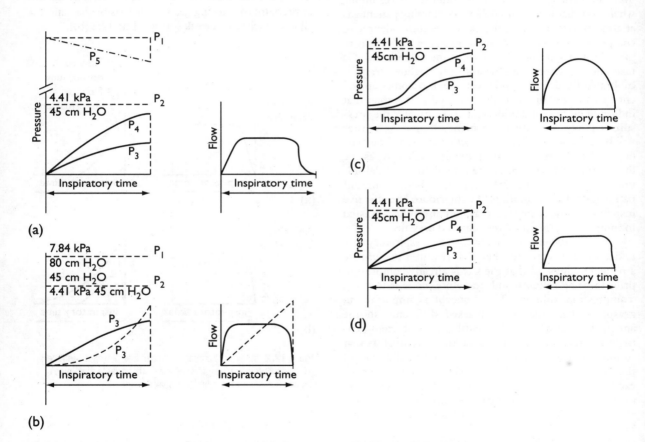

Figure 12.3 Inspiratory characteristics of high-powered ventilators. (a) Constant high-pressure generation (P_1) well in excess of that required to ventilate abnormal lungs (heavyweight pipeline gas supply) with fixed-performance flow restrictor. High-pressure generation produced by a bellows compressed by powerful springs provides a gradually declining pressure as the bellows empties (P_5 above). However, this is insufficient to affect the performance of the ventilator which develops pressures and flows as if it were constant high-pressure generation. (b) Constant high-pressure generation using a varying orifice flow-restrictor (electronically controlled to provide different inspiratory flow patterns from the same ventilator). (c) Increasing high-pressure generation (no flow restrictor required) bellows compressed by a sinusoidally applied power source (i.e. electric motor driving a crank). (d) Increasing pressure generation (no flow restrictor required) bellows compressed by a linear power source (i.e. bag in bottle). P_1, high constant pressure generated; P_2, safety valve release pressure; P_3, pressure rise downstream of restrictor as a result of flow to normal lungs; P_4 as above but to abnormal lungs; P_5, gradually declining high pressure.

Great store has been placed on the ability of different flow waveforms to increase ventilatory efficiency in various clinical situations. However, in anaesthetic practice the claimed advantages are less demonstrable.

Classification of Ventilators According to Cycling

Intermittent automatic ventilation of the lungs consists of two phases: inspiratory and expiratory. A ventilator is said to *cycle* between the two phases.

Inspiratory Cycling

During the inspiratory phase, the ventilator delivers a *volume* of gas into a patient's lungs. This takes place over a period of *time* producing an increasing airways *pressure*. There may also be a change in the pattern of *flow* (inspiratory waveform) at some stage in inspiration. However, the ventilator design allows only one of these to terminate the inspiratory phase when its predetermined value is reached. As all four variables are present in every inspiratory phase, it is sometimes difficult to decide which is the principal determinant of inspiratory cycling.

Volume cycling. A ventilator that uses this method of inspiratory cycling recognizes the point at which a predetermined volume of gas has left the ventilator and switches its internal mechanism to allow exhalation to occur. Many volume-cycled ventilators have a variable performance restrictor, which slows down the inspiratory gas flow, introducing some element of timing during inspiration. However, volume remains the primary determinant of inspiratory cycling.

Time cycling. Ventilator cycling may be achieved using mechanical, pneumatic or electronic timers to operate the cycling mechanism that function independently of the delivered tidal volume. This increases the sophistication of the ventilator. For example, it may allow the tidal volume to be delivered early in the inspiratory cycle, followed by a pause to allow better distribution of the gas prior to the start of the expiratory phase. Time cycling is now incorporated in most modern ventilators.

Pressure cycling. Pressure-cycled ventilators sense a predetermined airway pressure in order to terminate the inspiratory phase. However, if the airway resistance increases and/or compliance of a patient deteriorates, a pressure-cycled ventilator will deliver a reduced tidal volume at the preset cycling pressure. The performance of these ventilators is thus very variable.

Flow cycling. Recognition of flow pattern changes has been used to cycle ventilators (Bennett PR2 ventilator). However, this method is rarely employed nowadays.

Expiratory Cycling

The expiratory phase may be similarly terminated by one of the above-mentioned variables. For example:

- *An expiratory volume-cycled* ventilator may have a mechanism for terminating the expiratory phase when the bellows has filled to the desired tidal volume required for the next inspiration.
- *An expiratory pressure-cycled* ventilator would be able to identify a selected airways pressure at the end of exhalation that would trigger the next inspiratory phase.
- *An expiratory flow cycled* ventilator would switch to the inspiratory phase when the desired flow rate at the end of exhalation was reached.
- *An expiratory time cycled* ventilator is the most versatile as the phase may extend beyond the end of exhalation, unlike pressure and flow cycling. Nor is it limited by the fact that the inspiratory bellows is full, unlike a volume–cycled ventilator. It is therefore the most popular method of controlling the expiratory phase and is achieved by using electronic or pneumatic timers within the ventilator to switch phases.

Further explanations are included in the individual ventilators mentioned below.

Ventilators may use one of the methods described above for inspiratory cycling and another for expiratory cycling, depending on the method of construction, and in some of them, limits may be set to one or more of the above functions.

Cycling Mechanisms in Ventilators

Gas flow to and from the patient from a ventilator (cycling) is usually controlled by a series of one-way valves that are operated and synchronized either mechanically, electronically or pneumatically. Alternatively, the ventilator may be valveless. Here, gas flow is controlled ingeniously by the physical phenomenon of fluidics.

Ventilator Controls (General Principles)

The three variables involved in setting the ventilatory parameters on a ventilator are traditionally arranged in the simple equation below:

Minute volume = tidal volume × rate (breaths per minute)

Armed with this equation, a user should be able to switch on and set up any ventilator in its basic mode for controlled ventilation. The equation can have only two preset variables, the third being dependent upon the other two. Hence a ventilator needs only to have two of the above variables assigned to knobs present on its control panel, i.e. it may have controls for tidal volume and rate (e.g. Blease 8200), minute volume and rate (e.g. Servo 900 series), or minute volume and tidal volume (e.g. Manley series).

The equation may be made slightly more complicated by the fact that tidal volume and rate are derived values (see below) and can be represented in a different form. For example, tidal volume is derived from the *inspiratory flow* delivered by the ventilator, and the *time* over which this is delivered. It may be expressed in the equation:

$$\text{Tidal volume} = \text{inspiratory flow rate} \times \text{inspiratory time}$$
$$\text{e.g.} = 0.5 \text{ litre/s} \times 2 \text{ s}$$
$$= 1 \text{ litre}$$

Hence a ventilator may have no tidal volume control, but will have a flow control and an inspiratory time control to perform the same function.

Rate is derived from the cycle time and expressed as the number of complete *cycles* per *minute*. It may be expressed in the equation:

$$\text{Rate} = \frac{\text{time (1 min)}}{\text{cycle time}}$$

For example, if the inspiratory time is 2 s and the expiratory time is 4 s, then:

$$\text{Rate} = \frac{1 \text{ min (60 s)}}{(2 \text{ s} + 4 \text{ s})} = \frac{60}{6}$$

$$= 10 \text{ cycles/min}$$

Hence a ventilator that has no rate control knob will have an inspiratory and expiratory time control to perform the same function.

Classification of Ventilators According to Application

The miscellany of ventilator designs available and principles upon which they work is a result of (a) the wide spectrum of applications for which they are required and (b) efforts to harness the different power supplies that have been made available. However, there are four principal types of ventilator, which are classified here according to their application in clinical practice:

- mechanical thumbs;
- minute volume dividers;
- bag squeezers;
- intermittent blowers.

Mechanical Thumbs

The most common source of pressurized gas is that found in cylinders. This may be administered to a patient most easily as a continuous flow into the simplest of breathing systems, the T-piece (Fig. 12.4a). In Fig. 12.4b, the anaesthetist's thumb occludes the open end of the T-piece. The force of the fresh gas flow (FGF) inflates the patient's lungs until the anaesthetist removes the thumb from the open end, which allows expiration to occur (Fig. 12.4c). By rhythmical application of the thumb to occlude the T-piece, intermittent positive pressure ventilation (IPPV) is achieved.

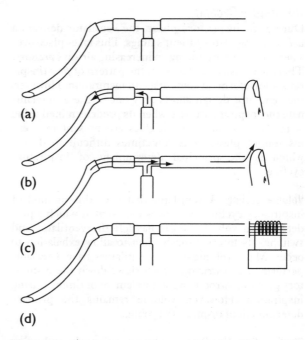

(a)

(b)

(c)

(d)

Figure 12.4 The T-piece principle and the 'mechanical thumb' (see text).

This is, therefore, a ventilator, that operates on the mechanical thumb principle. In ventilators such as the Sechrist (Fig. 12.5) the anaesthetist's thumb is replaced by a pneumatically operated valve, the cycling of which is determined by the settings on the ventilator controls. These ventilators are most useful in neonatal and infant ventilation as the breathing system components may be made small and with a low internal volume and hence compliance. As the FGF is diverted into the patient's lungs, it must be sufficiently high (equal to the mean inspiratory flow rate) to provide adequate ventilation. Also, since it continues to flow (out of the T-piece) at the same rate during exhalation, this becomes very wasteful when very high flows are required for larger patients.

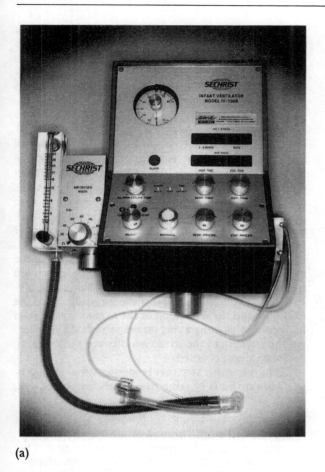

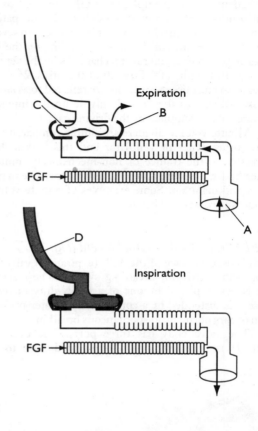

Figure 12.5 (a) The Sechrist paediatric ventilator. (b) Schematic diagram of the 'mechanical thumb'. A, patient connection; B, expiratory valve; C, deflated pneumatic valve; D, gas supply tube to pneumatic valve, which is now inflated.

Minute Volume Dividers

A more economical method of using a continuous source of pressurized gas is to feed it into a ventilator system (Fig. 12.6) to be collected by a reservoir (R), which is continually pressurized by a spring, a weight or its own elastic recoil. Two valves, V_1 and V_2, are linked together and operated by a bistable mechanism. When V_1 opens, V_2 closes and causes the reservoir to discharge gas to the patient, i.e. this is the inspiratory phase. When V_1 closes, V_2 opens and expiration is permitted, allowing the reservoir bag to refill in preparation for the next breath.

Figure 12.6 The principle of minute volume dividers (see text).

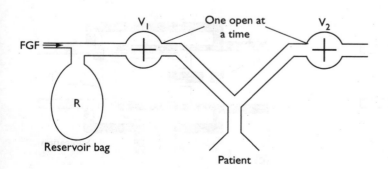

All of the driving gas that is supplied is delivered to the patient. If, for example, the FGF delivered to the ventilator is 10 litres/min, this is delivered to the patient as the minute volume. However, it is divided into several inspiratory volumes of 'breaths' depending on the settings on the volume and rate mechanisms on the ventilator, e.g. 10 breaths of 1 litre, 20 of 0.5 litres, 25 of 0.4 litres or so on. These ventilators are referred to as *minute volume dividers* as they merely divide up the intended minute volume supplied by the driving gas.

Minute volume dividers are simple compared with many other types of ventilator and this makes them attractive to the trainee or non-mechanically minded anaesthetist. They are also relatively inexpensive to purchase and maintain. Some examples of minute volume dividers are described below.

The East-Freeman Automatic Vent (Fig. 12.7)

This is used in place of the APL (expiratory) valve in a Mapleson A (Magill) breathing system. The reservoir bag is best replaced by one of a heavy-duty material, since it is distended by a considerably greater pressure than occurs normally in spontaneous breathing.

The valve body has three ports. The upstream port (I) is connected via a corrugated hose to the reservoir bag. Its aperture is occluded by the seating (S) on the closed end of the bobbin (B), which also carries at its centre a small magnet (M₁). The latter is attracted by another magnet (M₂) so that in the resting state the port is closed. Note that there is a gap (G) between the open end of the bobbin and the patient port (P) so that the patient may exhale via the expiratory port (E).

The FGF fills the reservoir bag and distends it until the pressure within it is sufficient to overcome the attraction between M₁ and M₂ and forces B off S. B then moves downstream until it closes G. At the same time, gases pass from the pressurized reservoir via the hose through holes in the periphery of the closed end of B, and thus to the patient. (G being closed, they cannot escape via the expiratory port.)

As the reservoir empties, the pressure falls and the mutual attraction of M₁ and M₂ returns B to its closed (resting) position. The expiratory phase then starts.

The only adjustments that can be made are to the FGF rate and the separation of the magnets, which can be altered by twisting a ring on the valve body. By altering the strength of the attraction between the magnets, the tidal volume is varied.

The Automatic Vent may be sterilized by cold methods, but care must be taken to avoid the ingress of grit,

Figure 12.7 (a) The East–Freeman Automatic Vent. (b, c) (Working principles. I, upstream port; P, patient port; E, expiratory port; B, bobbin; S, seating; M₁, M₂, magnets; G, gap that allows the exhaled gases to escape via the expiratory port. (See text.)

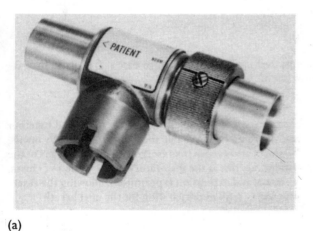

(a)

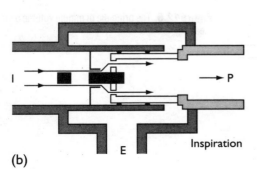

(b)

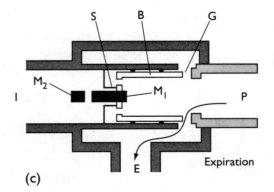

(c)

which could cause it to jam. A smaller reservoir bag should be used when treating children.

The Flomasta (Fig. 12.8)

The Flomasta is a considerably more sophisticated, yet very compact, minute volume divider, which is mounted directly on the common gas outlet of an anaesthetic machine. A driving gas pressure of 70–420 kPa (10–60 psi) is required. The single control knob (G) has several settings: the function of the valve in each mode will be described separately. The reservoir bag is enclosed in a rubber harness, partly to avoid overdistension and partly to achieve the appropriate volume/pressure characteristics.

During *automatic ventilation* the fresh gases enter via the inlet (A) and pass into the reservoir bag (B). The pressure within this part of the system rises until it is able to open the inspiratory valve (K) against the resistance of the spring (N). When K opens, the gases pass via the inspiratory limb (C) to the patient, but their escape via the expiratory limb (D) is prevented by the expiratory valve (J) (which is connected by the spindle (L) to the disc (V) of the inspiratory valve (K)), which is closed. The gases therefore pass around V, through a narrow orifice (W), and this maintains a relatively high pressure under V until the end of inspiration. As the patient's lungs become distended and the flow through W diminishes, so the pressure difference across V is reduced, and N successfully opposes the upward movement of V. K then closes and J opens, allowing the expired gases to pass to the atmosphere through the outlet (F). From here they may be metered by a spirometer and led to a scavenging system. The point at which inspiration ends depends on the tension in N, which in turn is controlled by setting the control knob to one of the 'auto' positions (1, 2, 3, 4 or 5).

During *manual or assisted ventilation* the inspired gases pass through K, raising V and thus closing J. When manual pressure on the reservoir bag is relinquished, K closes and J opens, allowing the expired gases to escape.

During *spontaneous respiration* gases are drawn by the patient through valve P, past the non–return valve (R). At this stage the patient cannot inhale via D because the non–return valve (H) prevents this. During expiration valve P closes, H opens, and the patient may exhale through the expiratory port.

As optional extras, an airway manometer may be inserted into a small socket that is otherwise occupied by a blanking plug, and a Wright respirometer may be directly attached to the exhaust outlet, which has a cage-mount (23 mm) taper.

The Flomasta may be autoclaved, provided that the respirometer and manometer are first removed. The manometer is not likely to become contaminated when in use, since it is in the inspiratory port.

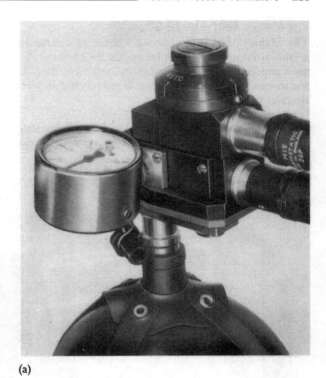

(a)

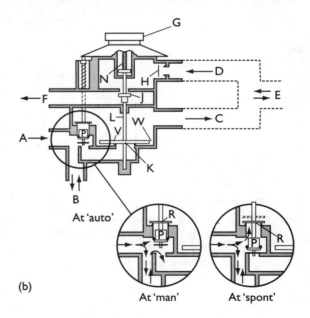

(b)

Figure 12.8 (a) The Flomasta ventilator. (b) Working principles. A, fresh gas inlet; B, reservoir bag; C, inspiratory limb; D, expiratory limb; E, patient; F, expired gas outlet; G, control knob. *For automatic and manual assisted ventilation:* K, inspiratory valve; V, disc of inspiratory valve; L, valve spindle; J, expiratory valve; N, spring; W, narrow orifice. *For spontaneous ventilation:* P, inspiratory/expiratory valve; R, H, non-return valves. (See text.)

The Manley MP3 (Fig. 12.9)

The Manley MP3 is the current version of a range of minute volume divider ventilators that have become the most popular of this type used in anaesthesia in the UK and in many other parts of the world as a result of its size, simplicity and reliably.

Mode of operation *Inspiratory phase*. At the beginning of this phase, the main bellows (B_2) has filled to the predetermined tidal volume. A lever (D) on top of the bellows housing trips a bistable mechanical linkage that operates the valves in the gas pathway so that:

- the valve V_1 closes and diverts the FGF to a storage bellows B_2;
- the valve V_2 opens and allows the weight on top of the bellows to expel the contents into the inspiratory pathway;

Figure 12.9 (Caption opposite.)

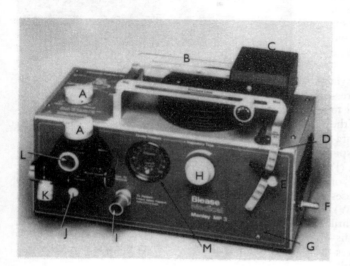

(a)

(b)

Pilot line

Mechanical link

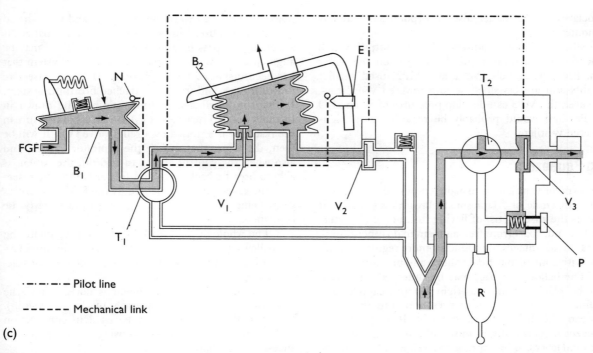

(c)

Figure 12.9 (a) The Manley MP3 ventilator. A, control taps; B, slide; C, sliding weight; D, stroke volume selector; E, catch; F, gas inlet; G, alternative position of gas inlet; H, inspiratory time control; I, to patient; J, tap release knob; K, to bag; L, from patient; M, airway manometer. (b,c) Working principles of the Manley MP3 ventilator. (b) Inspiration; (c) Expiration. B_1, reservoir bellows; B_2, main bellows; C, bellows weight, V_1, V_2, V_3, valves; T_1, inspiratory limb auto/manual tap; T_2, expiratory limb auto/manual tap, P, APL valve; W, trip lever for main bellows; N, trip lever for reservoir bellows; E, tidal volume catch for main bellows; R, reservoir bag.

- the valve V_3 closes in the expiratory pathway so that the inspiratory gas is directed to the patient.

Tidal volume. This is set by adjusting a sliding catch over the calibrations on the lever D. Without the storage bellows B_1, the fresh gas would supplement that in the main bellows B_2 during inspiration, and so deliver an unknown tidal volume.

There is a weight that slides along a lever attached to the top of the bellows. By sliding the weight closer to, or further away from, the hinge, the moment of force it exerts on the bellows causes the inspiratory pressure (within the bellows) to be altered.

During inspiration, the FGF is diverted into the spring-loaded storage bellows B_1, which expands, and when full trips the other lever (N) on the bistable mechanism. This in turn reverses all the valve positions and initiates the expiratory phase.

Expiratory phase:
- V_3 opens, allowing the patient to exhale through the expiratory pathway;
- V_2 closes preventing exhaled gas returning to the main bellows B_2;

- V_1 opens allowing the contents of the storage bellows and the FGF to enter the main bellows.

Cycling controls. The *inspiratory phase* is determined by the *time* taken to fill the storage bellows B_1 to the predetermined volume required to trip the lever D. The latter can be altered by adjusting the position of the trip lever with the 'inspiratory phase control'. Also, a high FGF will fill the bellows more rapidly and so shorten the inspiratory time.

The *expiratory phase* is *volume cycled* and may be altered by adjusting the *tidal volume catch* that regulates the degree to which B_2 is filled before the bistable mechanism is tripped to initiate inspiration.

Spontaneous respiration. When the ventilator is used in the mode for spontaneous breathing (by turning the taps T_1 and T_2), fresh gases pass directly to the patient, and the expired gases pass through tap T_2 to the reservoir bag (R) and finally escape via the expiratory valve (E). It therefore behaves as a Mapleson D system and will require the appropriately higher gas flows to avoid rebreathing.

Other features. The expiratory unit, complete with a condensation trap, may be detached very easily and autoclaved. This model also incorporates an airway manometer.

The ventilator produces a power output which depends on the position of the weight on the slider arm. Previous models (MN2 and MP2) used smaller weights and are classified as low-powered ventilators. However, the MP3 can develop pressures of 50 cmH$_2$O (5 kPa) and would probably be regarded as a high-powered ventilator.

Bag Squeezers

This type of ventilator is usually employed in conjunction with circle or Mapleson D breathing systems. It relieves the anaesthetist of having to squeeze the reservoir bag and, apart from freeing them to do other things, offers the advantages of producing more regular ventilation, with controllable tidal volume and pressure.

The bellows (or bag) may be squeezed pneumatically by placing it in a gas-tight Perspex canister and feeding driving gas (under pressure) into the space between the bellows and canister. It may also be squeezed mechanically, by means of a motor and suitable gears and levers, or by a spring or a weight (which may be adjusted to vary the pressure produced).

The Manley Servovent

Although the Manley Servovent (Fig. 12.10) bears a superficial resemblance to some of the minute volume dividers described above, it does, in fact, operate on an entirely different principle and is a bag squeezer. The driving gas, which may be compressed air or oxygen at a pressure of 300–400 kPa (45–60 psi), is kept entirely separate from the patient circuit. Cycling is by a pneumatic logic device with controls for on/off, expiratory time and inspiratory flow rate. It is, therefore, time cycled. There is also a tidal volume control, which permits a maximum of 1300 ml. During the expiratory phase, the piston (P) of a pneumatic cylinder is driven by the driving gas and opens, via levers, the bellows (B). During the inspiratory phase, P is returned by a pair of springs (S) and B closes, driving the gas to the patient. The inspiratory flow rate control operates by varying a flow restrictor which 'strangles' the exhaust from the cylinder, thus slowing down its return movement and determining inspiratory time.

Within the breathing attachment there is a diaphragm-operated valve (V$_1$), which is closed during inspiration by pressure from the control unit. Thus, during the inspiratory phase the gases from the bellows can pass only to the patient (or to atmosphere via the safety valve). The airway pressure is shown on a manometer (G). Because the piston that compresses the bellows is powerful, the ventilator is classified as high-

powered. During expiration, V$_1$ opens and the exhaled gases from the breathing system (to which the patient is attached) can pass into the reservoir (R). They may be augmented by more gas from the breathing system that has been displaced by the FGF. As B opens, gases are drawn from R and from the attached breathing system. If there is insufficient volume, air may be drawn in through a non-return valve (V$_3$). An excess of pressure in the reservoir is emptied by a relief valve (V$_2$). It will be seen, therefore, that during the expiratory phase, and also when the control unit is turned off, the patient is able to breathe backwards and forwards into the reservoir, the gases being augmented by the FGF and excess gases being voided through V$_2$, which must *always* be kept open.

The whole of the breathing attachment, including the bellows, may be detached and sterilized by autoclaving. G is isolated by a bacterial filter, since it is not suitable for this treatment.

The driving gas requirement is fairly heavy (the manufacturers claim an average of 12 litres/min). However, this ventilator may be used in conjunction with a circle absorption system using a low (economic) anaesthetic gas flow rate.

The Penlon Nuffield 400 Series Ventilator

The Penlon Nuffield 400 (Fig. 12.11) is classified as a bag squeezer and is used to power Mapleson D/E and circle systems. It consists of a suspended bellows arrangement within a Perspex canister (the bellows is attached to the top of the canister and travels downwards during filling as opposed to a rising bellows arrangement in which the bellows is attached to the base of its canister and travels upwards during filling). The control unit for the ventilator is also positioned on the top of the bellows and canister. It may be used in either of two modes.

Auto mode The drive unit is both powered and controlled pneumatically. When the manual/empty/auto control (17) is set to the auto position, this action moves the eccentrically positioned cam (18) to operate a valve (1). This allows driving gas from a compressed gas source at 290–650 kPa (42–95 psi) to enter the drive unit via a pressure regulator (2) and simultaneously supply a spool valve (3) and a logic circuit that controls inspiratory (4) and expiratory timers (5). The spool valve has a bias position in the expiratory phase position when signals are received simultaneously from the inspiratory and expiratory timers. This prevents the spool sticking in a mid position at any time in the cycle. The adjustable timers provide alternatively pulsed signals to change the position of the spool valve (3) and so control the inspiratory and expiratory phase times.

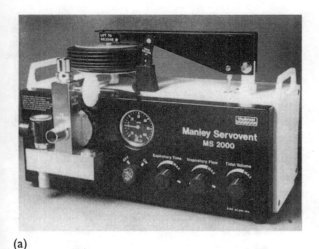

(a)

Figure 12.10 The Manley Servovent ventilator. (b) Working principles (see text). The portion to the right of the dotted line is detachable for sterilization. (P, piston rod; S, spring.)

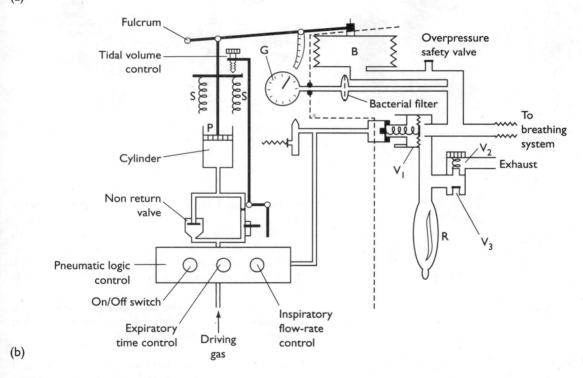

(b)

Inspiratory phase Driving gas passes across the spool in the 'open' position to an adjustable flow control (needle) valve (6). From here, it enters the bellows canister through an inflating valve (10). At the same time a piston in the inflating valve is activated by the driving gas and closes the driving gas exhaust port (20). The driving gas entering the canister compresses the bellows, displacing patient gas contained in the bellows out into the patient breathing system connection port (8). The driving gas also acts on a spill valve (15), preventing patient gas from escaping via the exhaust port during this phase. A fixed

setting relief valve (4.4 kPa/45 cmH$_2$O) is built into the canister lid to protect the canister against excessive driving gas pressure.

Expiratory phase When the spool is moved to the expiratory position, the driving gas contained in the bellows canister is exhausted to atmosphere via a port (21). The suspended bellows is dragged downwards by a small weight in the bellows base, allowing patient breathing system gas to re-enter the bellows. When the bellows is maximally filled, surplus breathing system gas is

(a)

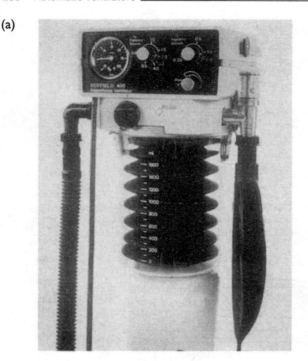

(b)

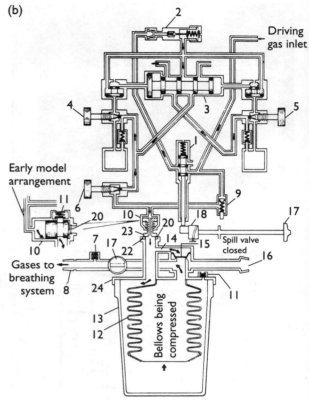

(c)

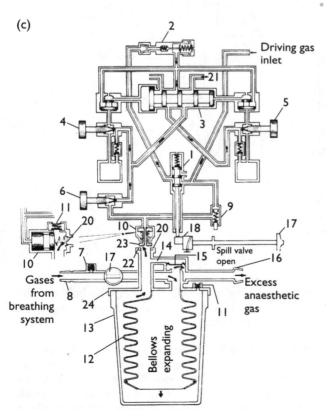

Figure 12.11 (a) The Nuffield 400 series ventilator. (b) Auto mode – inspiratory phase. (c) Auto mode – expiratory phase.

dumped through the now opened spill valve (15) to the atmosphere.

The ventilator is controlled for rate by the two pneumatic timers, which are calibrated in seconds. Inspiratory tidal volume is controlled by the needle valve (6) and can be read off the calibration scale on the bellows canister.

The ventilator is classified as an inspiratory and expiratory time cycled high-powered ventilator, which functions as a 'bag squeezer'.

Manual mode In the manual mode, the drive unit and bellows arrangement are isolated from the patient breathing system which is now connected directly to a reservoir bag and an optional APL valve attached to the ventilator.

The bellows The suspended bellows arrangement, while allowing convenient placement of the controls at the top of the ventilator housing, has some drawbacks. Prior to connecting a breathing system, the suspended bellows will be full of air that may need to be purged. An 'empty' setting between the auto and manual modes can be used to compress the bellows and lock the bellows closed in order to purge the air.

Also, the suspended bellows uses an internal weight to drag it downwards during the expiratory cycle. If there were a leak in the bellows, driving gas could enter the expanded bellows during the inspiratory phase and produce large delivered tidal volumes in excess of those anticipated. (Rising bellows arrangements are safer in this respect.) However, a bellows leak may be detected by using the 'empty' setting to compress the bellows. A gas-tight bellows remains compressed, but a leaky bellows

sucks in air through the leak and gradually expands. This test should be performed as part of the 'cockpit drill' prior to the start of any anaesthetic.

The Blease 8200s

The Blease 8200s (Fig. 12.12) represents a type of 'bag squeezer' that is controlled by a microprocessor. The latter increases greatly the range of ventilatory parameters available.

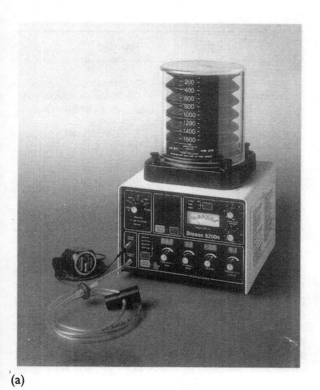

(a)

Figure 12.12 (a) Blease 8200s ventilator; (b) Working principles. A, drive gas input port (270–760 kPa (36–101 psi)); B, input gas filter (5 μm) and water trap; C, low supply pressure transducer (270 kPa); D, input pressure regulator; E, solenoid flow control valve; F, non-return valve; G, flow sensor; H, expiratory valve; J, solenoid dump valve; K, bellows assembly; L, pneumatic valve; M, microprocessor; N, patient gas expiratory port; R, driving gas exhaust.

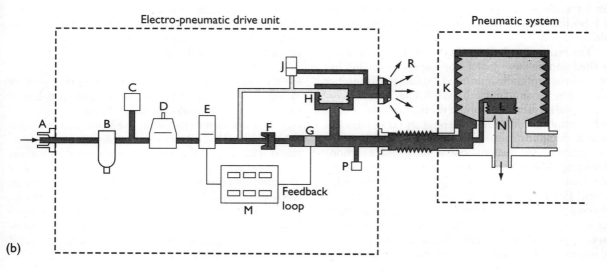

(b)

Inspiratory phase Driving gas from a pressurized source A (270–760 kPa (36–101 psi) is passed through a filter (B), a regulator (D) (set at 259 kPa (34.5psi)) and fed through a solenoid flow control valve (E) and flow sensor (G) to an airtight canister (K). The latter contains a rising bellows arrangement. The flow of the pressurized gas to the canister is controlled by a microprocessor (M). The latter is linked to the flow sensor and solenoid so that all three form a feedback loop providing a much wider variety of inspiratory flow rates and cycling times than a pneumatically controlled ventilator. As the driving gas enters the canister it also supplies a small pneumatic valve (L), causing it to occlude the expiratory port (N) in the patient circuit. This ensures that when the bellows is compressed, all the patient gas contained within passes to the patient.

Expiratory phase At the end of the inspiratory phase, the microprocessor instructs the flow control valve (F) to close and a second (solenoid) valve (J) to open. This opens the driving gas pathway to the atmosphere and causes the pressure within to fall. The reduced pressure permits the expiratory valve (H) in the ventilator gas pathway to open so that driving gas can escape from the canister when the bellows fills with exhaled gas. When the latter is full, it forces the pneumatic valve (L) open so that any excess gas is vented to the atmosphere via the scavenging attachment. During this phase, the bellows behaves as a reservoir bag, allowing spontaneous respiration to take place if desired. Both phases are time-cycled by the microprocessor.

Ventilator controls The front of the ventilator casing houses several panels. The top left hand panel has a single knob that when turned from the OFF position counter-clockwise passes through a standby mode (powering) the ventilator and alarm systems to the ON position for adult ventilation. Clockwise rotation from the OFF position sets up the ventilator for paediatric ventilation.

The main controls for setting ventilatory parameters are sited on the lower panel. The European version has two main control knobs, one for tidal volume and the other for rate. The version for use in the USA has a minute volume control in place of the one for the tidal volume. A third knob controls the inspiratory/expiratory (I/E) ratio and a fourth, the adjustable inspiratory pressure limiting system, controls the patient safety valve. All are non-interacting within the normal operating range. Above each control is an LED display indicating the value chosen. The value for the tidal volume is that nominally delivered by the bellows. However, if the optional spirometer is attached and placed close to the patient, then the display shows the actual tidal volume. This may include the additional effect of the FGF into the attached breathing system (especially if this is high). The range of the three main controls (tidal volume, rate and I/E ratio) can be extended by depressing the 'Range Select' button for at least 3 s. Gross adjustment of these controls may then set unattainable values in which case the offending parameter LED will flash and an alarm will sound until an appropriate value is chosen. Table 12.1 highlights the range selection available, including variables described below.

Table 12.1 Range selection for the Blease 8200s

	Normal	Extended
Minute volume		
Adult	4–20 litres/min	2–25 litres/min
Paediatric	4–20 litres/min	0.3–25 litres/min (also allows pressure limited ventilation in adults)
Frequency	6–40 breaths/min	2–100 breaths/min
Insp./exp. ratio	1:1 to 1:4	1:0.5 to 1:5
Pressure limit		
Adult	10–70 cmH$_2$O	10–70 cmH$_2$O
Paediatric	10–30 cmH$_2$O	10–30 cmH$_2$O
Pressure alarms		
High	10–70 cmH$_2$O	
Low	5–60 cmH$_2$O	

Paediatric ventilation The adult bellows can be easily removed and substituted by a smaller (300 ml) one. The paediatric mode should then be selected from the front panel of the ventilator, as this alters the range of respiratory rates available. However, for infants and neonates, a pressure-limited inspiratory phase is available. If the pressure limiter is adjusted to the peak inspiratory pressure required and the tidal volume set to a value greater than required, the inspiratory flow will reduce or cease in order to maintain the set pressure (even in the presence of a normal leak around the endotracheal tube), until the time-cycled inspiratory phase has been completed.

Alarms The airway pressures developed (either peak or mean) are displayed on a meter on the front panel, next to which are the knobs for the adjustable alarms for high and low airway pressure, the latter having a time delay of 30 s. This ignores transient low pressures associated with a normal expiratory pause even at respiratory rates as low as 2 per minute but recognizes a disconnection between the ventilator and the patient when the time delay has elapsed. The alarms are displayed on a separate panel that also includes machine-based alarms for low gas supply pressure, mains electricity failure, low back-up battery charge state and ventilator failure.

Classification The ventilator is a high-powered (capable of developing very high inflation pressures), time-cycled bag squeezer.

The Ohmeda 7800 (Fig. 12.13)

This is also a pneumatically driven, microprocessor-controlled bag squeezer. Although the microprocessor handles the driving gas in a somewhat similar fashion to that described above, the display and control knobs are somewhat different. Although three of the main operating knobs (for tidal volume, respiratory rate and inspiratory pressure limit) function in a similar manner, the fourth does not. On this ventilator, the latter is an inspiratory flow controller for the selected tidal volume to be delivered. Increasing the flow shortens the inspiratory time and vice versa. The respiratory rate knob, therefore, controls only expiratory time. The inspiratory/expiratory ratio is therefore a function of these two controls.

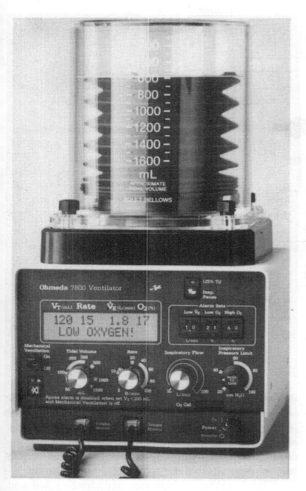

Figure 12.13 The Ohmeda 7800 ventilator.

There is an additional control (inspiratory pause) that holds the delivered tidal volume, prolonging the inspiratory time by 25%. This feature is said to allow redistribution of gas to those parts of the lungs that were slow to fill during the initial inspiration.

Displays The front panel houses a liquid crystal display (LCD). The normal display when the ventilator is switched on is: nominal tidal volume (i.e. the tidal volume delivered by the bellows into the attached breathing system), rate, expired minute volume and oxygen concentration in the breathing system (see below). Touching the front of the rate knob causes it to display the rate and the inspiratory/expiratory ratio.

Tidal volume Touching the front of the tidal volume knob causes the LCD to display the tidal volume (and rate) measured by the flow sensor. If the latter is placed between the breathing system and the patient (the most accurate location) it measures the actual tidal volume (inspired or expired, depending upon the direction in which the flow sensor is installed). This may include the volume delivered by the bellows (minus any leaks or losses) plus the additional effect of any fresh gas entering the breathing system in the inspiratory phase. It therefore often displays a greater value than the nominal tidal volume. The sensor is also often placed in the expiratory limb of a circle breathing system (for convenience). Here, it measures exhaled tidal volume (minus any leaks or losses) as well as some gas displaced from the breathing system by the ingress of fresh gas during the later part of the expiratory cycle. The latter statement needs further explanation. For example, at the beginning of the expiratory phase, the pressure exerted by the exhaled tidal volume closes the inspiratory valve in the circle. The exhalate passes undiluted through the expiratory limb and past the sensor. At the same time, fresh gas entering the circle cannot pass the closed inspiratory valve and is diverted to the ventilator bellows. When this is full, the fresh gas pushes the inspiratory valve open, enters the circle and moves towards the expiratory limb. The latter movement of gas will be recorded by the flow sensor in addition to the gas exhaled by the patient. The extra amount will depend on the FGF rate.

Alarms The ventilator is supplied with an oxygen fuel cell and flow sensor (see above), both of which are linked to the alarms and must be connected and functioning when the ventilator is switched on, otherwise the alarms will sound continuously.

The Oxford Mark 2 Ventilator (Fig. 12.14)

A bellows (B) containing the anaesthetic gases is operated by a pneumatic cylinder (C) that is powered by

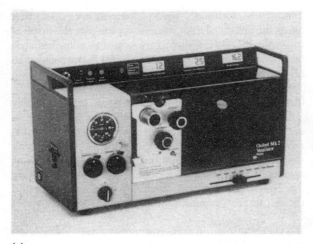

(a)

Figure 12.14 (a) The Oxford Mark 2 ventilator. Note the electronic digital readout of functions, including inspiratory and expiratory times and respiratory rate. (b) Working principles. B, bellows; C, power cylinder; S_1, main spool valve; S_2, second spool valve; T_1, T_2, trip valves; V, cylinder controlling expiratory valve. A third spool valve, connected in parallel with the other two, controls the electronic readout facility but has been omitted from the diagram for the sake of clarity. The portion to the right of the diagonal line is detachable for sterilization.

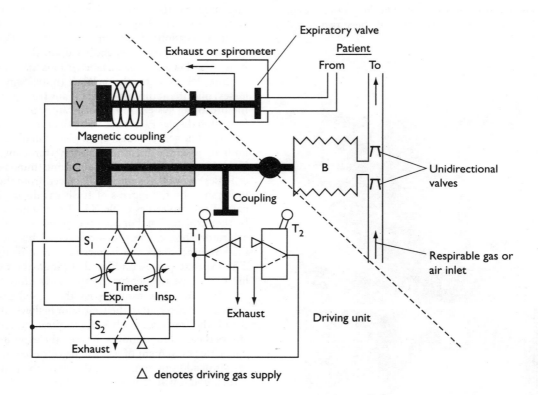

(b)

$\triangle$ denotes driving gas supply

compressed air and controlled by a pneumatic system. The direction of movement of the cylinder is controlled by a spool valve (S_1). A second spool valve (S_2) controls a smaller cylinder (V), which operates the expiratory valve of the breathing system. There is a lever on the piston rod of C that operates a trip valve (T_1 or T_2) at each end of its movement. The lengths of the inspiratory and expiratory excursion are thereby variable, altering the tidal volume of the ventilator (i.e. that volume of gas expelled from the bellows). The inspiratory and expiratory flow rates are adjusted by needle valves which 'strangle' the exhaust from the cylinder, thereby slowing its movement. The entire patient gas system may be removed from the ventilator for sterilization.

The ventilator is high-powered, time-cycled and may be used for both anaesthesia and intensive care.

The Servo 900 Series Ventilator

The Servo 900 Series ventilator is a sophisticated multi-mode ventilator (Fig. 12.15). Many of its functions are more relevant to an intensive care environment and are beyond the remit of this book. However, when used to ventilate anaesthetized patients it is most frequently used as a pneumatically driven, electronically controlled minute volume divider.

Fresh gas from the anaesthetic machine is fed into the low-pressure entry port sited on the side of the ventilator and is stored in a spring loaded 2-litre bellows. The spring load can be varied with the front panel key to a maximum working pressure of 11.8 kPa/120 cmH$_2$O although a much lower pressure of 5.88 kPa/60–65 cmH$_2$O is normally used. If the bellows is overfilled, excess gas is vented through a pressure-relief valve linked to this bellows. This pressurized gas supplies the inspiratory flow to the patient; hence in this mode, the FGF from the anaesthetic machine should be set slightly (12–15%) in excess of ventilatory parameters set up on the ventilator so that the bellows remains optimally filled.

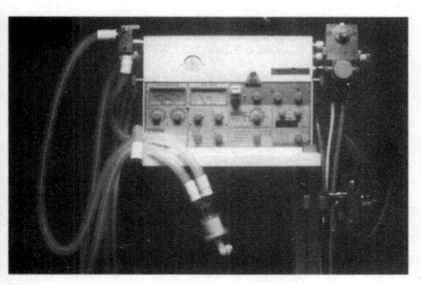

Figure 12.15 (a) The Servo 900 C Series ventilator. (b) Working principles: A, high pressure gas supply inlet; B, low pressure gas supply inlet; C, demand valve (this is tripped mechanically by the base plate of the bellows to maintain the bellows at two-thirds full); D, fuel cell housing; E, non-return valve on the low pressure gas inlet; F, inlet filter housing; G, spring-loaded bellows; H, overpressure safety valve (set at 120 cmH$_2$O); J, inspiratory pneumotachograph; K, inspiratory pincer valve; L, inspiratory pressure transducer; M, expiratory pneumotachograph; N, expiratory pressure transducer; O, expiratory valve.

(a)

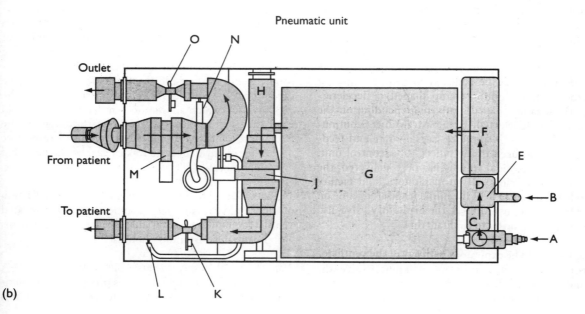

(b)

Alternatively, high-pressure gas (420 kPa in the UK) from a blender (nitrous oxide/oxygen) and a special high-pressure vaporizer may be fed into the bellows via the high-pressure inlet port, which is also sited on the side of the ventilator. Prior to entering the bellows, the gas passes through a demand valve which ensures that when any gas is removed from the reservoir bag it is immediately refilled from the blender and vaporizer. This extends the role of the ventilator from that of a simple minute volume divider to that of a machine that can respond to the extra gas demand caused by a patient breathing spontaneously, either with or between, controlled tidal volumes delivered by the ventilator (synchronized intermittent mandatory ventilation (SIMV) models 900C and E). It also allows a patient's respiratory efforts to be assisted by a variable amount when the 'pressure support' mode is selected (Servo 900C and D).

The ventilator is time cycled and so has a control switch for the cycling rate measured in breaths per minute. The inspiratory phase for each cycle is varied by an inspiratory time switch which can be supplemented by a variable end-inspiratory pause (pause time control switch). As the total cycle time is predetermined, any inspiratory adjustments are made at the expense of expiratory time. The other major parameter that can be adjusted is minute volume. The control knob for this is calibrated in litres/min.

The tidal volume delivered during each inspiratory cycle is therefore derived electronically from the settings for minute volume and rate set on the control panel, i.e.

$$\text{Tidal volume} = \text{Minute volume} \div \text{Rate}$$

Inspiratory phase When the electronically operated inspiratory valve (pincer action) opens, gas leaves the bellows and enters the patient's breathing system via a flow transducer. The pincer action of the valve is continuously adjusted via the machine electronics to produce a variety of inspiratory times, flow rates and patterns. The inspiratory flow may be adjusted to provide constant (square-wave), accelerating (ramp-shaped) or decelerating (reverse ramp shaped) patterns depending on the ventilatory mode selected. The flow transducer continuously measures the inspiratory gas flow rate and feeds this information back to the pincer valve control unit. When the desired tidal volume has been delivered, the inspiratory valve closes. If an inspiratory hold facility (variable from 0 to 33% of the initial inspiratory time on model 900C only) is required, the expiratory valve also remains closed in order to facilitate this.

Expiratory phase The expiratory pathway of the ventilator also contains an electronically operated pincer valve (the expiratory valve), a flow transducer and an airway pressure transducer. Exhalation occurs when this pincer

valve opens, allowing gas in the patient's lungs to escape through this pathway. The duration of this expiratory phase is again time cycled. The electronics linked to the flow transducer in the expiratory limb computes expired minute volume and provides the necessary information to the high and low expired volume alarms.

The airway pressure transducer in the expiratory limb (also linked to a high-pressure alarm) is used via the control panel to close prematurely the expiratory valve towards the end of expiration when a PEEP facility is required. It also senses spontaneous respiratory activity and allows the patient to trigger the ventilator to a degree permitted by the settings on the trigger sensitivity control.

Control panels The front panel on the machine is divided into two sections:

Panel for setting ventilatory parameters This main section houses the controls for setting ventilatory parameters as described above, i.e. minute volume, respiratory rate, flow pattern, inspiratory time, inspiratory hold and PEEP.

Alarm panel The various alarms (see above) for high and low airways pressure and expired minute volume are grouped together with visual display meters for these.

The ventilator, in the anaesthetic mode described above, is classified as a high-powered ventilator which is used as an inspiratory and expiratory time-cycled minute volume divider.

Alternative ventilatory modes The Servo 900C supports several other ventilatory modes (intermittent mandatory ventilation (IMV), synchronized intermittent mandatory ventilation (SIMV) and pressure support) which increases the capabilities of these ventilators beyond that of a minute volume divider. These are not described here as these modes are mostly used in an intensive care environment and are outside the remit of this book. The exception to this is the 'Pressure Control' mode on the 900C model, which allows the ventilator to be used in paediatric anaesthesia. In this mode the lungs of the patient are ventilated to a desired pressure irrespective of the size of any deliberate leak caused by the uncuffed endotracheal tube.

The Servo 900D The Servo 900D is a scaled-down version of the 900C ventilator, losing some of the sophisticated ventilatory modes, the variable inspiratory waveforms and the variable inspiratory hold facility.

Manual ventilation/spontaneous respiration (all models) A manual ventilation mode setting is provided on the control panel. However, in order to function this requires the fitment of a dedicated accessory consisting of bag mount, reservoir bag and a one-way valve to the inspiratory limb of the patient breathing system. In this mode the ventilator supplies gas to the reservoir bag until the pressure within it reaches 0.4 kPa/(4 cmH$_2$O) as measured by an inspiratory pressure transducer, at which time gas flow ceases. If the patient makes a respiratory effort, the expiratory valve closes, gas is withdrawn from the reservoir bag and fresh gas enters the lungs. The ventilator senses the pressure drop in the bag and replenishes the lost gas. When the patient exhales, the one-way valve in the bag mount accessory prevents expired gas contaminating the inspiratory limb, and so gas escapes through the expiratory valve, which now opens.

If the bag is manually compressed, the expiratory valve closes in response to the pressure rise and gas in the bag is directed to the patient. When the bag is released, the ventilator senses the pressure drop in the bag and replenishes the lost gas. The sequence of events in expiration is the same as described above during spontaneous respiration.

The M&IE Carden Electrovent Ventilator

This ventilator (Fig. 12.16a), also classified as a high-powered bag squeezer, consists of:

- an electronic control unit that supplies driving gas;
- a valve box that contains various valves and a venturi injector that allows driving gas to entrain supplemental air;
- a Perspex canister containing a rising bellows arrangement;
- a mode block that allows the bellows to be attached to different breathing systems.

Electronic control unit (Fig. 12.16b). Pressurized gas (air or oxygen) at 320–420 kPa (45–60 psi) enters the gas power inlet and passes to a solenoid valve. The latter is electronically opened and closed by a timing circuit that is adjusted by two control knobs on the front panel. There are two versions of the control unit. In version A, one knob (calibrated in seconds) adjusts inspiratory time and the other (also calibrated in seconds) the expiratory time. In version B, one knob alters the inspiratory ratio and the other the number of respiratory cycles (calibrated in breaths per minute, BPM). Both ultimately achieve the same aim.

When the solenoid opens, the gas flows through it and through an adjustable flow control valve to the valve box. The flow control valve exerts a degree of control on the delivered tidal volume and so is labelled 'Volume Control' on the front panel. It is not calibrated. This is explained in more detail below.

The valve box This device (Fig. 12.16c) is the interface between the control unit and the bellows unit. Pressurized gas from the control unit enters the valve box and passes through a venturi. The latter entrains ambient air from a non-rebreathing valve 'B'. The mixture of control unit gas and entrained air becomes *the driving gas* for the ventilator and passes through a non-rebreathing valve 'A' to supply the Perspex canister. When the control unit switches to the expiratory phase, driving gas flow ceases and allows gas in the canister to escape through the valve 'A' (in the valve box) to an exhaust port, driven by the bellows, which re-expands as it fills with exhaled patient gas. The valve box is a self-contained unit that fits inside the control unit but which can easily be removed for autoclaving.

A self-inflating bag can also be attached to the manual air inlet on the valve box to provide an alternative method of bellows compression when the ventilator is switched off, or if there is a failure of the driving gas.

The delivered tidal volume is dependent on two factors:

- *The flow through the venturi.* When the 'volume' knob on the control unit is turned clockwise, it increases the pressure (and flow) of driving gas to the venturi injector. This in turn causes a greater amount of air to be entrained. The increased flow of the air and driving gas enters the canister and displaces a larger volume from the patient bellows.

- *The compliance of the patient's lungs.* If these are easy to ventilate, the same venturi driving pressure entrains more air, which in turn displaces a greater volume from the bellows to the patient. As compliance can vary in an individual patient as well as from patient to patient, the 'volume' knob cannot be calibrated for tidal volume. Occasional adjustment may be necessary during use if lung compliance and airways resistance change during use.

The bellows unit (Fig. 12.16d,e). This consists of: (1) a Perspex canister and rubber bellows that can be supplied either as 1500 ml capacity items for use in adults or 750 ml ones for use in children; and (2) a bellows base into which the items above fit. Also, at the back of the base, there are two connections, one to the valve box for the driving gas and the other for the measurement of pressure in the breathing system. At the front of the bellows base there is a connection for a 'mode block' that links the bellows to an attached breathing system.

The mode block (Fig. 12.16d,e). There are two types of mode block. One has a single connector allowing to and fro movement of gas and allows the bellows to be used as a 'bag squeezer' for circle and Mapleson D/E systems (Fig. 12.16d). The other has three connectors and

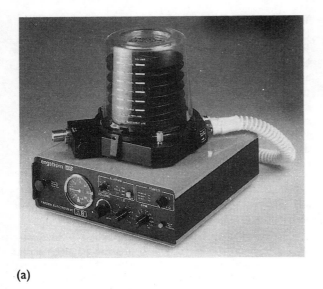

(a)

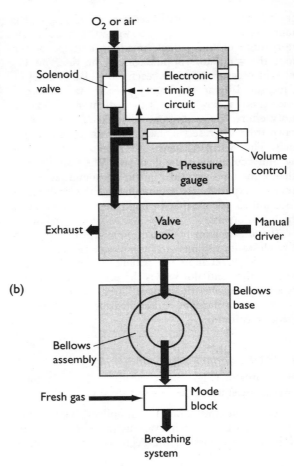

(b)

Figure 12.16 (Caption opposite).

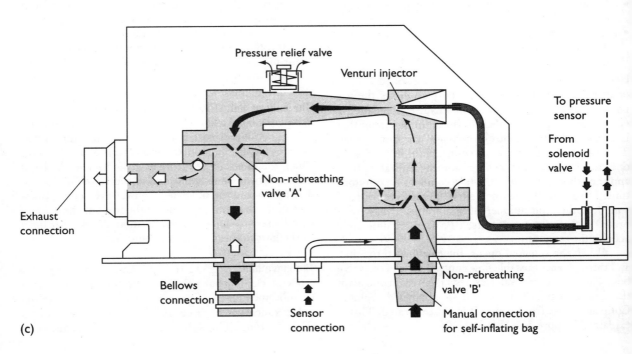

(c)

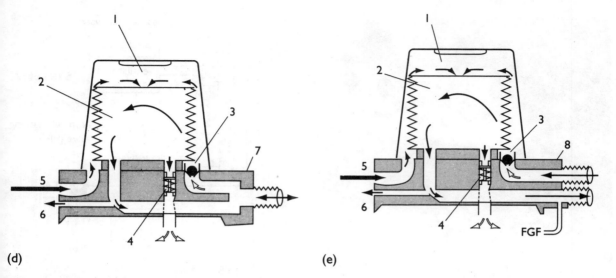

(d)   (e)

Figure 12.16 (a) The M&IE Carden Electrovent ventilator. (b) Schematic diagram of component layout. (c) Valve box operation (black arrows denote inspiration and white arrows expiration). (d) Schematic of bellows operation of to and fro mode block. 1, driving gas; 2, breathing gas; 3, PEEP valve (lifts at 2.4 cmH₂O); 4, pressure relief valve (65 cmH₂O); 5, bellows connector (from valve box); 6, pressure sensor connector (to valve box); 7, to and fro mode block. (e) Schematic of bellows operation of A mode block (8).

converts the bellows to an 'enclosed' Mapleson A system (Fig 12.16e). Two are wide-bore 22 mm breathing system connections and the third is a small-bore fresh gas feed. The working principles are described below.

To and fro mode (Fig. 12.16d)

Inspiratory phase Driving gas supplemented with entrained air enters the bellows canister and displaces an equal volume of patient gas contained in the bellows through the single bellows connection and into an attached patient breathing system. The pressure within the canister also closes a weighted one-way valve (see below).

Expiratory phase When the driving gas flow ceases, the main valve (non-rebreathing valve 'B') closes and the natural compliance of the patient's lungs pushes breathing system gas back into the rising bellows. When the bellows is full and the pressure therein exceeds 0.20 kPa (3 cmH₂O), the weighted one-way valve is lifted and excess gas vented into the canister where it escapes with driving gas through the valve box to the exhaust port.

'A' mode (Fig. 12.16e)

Inspiratory phase At the first inspiratory phase, it is convenient to assume that the fresh gas from the small-bore connection has filled the bellows completely and this is passed to the patient via the 'inspiratory' connection of the mode block.

Expiratory phase Exhaled gas pushes that gas left in the 'inspiratory' limb (which has the lower resistance) back to the bellows, which fills with a combination of this and fresh gas. When the bellows is full, the remainder of the exhaled gas is diverted to the other limb where it exits the weighted one-way valve (the cause of the higher resistance in this limb) in the canister, on its way to the exhaust system.

Safety features The control unit has two mechanical over-pressure relief valves fitted to prevent barotrauma to a patient.

The Cape TC50 Ventilator

This is a 'bag squeezer' type ventilator (Fig. 12.17a) that is often used by the Armed Forces in field hospitals. It consists of a bellows unit whose travel is controlled by a mechanical arm linked to a variable-speed, low-geared, low-voltage electric motor (Fig. 12.17b).

Inspiratory phase The mechanical arm linking the electric motor to the bellows has two components. When the electric motor is switched on, it causes the crank to rotate. This pushes the inner rod of the mechanical arm forward until it engages the outer arm. At this stage the mechanical arm starts to compress the bellows. The speed of the electric motor controls the cycle time and is adjusted by a knob on the front panel of the machine. The ventilator can therefore be regarded as time cycled. As the motor is powerful, the machine is capable of

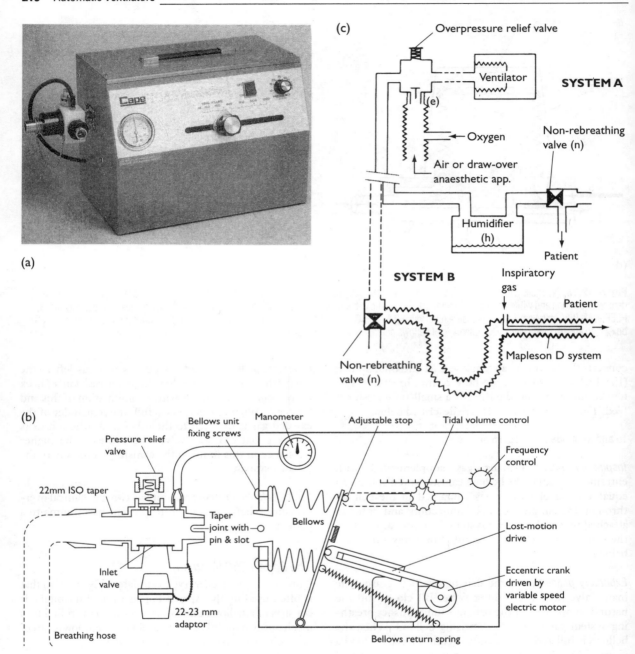

Figure 12.17 (a) The Cape TC50 ventilator. (b) Working principles (see text). (c) Ventilatory modes: (upper) non-rebreathing system; (lower) Mapleson D system.

generating high pressure (high–powered ventilator) and when connected to a patient breathing system requires the fitment of a safety valve.

Expiratory phase At the end of the inspiratory phase, the mechanical arm retreats as a result of the rotary action of the eccentric crank. The bellows is re-

expanded by the spring to a point fixed by the tidal volume control, which acts as a mechanical stop (see Fig. 12.18b). At this point the two components of the mechanical arm separate, allowing the crank to complete its rotation to be ready for the next inspiration. The mode of operation of the arm is referred to as a 'lost motion drive'.

Inspiratory/expiratory ratio. The inspiratory/expiratory ratio varies according to the tidal volume selected from 1–8 at a minimum tidal volume setting to 1–2 at the maximum volume selected. For example, at low tidal volume settings, the inner rod of the mechanical arm has a long free travel before it picks up the outer arm in order to compress the bellows. This effectively delays the inspiratory phase and prolongs the expiratory phase.

The ventilator is usually supplied with a 'gas entrainment block' for direct connection to the bellows port and this includes an overpressure relief valve (factory preset at 45 cmH_2O). The block has an outlet port which may then be connected to an appropriate breathing system (see below). As the electric motor is powerful, the ventilator is regarded as being high-powered. The cycling rate is controlled by the speed of the electric motor, which can be varied. It is therefore time-cycled.

Ventilatory modes (Fig. 12.17c)

- Non-rebreathing system (System A). Bellows excursion entrains respirable gas from the valve inlet (e) and then directs it into the breathing system, which has a non-rebreathing valve (n) positioned close to the patient. The respirable gas can be either air, or with a suitable attachment, an air and oxygen mixture, with or without anaesthetic agents from a draw-over system (Triservice, see Chapter 30). A humidifier (h) may also be added for intensive care situations. The ventilator with this system in use is popular with the Armed Services for anaesthesia and intensive care applications under battlefield conditions.
- Mapleson D system (System B). The non-rebreathing valve may alternatively be connected directly to the entrainment valve block and then attached via a suitable length of hosing to the reservoir bag port of a Mapleson D system so that it behaves as a 'bag squeezer'.
- Some interesting 'home-made' attachments have been described to allow the ventilator to be used in a circle system. These have been mainly for use in developing countries where the availability of volatile anaesthetic agents and compressed gases is at a premium. However, there is no purpose-built device made by the manufacturers.

Intermittent Blowers

These ventilators are driven by a source of gases or air, at a pressure of 300–400 kPa (45–60 psi). The driving gas is normally delivered to the patient undiluted but, it may be passed through a venturi device so that air, oxygen or anaesthetic gases may be added to it.

The Pneupac and Penlon Nuffield 200 Series Ventilators

These range from a small portable resuscitator (Pneupac) to an anaesthetic ventilator (Nuffield series 200), but since they all have a similar working principle they will be described together. Each consists of a *control unit* and a *patient valve*. The control units differ in the extent to which their inspiratory timers, expiratory timers and flow control knobs can be altered. For instance, the Pneupac model 2R (child/adult, Fig. 12.18) and Model 1 (infant/child, Fig. 12.19) has a single knob for 'Tidal Volume Cycling Rate' and 'I/E Ratio', which is actually the variable restrictor in the inspiratory timer. Since the flow rate is constant, when the inspiratory time is lengthened, the tidal volume is increased, the cycling rate is reduced and the I/E ratio is

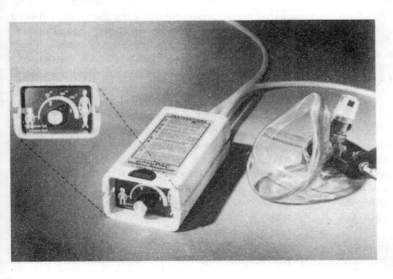

Figure 12.18 The Pneupac child/adult ventilator.

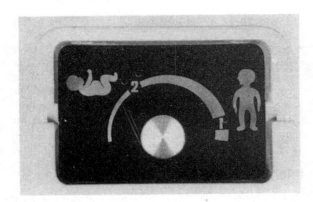

Figure 12.19 The Pneupac child ventilator.

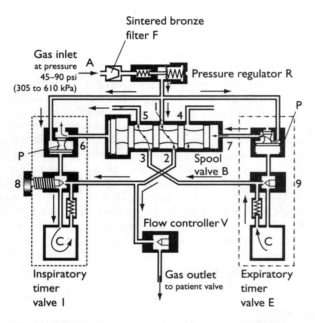

Figure 12.20 The Pneupac control module. A, point of entry of driving gas; F, filter; R, pressure regulator; B, spool valve, with ports 1–5; I, inspiratory timer; 8, variable flow restrictor; 9, fixed flow restrictor; P, pistons; C, capacitors; E, expiratory timer; F, flow controller. (See text.)

prolonged (and vice versa). The adult version (model 4R) has no adjustable controls so that it delivers a fixed tidal volume and rate based on conventional cardiopulmonary resuscitation values. In the Penlon Nuffield 200, both the inspiratory and expiratory timers are adjustable as well as an inspiratory flow rate control so that a wider range of ventilatory parameters can be selected.

The Pneupac ventilator The control module (Fig. 12.20) consists essentially of a spool valve (B) and two timers,

one for the inspiratory phase (I) and the other for the expiratory phase (E). The spool valve has five ports and there is a pneumatic actuator at each end. Each timer contains a piston (P), which is driven by gas entering at a constant flow via a flow restrictor into the capacitor (C), until such time as the pressure becomes high enough to actuate the piston. When this happens, driving gas is delivered to the end of the spool valve, driving the spool to the opposite end.

The driving gas, which may be oxygen, a nitrous oxide–oxygen mixture or compressed air at a pressure of 305–610 kPa (45–90 psi), enters the control module at A, passes through a filter (F), a pressure regulator (R) and then to port 1 of the spool valve (B). When the spool is to the left-hand side of the control module, the gas passes from port 1 to port 2 and then on via a flow controller (V) to the patient valve. This is the inspiratory phase. From port 2 the gas also passes to the inspiratory timer (I), where it is controlled by the flow restrictor (8), which, on the inspiratory side, is variable. As the inspiratory flow rate is constant, this control determines the tidal volume. At the end of the time determined by the setting of 8, the timer operates and the gas passes via port 6 to the actuator at the left-hand end of B, driving the spool to the right-hand side of the control module. This is the end of the inspiratory phase. The driving gas entering B at port 1 now leaves by port 3 and passes to the expiratory timer (E). The sequence of events now repeats itself, except that there is a fixed restrictor (9) in the expiratory timer and therefore a constant expiratory time. When the expiratory timer operates, the gas passes to B by port 7, driving the spool back to the right-hand side of the control module, initiating the next inspiratory phase. Trapped signals (Chapter 2) are vented at ports 4 and 5.

The Nuffield anaesthesia ventilator, Series 200 (Fig. 12.21). This is an elaboration of the Pneupac ventilator with the addition of variable inspiratory and expiratory timers and a variable inspiratory flow rate control. There is also an airway manometer and an On/Off switch.

The patient valve may be connected to the control module by a long narrow-bore tube, as in the Pneupac ventilator (Fig. 12.22), or it may be attached directly to the control module, as in the Penlon A-P. It contains a piston (P), which in the resting state, under the control of the spring (S), closes the inspiratory port and opens the expiratory port to permit exhalation. During inspiration the pressure of gas from the control module acts on P with sufficient force to overcome S and so close the expiratory port and open the inspiratory port to the patient.

The Pneupac patient valve, in a special metal form, may be autoclaved, but the more commonly supplied plastic version should not be subjected to temperatures

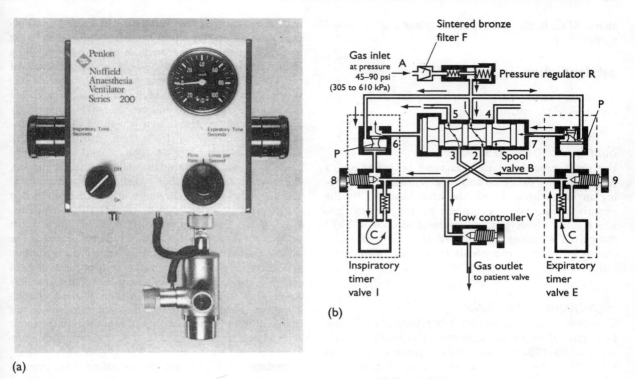

(a)

(b)

Figure 12.21 (a) The Penlon Nuffield anaesthetic ventilator. (b) Schematic diagram. Key: as Fig. 12.20. The mechanism of this is similar to that of the Pneupac. There are both variable inspiratory and expiratory timers, an airway manometer and a variable flow restrictor that controls the inspiratory flow rate.

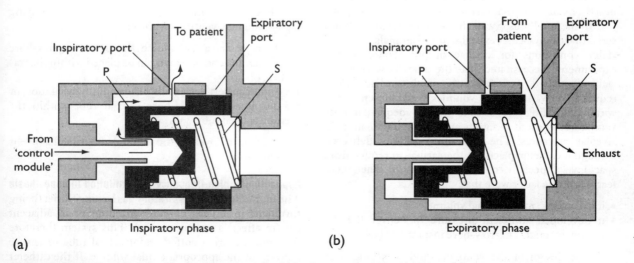

(a)

(b)

Figure 12.22 Working principles of the Pneupac patient valve: (a) inspiratory phase; (b) expiratory phase. P, piston; S, spring. (See text.)

above 90°C. It may be sterilized by any cold chemical agent.

Jet Ventilation

There are two ways in which a high-pressure jet of gas may be used to ventilate a patient:

Simple Jetting (Short Term)

For short procedures such as rigid bronchoscopy, a patient may be paralysed and then ventilated by applying an intermittent jet via the bronchoscope. By the venturi effect, air is entrained by the driving gas, which is usually oxygen, at a pressure of up of 420 kPa (60 psi). The jetting may be delivered via a manually controlled device. Anaesthesia is normally maintained intravenously.

High-Frequency Ventilation

Conventional intermittent positive pressure ventilation, i.e. at rates of 10–30 cycles per minute and with tidal volumes of 50–1000 ml, frequently depresses, as well as produces fluctuations in, cardiac output. During inspiration, the resultant increased alveolar pressure compresses the pulmonary vascular bed and forces the blood contained therein towards the left side of the heart, resulting in a greater stroke volume and a short-lived increase in cardiac output. The compressed pulmonary vascular bed subsequently provides an increased resistance to blood flow, a fall in the blood supply to the left side of the heart and a reduction in cardiac output. During exhalation, the resultant reduction in alveolar pressure causes blood to refill the pulmonary vascular bed preferentially rather than supply the left side of the heart, a manoeuvre that further reduces cardiac output.

In the late 1960s, Swedish researchers, conducting a series of cardiovascular experiments in animals, required stable conditions for cardiac output. However, the experiments necessitated that the animals were artificially ventilated. To achieve the stable cardiac output required, very small tidal volumes were chosen, along with high cycling rates so as to provide adequate minute ventilation without a significant rise or fluctuation in alveolar pressures. The inspiratory gas was delivered through a catheter placed at the carina (to reduce dead space), via a specially constructed ventilator. The salient features of the latter were that:

- it had a very small internal volume;
- it developed sufficient pressure to deliver the gas rapidly through a narrow-bore inspiratory hose.

The design of the ventilator and breathing hose proved to be the most significant factor, as its small internal volume ensured that the very small desired tidal volume was delivered efficiently, and not reduced by being absorbed in the internal volume of the system. (The internal volume of the wide-bore breathing hoses of most conventional ventilators partially absorbs inspiratory gas as a 'compression volume', reducing its speed of delivery and its intended volume.) It soon became apparent that, provided the design principles of the equipment were adhered to, the system provided effective ventilation in humans. The technique not only reduced alveolar pressures, minimizing falls in cardiac output, but also produced further benefits over conventional IPPV (see below). Furthermore, it was discovered that the inspiratory gas could be delivered (with some modification) via more conventional methods such as an endotracheal tube, rather than a catheter placed at the carina. Further investigation revealed that the technique was effective over a wide range of both respiratory rates (60–400 cycles per minute) and tidal volumes (mostly lower than the anticipated anatomical dead space). However, the mechanism by which gas transport occurs is the subject of much debate and is not within the remit of this book.

Advantages of high-frequency ventilation The claimed advantage over conventional ventilatory techniques is efficient alveolar ventilation but with a substantial reduction in mean airway and alveolar pressures. As previously mentioned, this results in:

- a minimal disturbance of cardiac output, and subsequent renal function;
- a reduction in leaks from broncho-pleural fistulae, often with an improvement in gas exchange;
- a more comfortable method of providing ventilator support for patients in the intensive care unit.

The most commonly used methods of applying high-frequency ventilation are via:

- a high-pressure gas source through a narrow-bore catheter, the end of which can be placed within the trachea; or
- a cannula inserted coaxially in an endotracheal tube; or
- a purpose-built, fine-bore coaxial tube within the endotracheal tube wall.

The term covering the methods described above is 'jet ventilation'.

Application of high-frequency jet ventilation in anaesthesia The high velocity of inspiratory gas leaving the jet (being turbulent) produces forward entrainment of adjacent gas (in effect, a venturi device). This system therefore does not require a cuffed endotracheal tube to ensure delivery of the appropriate tidal volume. If the catheter is placed distal to a disrupted airway (for example, during a tracheal resection), adequate ventilation may still be achieved. Furthermore, the small-bore delivery tubes improve surgical access in both pulmonary and laryngeal surgery. Also, the low delivered tidal volumes reduce lung movement, again improving surgical access as well as reducing alveolar pressures, which in turn reduces the risk of barotrauma and gas leaks from broncho-pleural fistulae.

The lower alveolar pressures minimize the adverse effect of positive pressure ventilation on the central venous pressure and cardiac output, with reported benefits in cardiac and neurological surgery.

Apparatus problems associated with high-frequency jet ventilation

Inhalational anaesthesia Current jet ventilation systems (the most popular method) do not readily lend themselves to providing inhalational anaesthesia. Although a nitrous oxide and oxygen mixture can be used with the ventilators (via a high-pressure blender) there are no commercial high-pressure vaporizers available for the addition of inhalational agents. Furthermore, as the jet may sometimes act as a venturi, entrained gas in any attached breathing system needs to be of the same composition as the driving gas in order to guarantee a suitably inspired oxygen concentration.

Humidification Conventional hot-water or condenser humidifiers are impractical for use with high-frequency ventilation, as they have too high an internal volume. The small delivered tidal volumes with high-frequency ventilation get 'lost' in the humidifier and are not delivered to the patient. However, warmed distilled water or saline can be fed into the jet line by a peristaltic pump. As this emerges from the jet it is atomized to provide a degree of humidification, which can be varied by adjusting the speed of the pump.

Measurement of delivered tidal volumes The high respiratory rates and small tidal volumes make conventional measurement of ventilatory functions (expired tidal and minute volumes, and end tidal carbon dioxide) very difficult. A much higher reliance is placed upon blood gas measurement in this situation.

Acutronic VS 150s

This is the anaesthetic version of a range of high-frequency jet ventilators (Fig. 12.23). It is based around a high performance, electronically controlled solenoid valve capable of frequencies up to 500 cycles per minute. The ventilator has three main controls. One alters the rate, another alters the I/E ratio (by altering the percentage of the cycle that is inspiration) and the

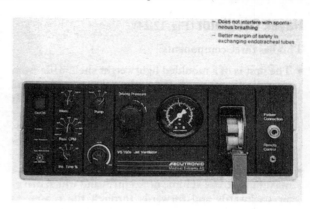

Figure 12.23 The Acutronic VS 150s jet ventilator.

third operates a needle valve that controls the output pressure of the driving gas. The delivered tidal volume/minute volume depends on a combination of all three settings. The unit is capable of delivering up to 60 litres/min.

The ventilator also incorporates a variable speed roller pump that delivers fluids (normal saline or water) to the jet. This mixes with the jetted gas as a nebulized spray to provide humidification.

Safety features The jet line is linked to a pressure transducer that measures the end-expiratory pressure. A factory set upper limit is set at 40 cmH$_2$O. At this pressure the solenoid valve closes until the pressure drops to a safe limit (5–8 cmH$_2$O).

NEGATIVE PRESSURE VENTILATION

A patient's lungs may also be inflated by encasing the patient in a gas-tight container from the neck downwards (tank cuirass) or by a smaller device that surrounds the patient's thorax only (thoracic cuirass), and applying an intermittent subatmospheric pressure (*negative pressure ventilation*). The thorax is 'sucked outwards' during the inspiratory phase causing air/respirable gas to enter the lungs. Exhalation is achieved either by the elastic recoil of the latter or by applying positive pressure to the cuirass.

This method had many attractions: it is non invasive; the patient does not require intubation either orally, nasally or through a tracheostomy; and unlike positive pressure ventilation, it does not reduce cardiac output. The smaller of the two types (thoracic ciurass) has been used in anaesthesia to ventilate patients requiring laryngoscopy and laser therapy without having to use conventional endotracheal intubation.

Hayek Oscillator (Fig. 12.24)

This has three components:

- The first is of a moulded lightweight shell made from clear plastic with soft foam edges that provide a seal around the anterior chest wall and upper abdomen. It comes in three sizes: one for infants, one for larger children and one for adults. Each version has appropriately sized wide-bore tubing that links it to the second component, the power unit.
- The power unit houses a diaphragm pump that has a maximum stroke volume of 3.5 litres and which drives air backwards and forwards through the tubing to intermittently evacuate the shell when it is attached to a patient. A second pump can be used to vary the baseline pressure of the driving gas below atmospheric. This determines the negative end-expiratory pressure within the shell and hence the functional residual capacity of the lungs.
- The third component (the control unit) sets the frequency (8–999) of oscillations per minute, the inspiratory pressure (up to -70 cmH$_2$O), the expiratory pressure (-70 to $+70$ cmH$_2$O) and the inspiratory/ expiratory ratio (6:1 to 1:6). It receives information from a pressure transducer (connected to the shell) so that it can automatically compensate for any alteration in performance.

Although it can function at conventional rates and tidal volumes, it is designed to work in its higher frequency range and with correspondingly smaller tidal volumes.

FURTHER READING

Adams AP, Henville JD (1977) A new generation of anaesthetic ventilators, the Pneupac and Penlon A-P. *Anaesthesia* **32**: 34–40.

Blease 8200S User and Maintenance Manual (1994). Chesham, Bucks, UK: Blease Medical.

Carden Electrovent Ventilator, Operator's Manual Tech Pub. 085 (1992). Sidcup, Kent, UK: Engström MIE Ltd.

Dilkes MG, Broomhead C, McKelvie P, Monks PS (1994) A new method for upper airway laser surgery. *Lasers in Medical Science* **9**: 55–58.

Editorial (1986) High frequency ventilation. *Lancet* **March**: 477–479.

James MFM (1978) The use of a Cape Minor ventilator with the circle absorber system. *Anaesthesia* **33**: 945–949.

Jones PL, Hillard EK (1977) The Flomasta, a new anaesthetic ventilator. *Anaesthesia* **32**: 619–625.

Mushin WW, Rendell-Baker L, Thompson PW, Mapleson WW (1980) *Automatic Ventilation of the Lungs*, 3rd edn. Oxford: Blackwell Scientific.

Ohmeda 7800 Anaesthesia Ventilator Operation and Maintenance Manual (1990). Hatfield, Herts, UK: Ohmeda.

Sjostrand U, Eriksson I (1980) High rates and low volumes in mechanical ventilation – not just a matter of ventilatory frequency. *Anesthesia and Analgesia* **59**: 8.

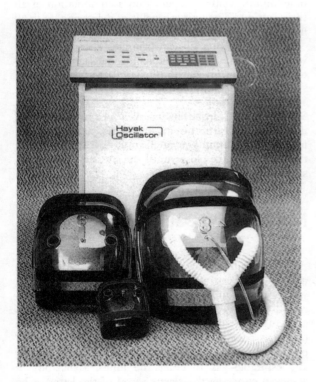

Figure 12.24 The Hayek oscillator with the infant, child and adult thoracic shells.

— 13 —

HUMIDIFIERS AND NEBULIZERS

INTRODUCTION

Humidity is the term used to describe the amount of water vapour present in air or in the gases concerned. The amount of water that a gas can carry depends upon its temperature. The graph in Fig. 13.1 shows the maximum amount of water that can be carried in air and how it varies with temperature.

For the rest of the chapter, unless otherwise stated, the humidity of air will be considered, but the same considerations apply to anaesthetic gases.

DEFINITIONS

The *absolute humidity* is the mass of water vapour actually present in a unit volume of air. It is usually measured in grams per cubic metre (g/m^3).

The maximum mass of water vapour that can be carried in a cubic metre of air at a particular temperature will be referred to in this book as the humidity at saturation (Fig. 13.1).

The *relative humidity* is the ratio between the absolute humidity and the humidity at saturation at the same temperature. It is usually expressed as a percentage.

Some examples will be considered to elucidate the important implications, since these are not always understood.

(1) Suppose that the temperature of air in a room is 15°C and that it has a relative humidity of 50%. From Fig. 13.1 it can be seen that the humidity at saturation at this temperature is about 13 g/ml; the actual amount of

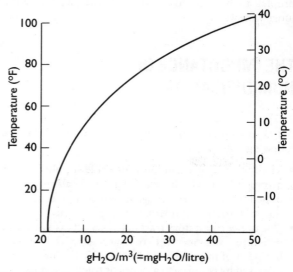

Figure 13.1 The mass of water that is carried at saturated vapour pressure in terms of grams of water per cubic metre of air.

water vapour in the air is therefore 50% of this, i.e. 6.5 g/ml.

At body temperature (37°C), the humidity at saturation is about 43 g/ml. Therefore, when the temperature of the air in the same room is raised to body temperature, its relative humidity is $(6.5/43) \times 100\%$, i.e. approximately 15%. If the air is to be saturated with water vapour within the body, the respiratory epithelium must vaporize $43 - 6.5 = 36.5$ g of water per cubic metre of room air inhaled. Since 1 m^3 is 1000 litres, 36.5 mg of water are required per litre of inspired air.

(2) If a humidifier saturates air at room temperature and then the air is warmed to body temperature, the absolute humidity is unchanged but the relative humidity falls to only about 30%.

(3) If air is saturated with water vapour at body temperature, i.e. in a 'warm' humidifier, and is then allowed to cool to room temperature before it reaches the patient, some of the water vapour will condense out and become liquid again. When the air is eventually rewarmed in the patient's respiratory tract, the relative humidity again will be only 30%. From this it will be seen that if the inspired air is required to have a relative humidity of 100% at body temperature, it will either have to be supersaturated at the lower temperature or will have to be maintained at body temperature after humidification. Supersaturation is achieved by adding to the air a mist or fog of minute droplets of water, which vaporize when the relative humidity falls. It should be understood that humidification refers to the addition to the air of water in the form of either vapour or nebulized droplets. The addition of excessive amounts of water in the form of droplets to the inspired air may lead to overloading of the lungs with water.

THE IMPORTANCE OF HUMIDIFICATION

Air or anaesthetic gases need to be humidified for the following reasons:

- Medical air, oxygen and nitrous oxide supplied either by pipeline or cylinder are dry gases. As already mentioned, this is to protect against corrosion, condensation and frost in cylinders, pipes, valves, etc.
- The upper respiratory tract normally acts as a heat and moisture exchanger (HME) increasing the relative humidity of inspired air to 100% at 37°C. This may be bypassed by endotracheal tubes or tracheostomies.

The atmosphere of the operating theatre, for which there is usually air conditioning, should be kept at a suitable level of relative humidity. This should be between 50 and 70%. Too high a humidity results in a most uncomfortable and tiring atmosphere for the staff, and too low a humidity can increase the risk of explosion due to static electricity. Ventilation and humidifying equipment used in operating theatres does not come within the scope of this book.

Consequences of Under-humidification

- The latent heat of vaporization of water is 2.43 MJ/kg. This energy will be used by the patient to saturate dry inspired gas. Yet more energy will be used to raise its temperature to 37°C. This may amount to up to a third of a neonate's basal heat production, with the possible fall in core temperature of more than 1°C per hour of ventilation with dry gases.
- There is a net loss of water from the patient in exhaled saturated gas.
- Dry gases cause the tracheal mucosa to become dry, inflamed and ulcerated and ciliary movement and mucus flow may also cease. Lung compliance will fall.

Disadvantages and Risks of Humidification

The potential risks of humidification include infection, water intoxication, mucosal cooling, mucosal heating, increase in dead space, and increased resistance to gas flow.

CLASSIFICATION OF HUMIDIFIERS AND NEBULIZERS

The various humidification devices used may be classified according to three criteria:

- Whether they produce water vapour or droplets of water, however small. The latter are generally referred to as nebulizers: the term humidifier refers strictly to the former only. There is a great deal of variation in the size of droplets produced by nebulizers and this will be discussed later.
- The source of energy. This may be either electric power, as in humidifiers and the ultrasonic nebulizer, or the power of a jet of air or gas in the venturi type, which may be used to humidify oxygen from the cylinder or pipeline. The 'bubble bottle', in which the gas is simply bubbled through water, is an example of a passive humidifier, as is the 'artificial nose' or heat and moisture exchanger (HME), which will be described below.
- The third classification is based on whether they are hot or cold. Those that are heated can produce air at body temperature, or even higher, that is saturated with water vapour. Needless to say, caution must be

Table 13.1 Efficiency of humidification systems

	Cold water	Hot water	Nebulizer	HME
Temperature (°C)	Ambient	36–38	23–36	<35
Relative humidity (%)	<100	100	>100	<<100
Absolute humidity (mg/litre)	15–20	42–47	177–1536	27–36
Compliance	Low	Moderate to high	Low	Low

taken to prevent scalding of the patient by air that has been heated to a temperature above that of the body. Some cold nebulizers produce such a profusion of droplets that even when the air has been warmed in the body to body temperature, the droplets are sufficient in mass to produce 100% humidity.

Nebulizers may also be used to administer drugs as an aerosol into the patient. However, unless the droplet size is very small, the drugs may not reach the alveoli as required, but be deposited in the bronchial tree and thus may be ineffectual. The scope for this type of administration of drugs is therefore limited unless there is close control of droplet size.

The four most commonly used humidifiers are:

- ambient temperature water vapour supplier. This usually consists of a water reservoir through which the gas is bubbled, e.g. use of a Boyle's bottle vaporizer;
- heated water vapour supplier or humidifier;
- nebulizer;
- heat and moisture exchanger.

The approximate efficiency of each of these systems is shown in Table 13.1.

Nebulizers

Whilst the heated water vapour humidifier and the heat and moisture exchanger are both sources of water *vapour*, nebulizers supply moisture in the form of water droplets. When considering nebulizers, thought must be given to the size of the particles of water. Too large a droplet will fall out of the 'mist' and be deposited on the breathing tube rather than passing down to the patient's lungs, while too fine a particle will be carried right down almost to the alveoli but will not sufficiently humidify the patient's tracheal and bronchial mucosa. The graph in Fig. 13.2 relates the size of droplets to the area of fall-out.

Ultrasonic nebulizers are useful for the dispersal of antiseptics when sterilizing anaesthetic machines and ventilators and some may be connected directly to the breathing system. However, problems have been experienced when using them for the humidification of gases, because the amount of water nebulized was excessive and virtually drowned the patient.

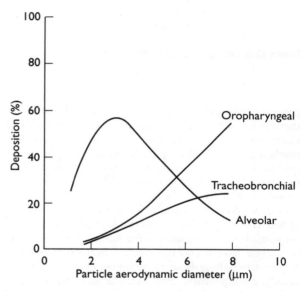

Figure 13.2 Droplet size and anatomical area of fallout. It can be seen that the type of nebulizer must be chosen according to the required fallout area. (Reproduced with permission from Clarke, SW. *Aerosols and the Lung: Clinical and Experimental Aspects*).

EXAMPLES OF HUMIDIFICATION EQUIPMENT

(1) A simple bottle humidifier (Fig. 13.3) may be used to humidify oxygen for administration to a patient in the ward situation. If the air passes over the surface of the water, a modest amount of vaporization takes place. Unless there is a very large surface area of water and a very low flow rate of gas, however, the air is by no means saturated with water vapour. Improvements to this type of humidifier may be made by either bubbling the air through the water or increasing the surface area with wicks immersed in the water, in the same way as in vaporizers for volatile anaesthetic agents (Fig. 13.4). To increase humidification further, the bottle may be heated (Fig. 13.5).

In the case of heated humidifiers, the temperature of the water must be thermostatically controlled. In

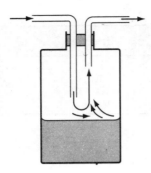

Figure 13.3 Simple bottle humidifier.

general two thermostats in series are used, so that if one thermostat were to fail the other would still cut off the electricity supply before a dangerous temperature was reached. After use, this type of humidifier may be sterilized by intentionally boiling the water inside it although modern units of this type usually have disposable water chambers (Fig. 13.5). The outlet and delivery tube from a heated humidifier should be lagged, if possible, to reduce the cooling that would result in condensation of some of the water vapour. Some heated water humidifiers even have a co-axial electric heater wire in the attached breathing hose to maintain the temperature. Ideally, a temperature sensor should be installed at the patient end of the delivery tube, in order to allow the

maintenance of maximum efficiency without the risk of scalding the patient.

Where the gases are bubbled through water, provision should be made to prevent the accidental reverse connection of the bottle, which would cause the water to be forced along the delivery tube to the patient.

(2) Water vapour or steam may be produced simply by boiling water. This is not a satisfactory method for use in conjunction with anaesthetic apparatus, but may be useful in the treatment of a patient, especially in his or her own home, by humidifying the whole atmosphere of the room. Simple steam therapy achieved by boiling water is not appropriate in hospitals and the danger of scalding the patient should be remembered.

(3) A jet of air or gases may be used to entrain water drawn up from a reservoir (Fig. 13.6a). As the water enters the jet it is broken up into a large number of droplets, i.e. it is nebulized. This principle is used in simple sprays for administering topical analgesics and is also used to humidify the inspired air in some ventilators. Such nebulizers create large droplets, but if these are made to impinge on a solid 'anvil' they are broken up into smaller ones.

(4) The water may also be broken up into a large number of small droplets by causing a fine jet to impinge upon one or more objects, such as pins, while subjected to a moving air stream (Fig. 13.6b).

(5) In ultrasonic nebulizers (Fig. 13.7), water is broken up into droplets or fine particles by a continual sonic bombardment generated by a high-frequency resonator.

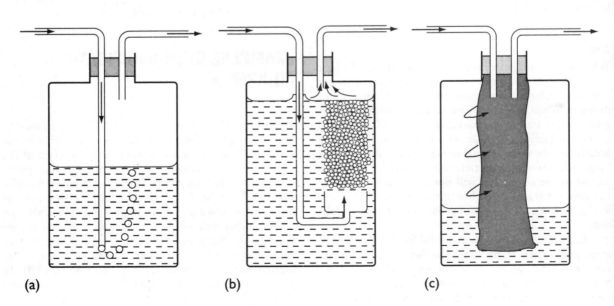

(a)   (b)   (c)

Figure 13.4 Methods of increasing humidification. (a) Bubbling gas through water; (b) using a sintered filter, which produces many small bubbles with consequent greater surface area, hence maximizing the rate of humidification; and (c) by immersing a wick.

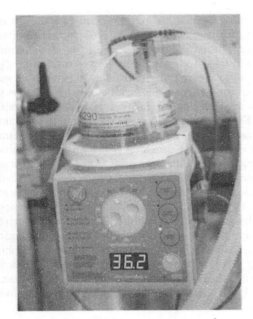

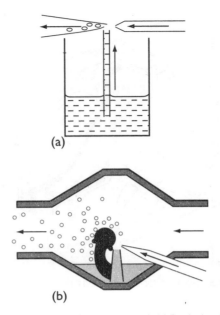

Figure 13.5 A Fisher & Paykel electrically heated humidifier. The vaporization chamber is disposable and may be fed continuously with sterile water. The heater has protective thermostats and a heating wire may be used inside the patient tubing to maintain the temperature up to the endotracheal tube.

Figure 13.6 The principle of the nebulizer. (a) Employing the Bernoulli effect, a jet of air may be used to draw a liquid up a small tube from a reservoir and to entrain it as droplets. (b) The droplets may be made to impinge on an 'anvil', so causing them to be broken up into still smaller droplets.

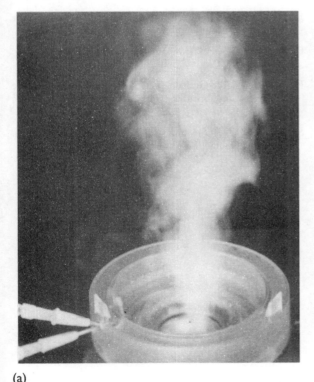

(a)

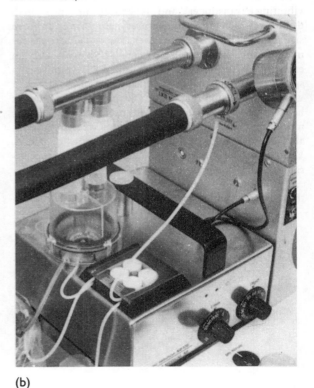

(b)

Figure 13.7 A cloud of droplets emerging from an ultrasonic nebulizer. This form of nebulizer is extremely efficient and there is a risk of drowning the patient! (b) The delivery of the correct volume of water by a peristaltic pump in the NB 108 nebulizer.

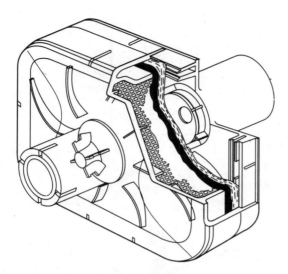

Figure 13.8 A typical disposable heat and moisture exchanging filter.

Two types of ultrasonic nebulizer require further comment. In one, a drop of water is allowed to fall on a vibrating 'transducer' and is broken up into small droplets (which one manufacturer claims are of uniform size, around 1 µm). In the other, the transducer is submerged and droplets of a variety of sizes, usually in excess of 1 µm, are produced. Since the volume of a sphere is proportional to the third power of the radius, it will be appreciated that a 2 µm droplet is eight times as heavy as a 1 µm droplet, and will therefore 'fall out' far more quickly. If the 'submerged' type of transducer is allowed to run dry, it may be irreparably damaged. Various measures to prevent such damage are incorporated in some models.

(6) Heat and moisture exchangers (HMEs) are of three types: condenser, hygroscopic and hydrophobic.

The purpose of the HME is to conserve the patient's own heat and moisture without external energy or water supply. The earliest type, the condenser HME, consists of a wire mesh screen in the path of the respiratory gases, as close to the mouth as possible. On exhalation, water vapour condenses on the wire mesh and this then evaporates again during the inspiratory phase. Hygroscopic HMEs are more efficient, as a greater proportion of expiratory water vapour is adsorbed into its element. This element may consist of paper coated with calcium chloride, glass fibre, or polypropylene coated with lithium chloride. The latest HMEs are of the hydrophobic type, which has a folded ceramic fibre element.

Both the hygroscopic and the hydrophobic types are much more efficient than the condenser type, which also suffers from the disadvantage that it provides no microbiological barrier. The hygroscopic and the hydrophobic types both provide some bacteriological protection, although the hydrophobic is said to be more efficient.

The construction of a typical HME is shown in Fig. 13.8.

FURTHER READING

Burton JDK (1962) The effects of dry anaesthetic gases on the respiratory mucous membrane. *Lancet* **Feb**: 235–238.

Clarke SW, Demetri P (1984) *Aerosols and the Lung*. London: Butterworth & Co.

Hedley RM, Allt-Graham J (1994) Heat and moisture exchangers and breathing filters (review article). *British Journal of Anaesthesia* **73**: 227–236.

Shelly MP (1993) *Intensive Care Rounds – Humidification*. Abingdon, Oxon, UK: The Medicine Group (Education).

—14—

EQUIPMENT FOR PAEDIATRIC ANAESTHESIA

Contents

INTRODUCTION

Various items of equipment required for paediatric anaesthesia have already been described in the appropriate chapters. It is important to understand the reasons why these differ from those employed for anaesthetizing adults. When selecting apparatus for paediatric anaesthesia, account must be taken of the respiratory physiological, anatomical and mechanical factors involved, which differ from those that present when adults are being anaesthetized. Even these may differ when comparing a neonate (up to 28-days old) to an infant (up to 1-year old) or a child (older than 1 year).

Difference in Respiratory Physiology Between Adults and Children

- Respiration in infants and neonates has a more sinusoidal pattern than in adults. The absence of an expiratory pause decreases the time in which fresh gas is able to flush away alveolar gas which is present at the end of expiration in all partial rebreathing systems (Mapleson A, D, E and F). This renders them all relatively less efficient during spontaneous respiration than in adults.
- Tidal volumes are small in infants and neonates so that any increased apparatus dead space may well become a high proportion of the tidal volume, with a significant effect on carbon dioxide elimination, oxygenation and the resultant increased work of breathing.
- Furthermore, any resistance to airflow caused by turbulence in breathing systems and angled connectors also increases the work of breathing. If the volume of the breathing system is high, this requires considerable kinetic energy expenditure in repeatedly reversing the direction of air flow within it.

Thus a system such as the Magill breathing system (Mapleson A), with high internal volume, relatively large apparatus dead space (see Fig. 14.1) and an APL valve providing expiratory resistance, is inappropriate in neonates and small infants. In fact, several adult breathing systems, even if scaled down, may not necessarily be suitable for infants and less so for neonates.

Anatomical Differences Between Adults and Children

The anatomy of the upper airway of a neonate, infant or child is different from that of an adult:

- Up to the age of eight or nine, the narrowest part is at the cricoid ring and not the larynx as in an adult. Hence tubes that pass easily through the larynx may well be too tight a fit at the cricoid ring.
- Since the diameter of the laryngeal and cricoid inlet of an infant is narrow and if intubation is to be carried

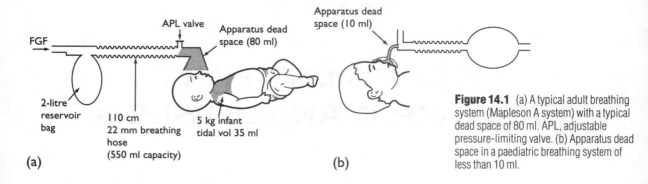

Figure 14.1 (a) A typical adult breathing system (Mapleson A system) with a typical dead space of 80 ml. APL, adjustable pressure-limiting valve. (b) Apparatus dead space in a paediatric breathing system of less than 10 ml.

out the tube will further reduce the effective diameter of this airway. A small reduction in the airway diameter of an already small air passage will greatly increase the resistance to flow (Poiseuille's law, *see* Chapter 1) and may provide too great a resistance to spontaneous respiration. Many anaesthetists would thus electively ventilate an infant who is intubated with a small endotracheal tube (2–3.5 mm internal diameter).

A similar situation arises when a tube that was too tight a fit is removed from a small airway. The resultant mucosal oedema and small reduction in airway diameter may be enough to cause severe respiratory embarrassment.

For these reasons, the material used and the design of the tube assume far greater importance in small children than in adults. For instance, some manufacturers' tubes have a greater internal diameter (due to thinner walls) than others of similar external diameter and may therefore be preferred when small tubes are required (Table 14.1). Similarly, plain tubes also provide a greater internal diameter than cuffed tubes of the same external diameter. This is because cuffed tubes have thicker (stronger) walls in order to reduce the possibility of inward herniation of the tube wall underneath the cuff site when the cuff is inflated. Plain tubes are thus almost always chosen when tubes of 6 mm internal diameter or less are required. In any case, the cricoid ring, being near circular in a child, provides a better fit, obviating the need for a cuff.

Table 14.1 Dimensions of some non-cuffed infant endotracheal tubes

Manufacturer	Int. diameter (mm)	Ext. diameter (mm)
Portex (silicone)	2.5	3.4
Sheridan (Ped-soft)	2.5	3.6
Portex (ivory)	2.5	3.6
Mallinckrodt (PVC)	2.5	3.6
Rusch (clearway)	2.5	4.0
Mallinckrodt (reinforced)	2.5	4.0
Portex (reinforced)	2.5	4.0
Rusch (rubber)	2.5	4.0
Portex (silicone)	3.0	4.2
Sheridan (Ped-soft)	3.0	4.2
Portex (ivory)	3.0	4.4
Mallinckrodt (PVC)	3.0	4.3
Rusch (clearway)	3.0	4.7
Mallinckrodt (reinforced)	3.0	4.7
Portex (reinforced)	3.0	4.7
Rusch (rubber)	3.0	4.7
Portex (silicone)	3.5	4.8
Sheridan (Ped-soft)	3.5	4.9
Portex (ivory)	3.5	5.0
Mallinckrodt (PVC)	3.5	4.9
Rusch (clearway)	3.5	5.3
Mallinckrodt (reinforced)	3.5	5.3
Portex (reinforced)	3.5	5.3
Rusch (rubber)	3.5	5.3

SPECIAL EQUIPMENT IN PAEDIATRIC ANAESTHESIA

The Anaesthetic Machine

A continuous flow machine is needed: intermittent flow or draw-over machines require too much inspiratory effort by the patient and are therefore unsuitable for small children. The single exception is that in dental-chair anaesthesia of short duration; varying flow machines, such as the McKesson intermittent flow machine, the AE or the Walton Five, may be used provided that the 'pressure' control is advanced sufficiently to give an adequate fresh gas flow (FGF) rate.

The vaporizer should be of a type that gives an accurate percentage of vapour, even when low flow rates are used. Nevertheless, in most instances a relatively high FGF rate is employed.

There should be a pressure relief valve at the end of the back bar, particularly where the regulated supply pressure to the anaesthetic machine is high, i.e. 420 kPa (60 psi).

Breathing Systems

Breathing systems for use with very small children should ideally:

- have minimal functional/apparatus dead space;
- be either valveless or fitted with very low resistance valves;
- have small internal gas volumes;
- be constructed in such a way as to minimize gas turbulence and subsequent flow resistance.

Mapleson D, E and F systems (see Chapter 8) are the most commonly used as they most closely meet the criteria for an ideal paediatric system. These are based

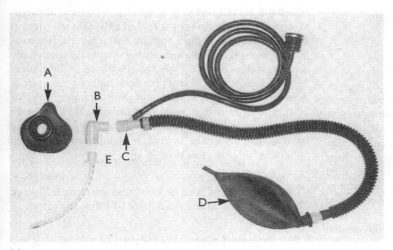

Figure 14.2 (a) Recent version of the Jackson Rees modification to Ayre's T-piece paediatric breathing system. A, Rendell–Baker paediatric facemask; B, right-angle connector; C, T-piece; D, reservoir bag; E, 15 mm ISO standard endotracheal connector. (b) A disposable lightweight plastic Mapleson E system.

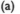
(a)

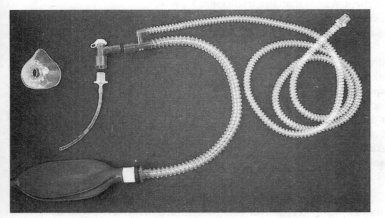
(b)

on modifications to Ayre's original T-piece system. The most commonly used of these is the Mapleson F (Jackson Rees modification, Fig. 14.2).

The three arms of the modified T-piece are employed as follows:

- One is supplied by a continous flow of fresh gas.
- Another is fitted with a suitable length of breathing hose that is attached to a distensible bag with an exit hole in its tail. This arm acts as both reservoir for the bulk of the inspired gas and also as the low–resistance expiratory pathway.
- The third arm is attached as closely as possible to the patient's airway. This is because its internal volume constitutes the apparatus dead space which should be as small as possible.

The low resistance to airflow as a result of the abscence of valves and the small apparatus dead space make it the preferred system for both spontaneous and controlled ventilation in paediatric anaesthesia.

Fresh Gas Flow Rates in D, E and F Systems

These depend on:

- the capacity of the reservoir limb;
- the metabolic status and size of the patient;
- the respiratory rate.

The capacity of the reservoir limb especially without a reservoir bag is important. It should contain a volume equal to or greater than the intended tidal volume. If it is less than the patient's tidal volume, air entrainment is possible at low FGF rates. In the extreme where the expiratory limb presents mainly as an orifice, then the FGF rate should be equal to the peak inspiratory flow rate to prevent air entrainment and dilution of inhaled anaesthetic gases.

As these systems do not include unidirectional valves to prevent exhaled gas mixing with fresh gas, the elimination of carbon dioxide is largely dependent on the flushing effect of fresh gas flowing through them. As carbon dioxide production increases with the size of the patient and metabolic state, so its elimination will require an increase in FGF.

The respiratory rate plays an important part in deciding the FGF rate in T-piece systems both for controlled and, more importantly, spontaneous respiration. A longer expiratory phase allows a greater time for fresh gas to: (a) flush downstream the expired gas entering the reservoir limb; and (b) to fill the proximal part of the system. This reduces or removes the presence of exhaled carbon dioxide in the initial portion of the subsequent inspiratory mixture. One formula that takes this into account is:

$$\text{FGF rate (ml/min)} = 15 \times \text{weight (kg)} \times \text{respiratory rate (per min)}$$

i.e. a 10 kg infant with a respiratory rate varying between 20 and 30 breaths per minute requires an FGF rate of between 3000 and 4500 ml/min.

These systems are discussed in greater detail in Chapter 8 (pp. 118–119).

Modifications to Ayre's T-piece Arrangement

Several methods of reducing the apparatus/functional dead space even further than Ayre's original T-piece have been described.

The Cape Town attachment (Fig. 14.3a). This directs fresh gas into the endotracheal/facemask connection. The functional dead space of this system has been shown to be less than the apparatus dead space owing to the continuous flushing action of the fresh gas.

Co-axial arrangement (Fig. 14.3b). A co-axial arrangement of the gas delivery tube, as in a Bain system, acts in a similar manner to the Cape Town attachment. It is worthy of note that the Bain breathing system is functionally similar to the T-piece. Only the resistance in the expiratory valve (when present) for spontaneous respiration and the increased compliance of the long outer limb (for intermittent positive pressure ventilation (IPPV)) make it functionally inferior for use in infants. When the valve is used as part of the system, it should not be used in children weighing less than 20 kg.

The Y-piece (Fig. 14.3c). Fresh gas entering a Y-piece reduces the functional dead space by a flushing effect.

The Bethune T-piece (Fig. 14.3d). In this system, the FGF enters the breathing system closer to the patient than in a traditional T-piece.

Jackson Rees T-tube (Fig. 14.3e). The T-piece is incorporated within an endotracheal tube. However, the T-piece has the same internal diameter as the tube and so has an increased resistance to flow when compared with a standard arrangement.

Some manufacturers produce compendia of fittings that may be connected up by the anaesthetist to form a variety of breathing systems. If these are used, it must be ensured that they are suitably assembled and that the basic principles, such as the reduction of dead space and the prevention of rebreathing without carbon dioxide absorption, are observed. They are capable of being assembled incorrectly, with dangerous consequences.

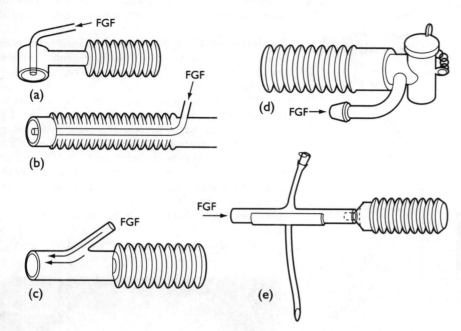

Figure 14.3 Modifications to Ayre's T-piece arrangement. (a) Cape Town arrangement; (b) co-axial arrangement; (c) Y-piece; (d) Bethune T-piece; (e) Jackson Rees T-tube. FGF, fresh gas flow.

Mapleson A Systems

The efficiency of this system in children depends not only on its ability to function as an A system (*see* Chapter 8) but in the ability of various commercial designs in minimizing the apparatus dead space, as well as decreasing the resistance to flow in any mechanical expiratory valve used.

The Magill configuration, with a standard APL valve placed between the patient and the FGF, increases the apparatus dead space (40 ml without facemask) and should not be used in children weighing less than 20 kg. (see Fig. 14.1). However, systems such as the Lack and the A configuration of the Humphrey ADE (*see* Chapter 8) deposit fresh gas much closer to the patient's airway (apparatus dead space 1.8 ml) and are consequently more effective.

The Humphrey A system modified to use 15 mm breathing hose has been used in paediatric patients weighing under 15 kg during spontaneous respiration. Fresh gas flow of approximately 123 ml/kg/min from the system has been shown to prevent rebreathing compared with 386 ml/kg/min for a traditional Mapleson F arrangement of the Ayre's T-piece.

In all versions of the Mapleson A system, if the standard 2 litre bag is replaced by a 1 litre bag, then respiratory movements will be more easily observed in small patients. This does not necessarily mean that the system becomes more efficient, however. Mapleson A systems should not be used for controlled ventilation in children because the required FGF to prevent rebreathing is high and unpredictable.

Mapleson B Systems

A refinement of the Mapleson B system for paediatric use is the Rendell-Baker system. Dead space is reduced by introducing the fresh gas through a chimney arrangement as near as possible to the patient (Fig. 14.4). Expired gas is vented via a second chimney to a smaller and lighter APL valve than would conventionally be used. Fresh gas flow rates for spontaneous respiration should be set at two to three times the anticipated minute ventilation (i.e. more than for a Mapleson A but slightly less than that required for a Mapleson D system).

Systems Utilizing Carbon Dioxide Absorption

In the days when cyclopropane, which is explosive and costly, was commonly used there was a preference for these systems. 'To-and-fro' absorption systems with a 'Waters' canister or similar device did not prove altogether satisfactory. This is because there was:

- a large dead space, which increased as the soda lime at the patient end of the canister became exhausted;
- and as the absorber had to be placed close to the patient's head, it was cumbersome and it increased the possibility of the inhalation of soda lime dust.

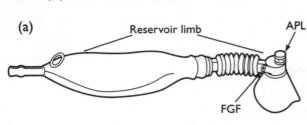

(a)

Reservoir limb

APL

FGF

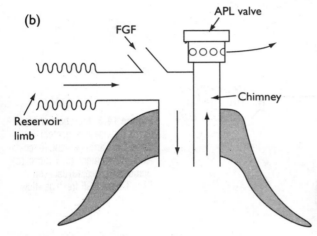

(b)

FGF

APL valve

Chimney

Reservoir limb

Figure 14.4 (a) Rendell–Baker system. (b) Working principles showing the 'chimney' and paediatric facemask which reduce the apparatus dead space.

Adult circle absorbers can be used for children, but it is preferable to use breathing systems with scaled-down components and tubing, in order to overcome the inertia of large volumes of gases. Special facemask mounts overcame the problems of weight and, by incorporating a chimney, reduced the dead space. More modern, lightweight plastic tubing and components, in which the need for antistatic precautions has been obviated by the use of non-explosive anaesthetic agents, lend themselves to more suitable breathing attachments for paediatric work. With the increasing awareness of atmospheric pollution and the use of scavenging systems, there may be a return of the popularity of low flow systems.

THE COMPONENTS OF A BREATHING SYSTEM

Reservoir bags These may be smaller than the usual 2 litre bag used for adults, 0.5 or 1 litre bags being the most popular. The capacity of the bag must be not less than the patient's tidal volume. The material of which it is constructed must not be too stiff and if it is to be used with a

Mapleson D or F system, which is valveless, it should have a tail that can be cut so that it becomes open-ended.

Reinforced breathing hose The new plastic hoses available are considerably lighter than the old rubber or neoprene ones. They therefore drag far less on the facemask or endotracheal tube. They may also be of smaller diameter; 15 mm smooth-bore hosing is now available with a reinforcing spiral attached to its outer surface. The smooth inner lining produces less resistance to flow when compared with corrugated hose of similar diameter. The lack of corrugation also makes it easier to clean and less likely to harbour infection. Some plastic hoses have the disadvantage that although they may be easily coiled up, they offer resistance to twisting along their long axis. This may cause them either to kink or to transmit the torque to an endotracheal tube, which may then be either displaced or sufficiently twisted to become occluded (Fig. 14.5).

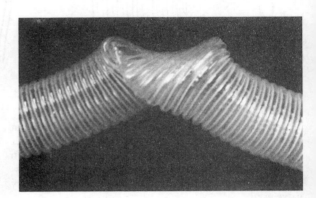

Figure 14.5 A lightweight corrugated hose may become twisted along its long axis and as a result become obstructed. This is because it is not flexible around its long axis.

APL (expiratory) valves The Heidbrink valve may offer too much resistance for an infant. There are several smaller, lighter valves, such as the Rendell-Baker (Fig. 14.4), made of plastic and having a chimney to reduce dead space.

AIRWAY MANAGEMENT DEVICES

Facemasks Facemasks for neonates and infants, an example of which is shown in Fig. 14.6 (see also Chapter 8), are usually anatomically moulded to fit the face as closely as possible. Considerable experience in the selection of a facemask of exactly the right size is required to achieve a good fit but without obstructing the nares.

Flaps and inflatable rims are not necessary, as the smooth, round and soft tissues of the patient's face usually facilitate a good fit. For larger infants and children a facemask with a flap, may be used.

Facemask mounts The mount or angle piece is constructed so that it also minimizes apparatus dead space. This is achieved by: (a) siting it on the mask so that it is positioned immediately over the airway; and (b) dividing the internal lumen into two so that one channel provides inspiratory gas and the other ducts away exhaled gas (Fig. 14.6).

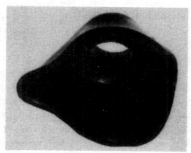

Figure 14.6 A paediatric facemask.

Pharyngeal airways Scaled-down versions of adult oropharyngeal and nasopharyngeal airways are manufactured in a range of sizes and patterns and are discussed in Chapter 9.

Laryngeal mask airways These are available in sizes to fit neonates, infants and children. Their use and

mode of insertion are again discussed more fully in Chapter 9.

Endotracheal connectors Prior to any standardization, connector sizes were left to individual designs (Magill connectors, 13 mm; Worcester, 12 mm; Metal Cardiff, 12 mm; Knight, 9 mm; Bennett, 14 mm). However, a 15 mm ISO connection size was standardized, which, although suitable for adults and large children, could be too cumbersome for infants and neonates. More recently, 8.5 mm connectors have become available for endotracheal tube sizes of 2–6 mm internal diameter, with adaptors to connect to the 15 mm standard if required. The Portex Mini-Link system shown in Fig. 14.7 is an example of this new system.

Endotracheal tube types

Magill pattern Magill tubes (Fig. 14.8a,b) are curved, parallel-sided and bevelled at the tip from left to right so that they would, if too long, pass down the right main bronchus. They are probably the most commonly used tubes and are supplied long, requiring cutting to length. They can be made of red rubber or thermoplastic and can be passed either nasally or orally. Of the two examples shown, one (a) has the 8.5 Mini-Link connector whilst the other (b) has the 15 mm ISO standard connector.

Armoured tubes (Fig. 14.8c). The armour is provided by a nylon or wire spiral embedded in the wall of the tube which prevents it from kinking when the tube is acutely angled. The inevitable thickness of the tube is often too

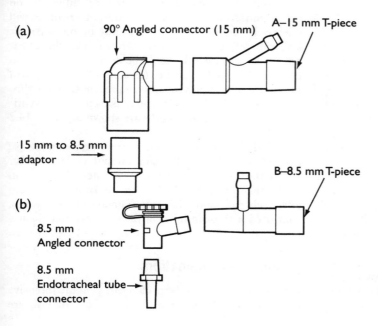

Figure 14.7 Paediatric breathing system connectors showing 15 mm ISO standard (a) and 8.5 mm Portex Mini-Link (b) systems with adaptors for interconnection of the two systems as required.

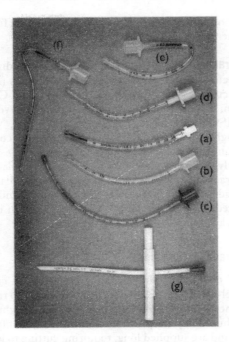

Figure 14.8 Disposable paediatric endotracheal tubes. a, Magill endotracheal tube with 8.5 mm connector; b, Magill endotracheal tube with 15 mm ISO connector; c, reinforced endotracheal tube; d, Cole endotracheal tube; e, oral RAE endotracheal tube; f, nasotracheal RAE endotracheal tube; g, Jackson Rees nasotracheal T-tube.

great for neonatal use. Formerly, armoured tubes were constructed of latex or red rubber, which perishes rapidly, but recently silicone rubber armoured tubes have been developed.

Cole pattern tubes (Fig. 14.8d). The body of a Cole pattern tube is relatively large, culminating in a shoulder leading to a small intratracheal section. The design minimizes the possibility of endobronchial insertion as the body is too large to pass through the larynx. However, the flow resistance of these tubes is greater than that of the parallel-sided variety because of turbulence at the shoulder. Furthermore, laryngeal damage caused by pressure from the shoulder can occur and the tube is not now in common use.

RAE (Ring, Adair and Elwin) pattern tubes (Fig. 14.8e,f). There are two separate versions of these tubes (named after their inventors, Ring, Adair and Elwin). The tube for orotracheal intubation (Fig. 14.8e) has a preformed bend on that part of the tube where it exits the mouth, so that the part housing the ISO connection passes down the chin and away from the face so improving surgical access to the mouth, nose and head of the patient. The nasotracheal version (Fig. 14.8f) is bent where it

exits the nose so that the part housing the ISO connection passes upwards to the forehead. It is used to improve surgical access in intraoral procedures. The main disadvantage of both designs is in the fixed length of the intraoral section. This is rarely too short but is occasionally too long and can enter a main bronchus to provide unilateral ventilation. Although it may be withdrawn into the trachea, the preformed curve no longer fits the face snugly and securing the tube becomes difficult. Also, the oral version of the tube in the smaller sizes has been known to kink at the point of maximum curvature, especially when used with a Boyle–Davis gag. Furthermore, because of their shape and length, tubes with internal diameters of 3 mm or less have appreciably more resistance to flow than equivalent-sized Magill pattern plastic tubes and should perhaps be used only with controlled ventilation.

Jackson Rees paediatric tube (Fig. 14.8g). This is intended for nasotracheal intubation. The proximal end is cross-shaped. One arm of the longitudinal section has a suction facility (sealed with a spigot) whilst the other is the actual nasotracheal tube. The transverse section behaves as the T-piece.

Orotracheal Intubation

Choice of the appropriate size of endotracheal tubes for infants and neonates is very important. Tubes must be of a size that, when inserted, allow a small leak when tested with positive-pressure ventilation. A tube that is big enough to compress the tracheal mucosa may well produce mucosal oedema resulting in a reduction in the airway size that can cause respiratory difficulty on extubation. Mucosal oedema of 1 mm in a neonate will effectively reduce the tracheal airway by 60%! An air leak is therefore essential to demonstrate that the tube is not too large. The leak should be detectable at inflation pressures of less than 2.5 kPa (25 cmH$_2$O). The length of the tube is also important so as to prevent the tube slipping down a main bronchus and causing unilateral ventilation. Tube sizes and lengths are shown in Tables 14.2 and 14.3.

Cuffed endotracheal tubes are undesirable for use in children aged under 10 years. The cuff and the thicker wall of the tube (designed to prevent internal herniation of the tube under the cuff when the latter is inflated) effectively reduce the internal diameter of these tubes, compared with plain tubes of the same external diameter.

Nasotracheal Intubation

Where intubation is to be prolonged, as in the Intensive Care Unit, nasal tubes may be preferable. Not only are

Table 14.2 Diameters of endotracheal tubes for various ages

Age of patient	Internal diameter of tube (mm)
Preterm	2.5
At birth	3.0 or 3.5
6 months	4.0
1 year	4.5
Over 1 year	According to formula: Age in years ÷ 4 + 4.5

From Jackson Rees, G. and Cecil Gray, T. *Paediatric Anaesthesia – Trends in Current Practice*. London: Butterworths (1981).

Table 14.3 Endotracheal tubes: correct lengths for given diameters

Nasal		Oral	
Diameter (mm)	Length (mm)	Diameter (mm)	Length (mm)
2.5	13.0	2.5	10.5
3.0	13.0	3.0	10.5
3.5	14.0	3.5	11.0
4.0	14.5	4.0	12.0
4.5	15.0	4.5	13.5
5.0	16.5	5.0	14.0
5.5	17.0	5.5	14.5
6.0	17.5	6.0	15.0
6.5	18.5	6.5	16.0
7.0	19.0	7.0	17.5
8.0	19.5	8.0	18.5

From Jackson Rees, G. and Cecil Gray, T. *Paediatric Anaesthesia – Trends in Current Practice*. London: Butterworths (1981).

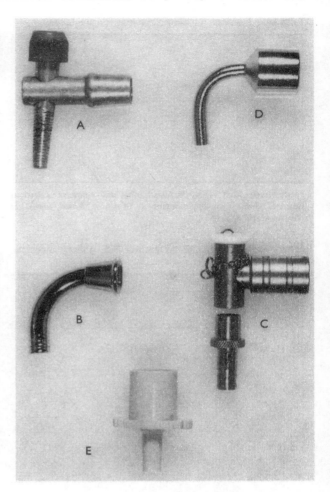

Figure 14.9 Paediatric endotracheal tube connectors. A, Cardiff; B, Magill; C, Oxford; D, Penlon; E, Portex.

they less restrictive of access to the mouth, e.g. for tube feeding, they are also less prone to movement within the trachea and thus to traumatizing the delicate mucosa in that area since they are splinted by the nose and nasopharynx.

Resistance to Gas Flow in Breathing Systems

Endotracheal connectors (Fig. 14.9). Most connectors for neonates have been shown to create turbulent flow at flow rates seen in clinical practice. Although the ISO standard (15 mm) connector is supplied with most endotracheal tubes, it is not the one with the least resistance to gas flow, as can be seen from Table 14.4. Of the now non-standard connectors, the curved versions were always thought to be better at creating laminar flow and reducing flow resistance. However, this is not necessarily the case. Curved connectors (Magill) perform no better than an angled Cardiff connector. Fifteen-millimetre connectors (ISO Tapers, Portex and Penlon cones) have higher resistances to flow even though they do not have a bend in

them. This is caused by turbulence at the junction with the taper used for attachment to an endotracheal tube.

Endotracheal tubes Resistance to flow in an endotracheal tube is proportional to its length (so a shorter tube is preferable). Its cross-sectional area is also important. The larger this is, the less the resistance will be. In small tubes the flow is usually turbulent and so is related to the radius multiplied by the power of 2 (see Chapter 1). Plastic tubes have been shown to have thinner walls than red rubber tubes of a similar internal diameter. It may therefore be possible to use plastic tubes half a size larger than red rubber tubes, with a corresponding reduction in flow resistance (Table 14.5).

The resistance of Jackson Rees tubes when measured between one side of the wide-bore cross-arm and the tracheal limb (with the suction port and the other

Table 14.4 Resistance of tracheal tube connectors (cmH$_2$O/litre/s)

Connector	Smallest ID (mm)	Fresh gas flow (litres/min)		
		1	3	5
Cardiff	2.6	9	20	30
Magill	2.8	12	22	32
Oxford	2.5	12	24	36
Oxford	3.0	5	10	15
Penlon 15 mm cone	2.5	21	30	44
Portex 15 mm cone	2.7	13	24	33

From Hatch, D. J. (1978) Tracheal tubes and connectors used in neonates: dimensions and resistance to breathing. *British Journal of Anaesthesia* **50**: 959–964.

Table 14.5 Resistance of endotracheal tube without connectors (cmH$_2$O/litre/s)

	Flow (litres/min)		
	1	3	5
2.5 mm			
Portex	19	21	23
Rubber	15	17	20
JR	45	74	106
3.0 mm			
Portex	8	11	12
Rubber	12	15	17
JR	24	35	47
3.5 mm			
Portex	4	5	7
Rubber	7	9	11
JR	18	26	30

JR, Jackson Rees.

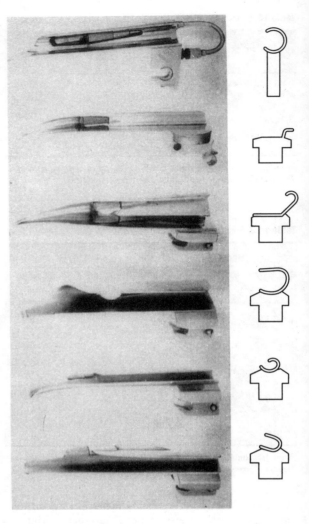

Figure 14.10 Straight laryngoscope blades for use in infants. From top: Anderson–Magill, Seward, Robertshaw, Oxford, Miller, Wisconsin. (Reproduced from Hatch and Sumner (1986) *Neonatal Anaesthesia and Perioperative Care*. Arnold, London.)

side of the wide-bore cross-arm occluded) was substantially greater than that of equivalent-sized Portex tubes.

LARYNGOSCOPES

When compared with an adult, the neonate has a more anteriorly placed laryngeal inlet that is more easily obscured by a relatively larger and more floppy epiglottis and tongue. The intubating view is improved by using laryngoscopes with either straight blades or less curved blades than those of an adult Mackintosh laryngoscope. The choice of paediatric laryngoscope and blades is extensive and selection is largely a matter of user preference. Some examples of laryngoscope blades are shown in Fig.14.10.

SUCTION EQUIPMENT

When treating neonates and infants, a relatively low-power vacuum should be used in spite of the fact that a very narrow catheter may be needed to aspirate viscous secretions. Too high a vacuum could result in pulmonary atelectasis. Damage to the delicate mucosa could result from the employment of a catheter with an inappropriate termination by performing a 'suction biopsy'. Paediatric suction catheters should have a limiting pressure vent in the handle that can be occluded or partially occluded by a thumb to control suction pressure, as well as having a tip with multiple side holes so that the suction tip does not attach itself to the tracheal wall.

VENTILATORS

Chapter 11 describes ventilators in general and includes automatic ventilators that may be used for children, infants and neonates. However, there are some practical points that should be considered here. In the latter two groups, controlled ventilation is administered through narrow-bore tubes and as small tidal volumes. In order to do this efficiently, a ventilator and breathing system should have a small internal volume (and thus a low compliance). The latter allows the pressure to rise rapidly at the beginning of inspiration to that required so that gas is pushed through to the alveoli efficiently.

Neonates

The simplest way to achieve IPPV in infants and neonates is to employ a T-piece system and intermittently occlude the expiratory limb with a thumb or with a ventilator, which performs the same function mechanically or pneumatically (T-piece occluder). The disadvantage of this system is that the inspiratory flow rate is limited to the FGF rate. This is suitable for neonates and infants, but is a great waste of fresh gas in children above 20 kg. T-piece occluders are therefore of limited value in the older child.

Children

Adding a bellows or bag to the expiratory limb (as in the Jackson Rees modification of the T-piece) allows much larger tidal volumes to be given. This is because FGF is augmented by gases that have been displaced from the expiratory limb as a result of the 'bag' being squeezed. This can be done in several ways:

- Some 'bag squeezer' ventilators have the ability to substitute the adult bellows for a paediatric version with a much smaller volume (e.g. Carden, Penlon Oxford, Penlon OAV and Ohmeda 7780 ventilators). This reduces the internal compliance of the system providing that narrow bore (15 mm) breathing hose is used.
- Alternatively, some adult 'bag squeezers' can be set up to deliver an inspiratory phase that is *pressure limited*. Firstly, a bigger tidal volume and at a higher flow than required is selected. As the driving pressure reaches a *preset safe limit*, before either of these values are reached, the flow either stops or reduces drastically (where there is a deliberate leak around

the tube), in order to maintain that pressure. The tidal volume delivered is thus dependent on the preset pressure.

The 'T'-piece can be replaced by a ventilator that employs a conventional unidirectional breathing system provided that:

- it has a low internal compliance;
- it accurately measures inspiratory tidal volumes;
- paediatric (15 mm) breathing hoses are used to reduce the compressible volumes of respiratory gases.

The Newton Valve (Fig. 14.11)

This is an ingenious device that consists of ventilator input port, a patient port and fixed orifice gas outlet. It can be attached to and driven by several low-compliance ventilators (i.e. Nuffield series 200) so that ventilator gas enters the valve and exits the fixed gas outlet. The patient port is connected to the expiratory limb of a T-piece (Mapleson E system) where it replaces the reservoir bag.

At the recommended FGF rate for the 'T'-piece, and at low ventilator gas flow rates, the pressure developed inside the valve (as a result of continuous leakage from the fixed orifice outlet) only partially dams the expiratory limb of the breathing system, and so acts as a partial 'thumb occluder', providing very small tidal volumes. At these tidal volumes the 'internal volume' of the valve (and hence compliance) is relatively high in relation to the delivered tidal volume and the performance of the ventilator may well be more variable than expected when used in infants with low or changing compliance. As the flow rate of driving gas into the valve increases, the valve becomes effectively a 'thumb occluder' when the gas into the valve equals the gas leaving it via the fixed orifice outlet. When the ventilator delivers an even greater flow into the valve, part of this gas enters the expiratory limb of the T-piece, driving patient gas backwards in the system, thus acting as a 'bag squeezer' delivering relatively larger tidal volumes. In the latter mode, however, it is heavily consumptive of driving gas (15–30 litres/min), which may be important in situations where cylinders only are used.

PAEDIATRIC SCAVENGING SYSTEMS

The absence of an APL (expiratory) valve in most paediatric breathing attachments precludes the use of adult-type collecting systems for scavenging. However, alternative systems do exist.

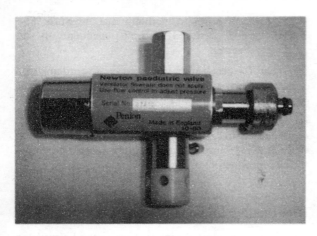

Figure 14.11 Newton valve, sectional view.

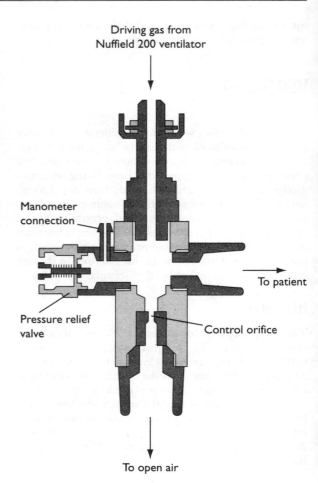

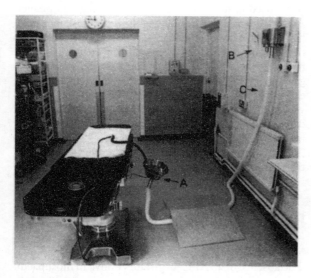

Figure 14.12 Howarth–Great Ormond Street collecting system. A, collecting dish with sieve base; B, junction with air-break system leading to extractor fan; C, wide-bore collecting hose.

- *The Howarth–Great Ormond Street Hospital collecting system* consists of a funnel arrangement (Fig. 14.12) into which the double-ended bag is placed. The base of the funnel, which has a plate with multiple perforations, is connected to a very wide-bore extraction hose that ducts the expired gas to a vacuum unit. This type of system would be classified as a high-volume, low-vacuum active gas scavenging unit. The very wide-bore extraction hose allows a high gas extraction

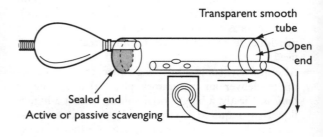

Figure 14.13 Diagram of a Stellenbosch collector.

rate (750 litres/min) at low gas velocities with a very low noise level.

- *Shrouding* the open tail of the reservoir bag: one of the most elegant is the system that is supplied with the Stellenbosch kit (Fig. 14.13).

- *Theatre air conditioning systems* that provide a laminar flow from ceiling to floor with sufficient force to change the air 25 times an hour (instead of the usual 20 times) are as effective as the paediatric anaesthetic gas scavenging systems described above.

FURTHER READING

Hatch DJ (1978) Tracheal tubes and connectors used in neonates: dimensions and resistance to breathing. *British Journal of Anaesthesia* **50**: 959–964.

Hatch DJ (1985) Paediatric anaesthetic equipment. *British Journal of Anaesthesia* **57**: 672–684.

Hatch DJ, Yates AI, Lindhahl SGE (1987) Flow requirements and rebreathing during mechanically controlled ventilation in a 'T' piece (Mapleson E) system. *British Journal of Anaesthesia* **59**: 1535–1540.

Perez Fontan JJ, Heldt GP, Gregory GA (1985) Resistance and inertia of endotracheal tubes used in infants during periodic flow. *Critical Care Medicine* **13**: 1052–1055.

—15—

EQUIPMENT FOR DENTAL CHAIR ANAESTHESIA

Contents

INTRODUCTION

Anaesthetic equipment is employed in the dental surgery (operatory) for two purposes:

1. To give *relative analgesia* (RA) which is a form of conscious sedation in which the patient remains awake, and does not lose any protective reflexes. This is administered by the dentist himself, sometimes in conjunction with local or regional analgesia by injection. Subanaesthetic concentrations of nitrous oxide in oxygen are used, and some machines are incapable of giving anaesthetic mixtures. Since the services of a specialist anaesthetist are not called for, the equipment for RA will not be discussed further in this book.

2. To administer general anaesthesia for the extraction of teeth or for dental conservation. While some cases may be of very short duration, others may be prolonged, for example 'whole-mouth dentistry' for mentally- or physically-handicapped patients. But, however short the duration of anaesthesia may be, all precautions must be taken, and all monitoring equipment and means of resuscitation must be available, as would be the case in the operating theatre.

In dental surgery special circumstances appertain, namely:

- the patient is required to be fit to leave for home within a short period of time;
- the induction of anaesthesia is often by inhalation;
- during the operation the anaesthetist must allow the dentist access to the open mouth, thereby sharing the air passages with him or her;
- many of the procedures are of such short duration that many practitioners feel that these can be performed without the use of a laryngeal mask airway (LMA) or endotracheal intubation.

These seemingly impossible requirements are met by the use of a nasal inhaler. For inhalational induction patients are instructed to keep their mouth closed so that they breathe through the nose. When anaesthesia is established the mouth is opened and a pack is inserted to prevent mouth-breathing and the inhalation of blood or dental debris during the operation.

It is not always possible to obtain a good fit between the inhaler and the face at the start of induction, so a high flow rate of gases must be available to prevent the inhalation of air rather than the anaesthetic mixture. It may be desirable to be able to make changes to flow rate and to the percentage of nitrous oxide and oxygen independently of each other, on a 'breath to breath basis' and with minimal manual manipulation. This is administered more conveniently by a machine that supplies inhalational agents using a single N_2O/O_2 percentage control rather than a more conventional continuous flow machine with separate flowmeters for each gas.

ANAESTHETIC MACHINES

Continuous Flow Machines for Dental Anaesthesia and Analgesia

A Boyle's machine can be used provided it has an anti-hypoxia system fitted (i.e. it cannot give less than 30% oxygen), but it may present difficulties. The maximum flow rate of nitrous oxide may be lower than is convenient and the manipulation of the flow control valves may require more movements of the hand than are desirable.

The Quantiflex MDM (Monitored Dial Mixer) machine (Fig 15.1) is designed for RA or GA. It has:

- flowmeters for nitrous oxide and oxygen controlled by a single dial. Note that the oxygen flowmeter is sited on the right of the bank as opposed to the sequence seen on many anaesthetic machines in the UK;
- a separate mixture control wheel that determines the percentage of delivered oxygen (from a minimum setting of 30% to a maximum of 100%);
- a nitrous oxide shut-off device that operates in the event of an oxygen supply failure. (The nitrous oxide supply also diminishes in proportion to the falling oxygen pressure.);
- an oxygen flush which bypasses the flowmeters and directs a flow of 50 litres/min into the breathing system connection;
- a connection (mount) for a reservoir bag. (This lies on the underside of the block housing the air entrainment valve and is not visible in the illustration provided.);
- a one-way check valve on the patient side of the bag mount to protect against the rebreathing of exhaled gases;
- an air intake valve that allows the patient to entrain air into the breathing system in the event of an oxygen supply failure;
- at the back of the flowmeter block, an auxiliary high-pressure oxygen outlet for connecting a demand valve or a resuscitator;
- a common gas outlet.

The McKesson MC1 and MC2 RA/GA machines (Fig. 15.2) both have features similar to the Quantiflex. However, the MC2 can be fitted with either a cage-mount vaporizer or a Selectatec backbar so that a volatile anaesthetic can be added to the breathing mixture. It

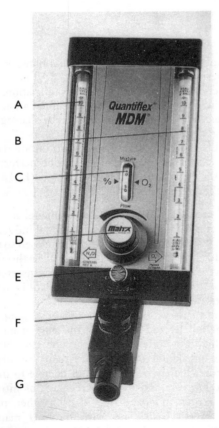

Figure 15.1 A Quantiflex MDM machine. A, Nitrous oxide flowmeter; B, oxygen flowmeter; C, mixture control wheel; D, flow control dial; E, oxygen flush; F, air entrainment valve – underneath the block housing this valve is the bag mount (not seen in this photo); G, common gas outlet.

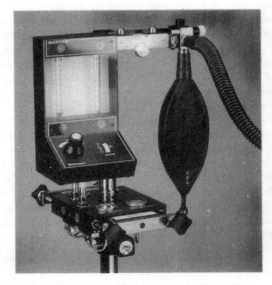

Figure 15.2 A McKesson MC2 RA/GA machine fitted with a Selectatec vaporizer station.

may then be used for the provision of general anaesthesia rather than relative analgesia. Both these machines give a minimum of 30% oxygen.

Intermittent Flow Machines

In dental anaesthesia these machines, which were used with *varying flow*, reigned supreme for many decades. They had no flowmeters. The two controls, which acted independently of each other, were for mixture (percentage of N_2O and O_2) and flow rate. In experienced hands these two could be controlled on a 'breath-to-breath' basis far more quickly and smoothly than with a continuous flow machine. They were ideal for the quick extraction of a single tooth. Examples are The McKesson Simplor, The Cyprane A E and The Walton Five. Many of these are still in use, but the latter two are declared obsolete by their manufacturers. The McKesson is still supported by McKesson GB Ltd. All three were discussed fully in earlier editions of this book.

NASAL INHALERS

There are two traditional types of nasal inhaler (or hood).

Single Hose

McKesson 900 nasal inhaler (Fig. 15.3). This is based on the now obsolete Goldman inhaler. Gases enter it via a standard 22 mm breathing hose, which passes over the top of the patient's head. They escape through an APL (expiratory) valve. The body of the mask has a stud on each side so that it can be held in place by a Connell-type harness.

McKesson Comfort Cushion inhaler (Fig. 15.4). The APL valve has been replaced with a connection to a scavenging hose. It is intended for both anaesthesia and relative analgesia. A head strap is available for securing it during longer cases.

Double Hose

The Matrx nasal inhaler (Fig. 15.5). This is constructed of grey (cold sterilizable) or blue (autoclavable) rubber

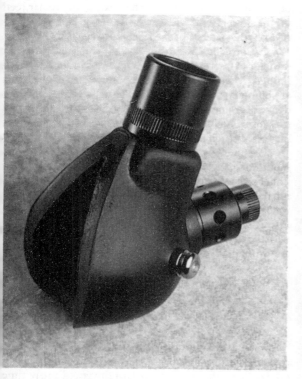

Figure 15.3 A McKesson 900 nasal inhaler.

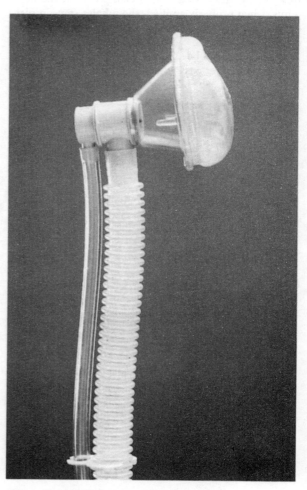

Figure 15.4 A McKesson Comfort Cushion inhaler.

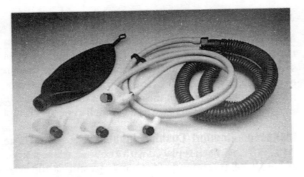

Figure 15.5 Matrx nasal inhalers.

and fits over the nose. It is quite flexible and can be widened or narrowed. The gases enter through two narrow tubes, one on each side of the inhaler, and exit through an APL valve sited on the front. The tubes pass round each side of the patient's head and are held together by means of a sliding clamp behind the head. Thus, when properly applied, the inhaler stays in place on its own, thereby freeing the anaesthetist's hands for other manipulations.

The mask can be supplied with wider-bore breathing hose for either passive scavenging or active scaveng-

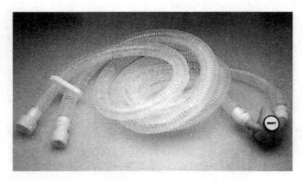

Figure 15.6 A Matrx passive scavenging nasal inhaler.

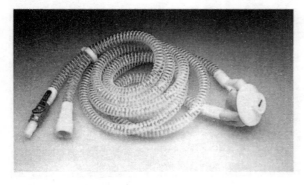

Figure 15.7 A Matrx active scavenging nasal inhaler.

ing. In these instances, fresh gases enter one limb only and escape via the other. In the passive scavenging system (Fig. 15.6), the APL valve has been removed and the expiratory limb fitted with a non-return valve adjacent to the mask.

In the active scavenging system (Fig. 15.7), the APL valve is replaced by a large cone which entrains any escaped gases that may have escaped around the inhaler.

AIRWAY MANAGEMENT DEVICES

Where obstruction of the upper airway may occur during a case of short duration, the employment of a purpose-made nasopharyngeal airway can be most useful (see Fig. 9.1d, p. 140). It should be made of a soft pliable material such as latex so as not to cause bleeding on insertion.

Operations of a longer duration (multiple extractions and conservation) may be better managed by a laryngeal mask airway and pharyngeal packing. This combination almost always provides a more patent airway with a greater degree of protection against tracheal soiling. However, the LMA may be temporarily displaced (causing airway obstruction) by excessive downward pressure on the lower jaw, a procedure commonly performed by the operator when extracting molar teeth in the lower jaw. Elevating the latter almost always restores the patency of the upper airway.

Nasotracheal intubation is still commonly used for difficult extractions, especially where intraoral access is limited. Many endotracheal tubes now have bevels that are blunted (Fig. 9.21b, p. 152) so as to reduce the incidence of traumatic bleeding from the nasopharynx during insertion. They may also be made from softer materials which may also reduce this complication.

A suitable pack must always be inserted into the mouth or pharynx in any dental procedure carried out under sedation or general anaesthesia so as to prevent the inhalation of dental debris. A strip of Gamgee may be used to advantage, but it must be at least 12 inches (30 cm) long. Specially designed pharyngeal packs are available for use with the laryngeal mask, oral and nasal endotracheal tubes and with relative analgesia (Fig. 15.8).

GAGS AND PROPS

The patient's mouth is frequently kept open with either a dental prop or a gag. Since the days of Hewitt (1857–1916) the prop has been reinvented many times and a typical set is shown in Fig. 15.9. A prop should be

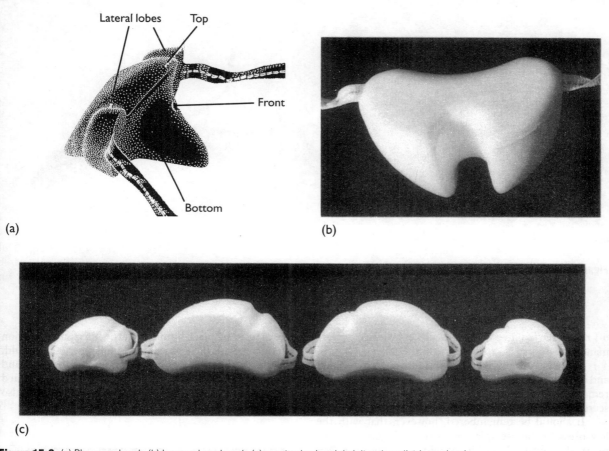

Figure 15.8 (a) Pharyngeal pack; (b) laryngeal mask pack; (c) nasotracheal pack (adult and paediatric versions).

attached to a length of cord or chain to facilitate its retrieval if it slips into the patient's mouth. Conveniently, three or four props of different sizes may be linked together by their chains.

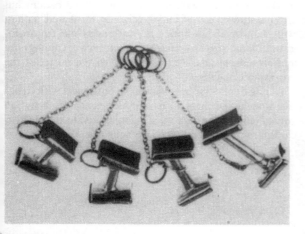

Figure 15.9 A set of mouth props.

Two popular versions of mouth gag are Mason's and Ferguson's gags (Fig. 15.10). The blades may be covered with plastic or rubber tubing to protect the patient's teeth from damage. The pieces of tubing should not be so short that they might fall off and be inhaled by the patient. Plastic tubing is more easily threaded onto the blade of the gag if it is first softened by immersion in boiling water; however, the use of plastic tubing may lead to problems with methods of sterilization.

SUCTION EQUIPMENT

In the dental surgery suction equipment should be of the high displacement type (see Fig. 24.3, p. 331). The high-pressure, low-displacement type, such as that produced by a hospital piped medical vacuum or a good quality portable electrically operated suction pump, may be satisfactory, but low-displacement types such as the foot-operated suction pump or the venturi type working

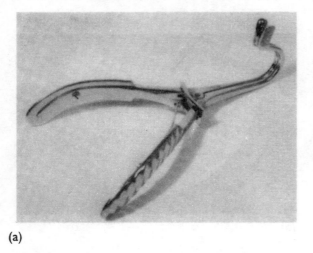

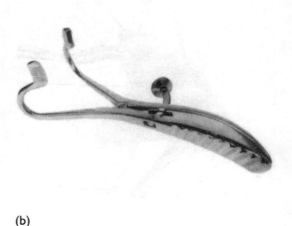

(a)   (b)

Figure 15.10 (a) Ferguson's mouth gag; (b) Mason's mouth gag.

off the water tap give far less than the desirable performance.

The sucker is used most commonly to remove blood and debris from the site of operation, and only seldom to remove regurgitated or vomited stomach contents, or secretions, from the respiratory tract.

It should be remembered, however, that with the low-pressure, high-displacement type of suction equipment, the nozzle should be of wide diameter, between 0.5 and 2 cm, and as short as possible. Long, narrow-bore suction catheters are inappropriate.

THE DENTAL CHAIR

The chair itself is justifiably included in this chapter since the ease with which the posture of the patient may be altered and, equally importantly, the security with which the patient, and the head in particular, may be maintained in the desired position are of paramount importance in the pursuit of safety during dental anaesthesia.

Whether the patient is anaesthetized and subjected to operation in the sitting, semi-recumbent or horizontal position is a matter for individual choice. Whichever is preferred there is no argument that the patient who col-

lapses must be placed quickly in the horizontal position preferably with the legs raised. The anaesthetist should, therefore, be familiar with the workings of the chair and also check before use that any electrical controls are turned on and functioning correctly. The anaesthetist should also know how to operate the chair in case of power failure.

MONITORING AND RESUSCITATION EQUIPMENT

Where general anaesthesia or sedation is employed in the dental surgery the level of monitoring should be the same as for inpatient anaesthesia. A pulse oximeter may be the minimum requirement for a sedated patient but an anaesthetized and endotracheally intubated patient will require, in addition, a continuous electrocardiogram, blood pressure measurement device, capnograph and an oxygen analyser connected to the outlet of the anaesthetic machine.

The dental surgery should be equipped with drugs that may be required for cardiopulmonary resuscitation and a defibrillator capable of being linked to the electrocardiogram so as to provide a synchronized output.

— 16 —

EQUIPMENT FOR LOCAL ANALGESIA

Contents

INTRODUCTION

Local anaesthetic drugs may be administered to a patient by placing them:

- topically (i.e. directly onto the skin or mucosa);
- by field block (i.e. infiltrating an area of tissue containing small nerve fibres or nerve endings using a hypodermic needle);
- by regional block (i.e. by placing the drugs adjacent to a major nerve pathway via a needle or catheter).

The latter two may be performed with greater safety and accuracy by using special equipment.

GENERAL CONSIDERATIONS

Needle Design

Length
The needle should be of sufficient length to reach its target.

Diameter
This will depend on several factors, such as:

- The viscosity of liquid that is required to pass through the needle. Aqueous solutions (local anaesthetics) will pass through very small diameters (29 gauge). However, if the technique involves an aspiration test to ensure the needle is not in a blood vessel, a larger diameter may be safer. Oil-based agents (for destructive nerve blocks) will only pass easily through much larger diameters (18 gauge). Table 16.1 shows the comparison of gauge size (G) to metric measurement. Note that all the sizes mentioned in this chapter refer to the external diameters of the equipment.
- The rigidity required of the needle for its insertion. The longer the needle the more flexible it becomes. This makes it more prone to deflection (especially if the tip has a bevel) so that it may not reach its intended target (e.g. needles for spinal anaesthesia). If the tissues through which it has to pass are tough, then the needle wall has to be stronger (i.e. thicker) to prevent deformation of the tip and buckling of the shaft. An example of such a needle is that used for epidural injection.

Table 16.1 A comparison of standard wire gauge sizes with a metric equivalent

30 G	27 G	26 G	25 G	23 G	22 G	21 G
0.3 mm	0.4 mm	0.45 mm	0.5 mm	0.6 mm	0.7 mm	0.8 mm

Shape

- The thinner the needle, the less is the tissue damage produced during insertion. For example, larger needles if passed through a blood vessel may cause bigger haematomas than smaller needles.
- Where needles are bevelled, the short type (Fig. 16.1) is allegedly preferable for use in a nerve block. The short bevel is blunter than that of a hypodermic-type needle and is less likely to penetrate and either cut a nerve bundle or deposit local anaesthetic within it. (Some preparations of local anaesthetics have been shown to be toxic to nerves when deposited in this manner, unlike those that are injected so that they surround the nerve bundle and diffuse into it.) However, this view is not universally held as many of the studies have been performed on animal preparations. Paradoxically, short-bevelled needles have been shown to cause more disruption to the choroid and retina than sharper needles when they have accidentally pierced the eyeball during peribulbar blocks.

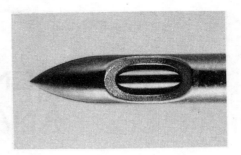

Figure 16.2 The Braun Pencan. This is an example of a pencil point (atraumatic) needle tip.

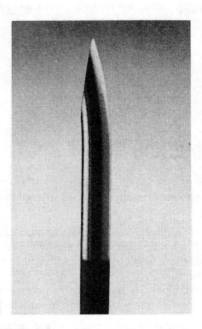

Figure 16.3 The Huber point.

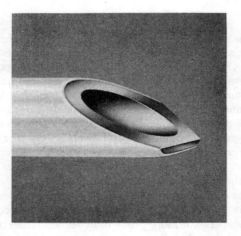

Figure 16.1 A short-bevelled needle for major nerve block. The tip has blunt leading edges and the shaft is coated in an insulating material so that only the bevel can transmit an electrical stimulus.

- Needles with a 'pencil point or bullet-shaped tip' and with a side port on the shaft (Fig. 16.2) are again allegedly preferable for nerve blocks as the tip separates rather than cuts tissue as it is advanced and the side hole makes intraneural injection much less likely. This type has also become very popular in spinal anaesthesia where the tip is said to produce a smaller dural puncture and as a consequence has resulted in a substantial reduction in post-procedure headache.
- Needles with a 'Huber point' (Fig. 16.3) have become deservedly popular for epidural anaesthesia. The bevel

is set obliquely to the shaft so that the tip of the needle is blunt. It will, therefore, pierce more rigid tissue during insertion (ligament), but tends to push away more pliant tissue (dura mater).

Hubs

These should all be fitted with a standard luer taper and lock. The former ensures that when a syringe is attached, it will form a leak-free fit. The latter prevents accidental spillage of toxic agents that may be contained in the syringe (e.g. phenol), especially if high pressure is required for injection. The hub may be made of clear plastic in order to aid the detection of blood or cerebrospinal fluid.

EQUIPMENT FOR SPINAL ANAESTHESIA

As this procedure must be carried out under the strictest of aseptic conditions, the various items used must be sterilized and wrapped either individually or in a suitable self-contained pack. The latter may be purchased commercially or prepared by the hospital's sterile supply unit. It may contain:

- items used to aid skin cleansing and disinfection (sponges, swabs and containers to hold small amounts of disinfectant);
- suitable draping that covers the areas around the site of injection that have not been treated;
- various hypodermic needles and syringes used to draw up the local anaesthetic agents.

The spinal needle is usually added to the opened pack just prior to performing the procedure. This allows the operator to choose a preferred size and type.

Types of Spinal Needle

Diameters These vary from 18 to 29 standard wire gauge (swg). They are all supplied with a close fitting metal stylet that fits into the lumen of the needle to strengthen it and to prevent tissue entering the lumen during insertion and blocking the needle.

Lengths The most common length is 10 cm, although 5 cm (for paediatric use) and 15 cm (for obese patients and for use through an epidural needle, see below) are available.

Shapes There are two distinctive shapes of needle tip. In one, the shaft is cut obliquely so that the needle and stylet form a bevel with a sharp cutting edge. The two common patterns of the cutting edge are the Yale and Quincke (Fig. 16.4) designs. In the other (see Fig. 16.2), the shaft ends in a point. As this is advanced, it tends to stretch and separate the tissue causing less trauma. The two common patterns of this type of tip are the pencil point (Whitacre) and bullet shape (Sprotte). As the needle tip is solid, a side port is cut into the lumen of the needle as close to the tip as possible to allow the local anaesthetic to be injected.

Practical Problems

- Diameters smaller than 23 gauge are prone to bend on insertion. This can be circumvented by passing them through an introducer (a shorter but slightly

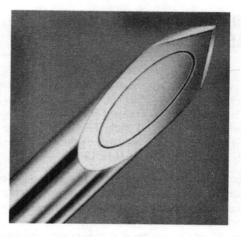

Figure 16.4 A Braun spinal needle with a cutting bevel (Quincke).

wider needle) which is inserted initially at the intended site.

- Although the bevelled tipped needles are easier to insert, the oblique face of the latter, when pushed through tissue, may cause the smaller-diameter needles to bend through an arc during insertion so that the tip may deviate away from the intended target. This effect is reduced when an introducer is used.
- The incidence, severity and duration of headache (thought to be related to the rate of leakage of cerebrospinal fluid from the dural puncture) is increased significantly with the larger-bore needles, especially if they have cutting bevels.
- As the internal diameter of the needle decreases, so does the flow back of cerebrospinal fluid. With the smallest-diameter needles this may take as long as 15 s to appear. This may dent the confidence of a less experienced operator.

Equipment for Continuous Spinal Anaesthesia

A very fine catheter (28 gauge) can be inserted into the dural space through a spinal needle (22 gauge) and left in situ as the spinal needle is withdrawn. As it is about 90 cm long, it can be secured to the patient's back so that its other end can be conveniently accessed for injection of local anaesthetic when the patient is lying supine. This end is attached to a luer locking device incorporating a bacterial/viral filter (0.2 μm). Using this method, the duration of anaesthetic action can be prolonged by repeated injection through the catheter. These kits have been very expensive to purchase owing to the high manufacturing costs for the very fine catheter, although they are now becoming more affordable.

EQUIPMENT FOR EPIDURAL ANAESTHESIA

As this procedure also must be carried out under the strictest of aseptic conditions, the various items used must be sterilized and wrapped either individually or in a suitable self-contained pack. The latter may be purchased commercially or prepared by the hospital's sterile supply unit. It may contain (Fig. 16.5):

- items used to aid skin cleansing and disinfection (sponges, swabs and containers for the disinfectant);
- suitable draping that covers the areas around the site of injection that have not been treated;
- various hypodermic needles and syringes used to draw up the local anaesthetic agents;
- An epidural catheter, bacterial/viral filter;
- epidural needle;
- specialized syringe to elicit loss of resistance.

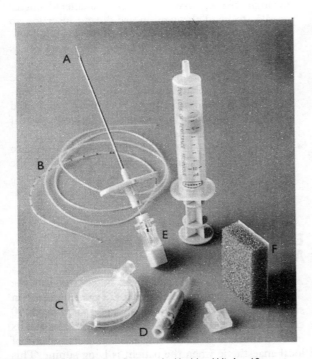

Figure 16.5 A combined Portex spinal/epidural kit. A, a 16 gauge 10.5 cm Tuohy needle with a Huber point, wings and with 1 cm markings on the shaft. Inserted into the needle (for demonstration purposes) is a longer than usual 26 gauge spinal needle (11.7 cm); B, a 19 gauge epidural catheter with multiple side holes and markings; C, a bacterial/viral filter with luer locks at both ends; D, a connector that fits on one end of the catheter so that it can be connected to the filter; E, spinal needle; F, fixing (anti-kinking) sponge for the catheter.

Epidural Needle

The Tuohy needle is the most common type used.

Diameters This is normally supplied as a 16, 17 or 18 gauge needle for use in adults as well as a 19 gauge version for use in children.

Lengths The standard version is approximately 10.5 cm in length (8 cm shaft and 2.5 cm hub) although a longer version (15 cm) is available for use in obese patients. Most have 1 cm markings on the shaft to show the depth of insertion from the skin. Also, there is a paediatric version that is 5 cm long with 0.5 cm markings. They are all supplied with a close-fitting stylet that fits into the lumen of the needle to prevent tissue entering the lumen on insertion and blocking the needle.

Shape The tip is curved (the Huber point, see Fig 16.3) causing the exit hole to emerge at an angle of about 20° to the shaft. The tip of the needle is also blunt so that it can pierce more rigid tissue during insertion (ligament), but tends to push away more pliant tissue (dura mater). This reduces the incidence of dural penetration by the needle when it is inserted into the epidural space. When a catheter is passed through the shaft it emerges at an angle that can be used to exert some degree of direction on it. If it impinges on the dura during initial insertion, it should do so at an angle that causes it to be deflected away. Some manufacturers supply a flange (wing) at the hub for a better grip during insertion.

Technique

The epidural space is normally identified by a loss of resistance technique. As the needle approaches the ligamentum flavum, the stylet is withdrawn and a low-resistance syringe attached to the hub. It can be filled with either air or saline. By applying pressure to the plunger as the needle is advanced, a resistance to injection can be felt, caused by the dense ligament surrounding the needle tip. As the latter enters the epidural space, the loose connective tissue allows the free injection of the contents of the syringe (the so-called 'loss of resistance').

The depth of the epidural space from the skin is then ascertained by calculating the number of marks on the shaft that have been inserted. The catheter, which is narrower than the needle, may then be fed into the epidural space, the optimal length inserted depending on the operator's preference and intended use for the technique. It has standardized markings (BS 6196), which consist of:

- a single marking at the tip;
- five single markings 1 cm apart from 5 to 9 cm;

- a double marking at 10 cm;
- four single markings from 11 to 14 cm;
- a triple marking at 15 cm;
- a quadruple marking at 20 cm.

Many catheters have a sealed tip with multiple side holes (through which the anaesthetic disperses) sited along a 2.5 cm length behind it. Therefore a minimum of 3 cm should be inserted to be sure that all the anaesthetic is deposited in the space. Some catheters, however, have a single exit hole at the tip.

When a suitable length of catheter has been inserted, the needle is then withdrawn and the catheter fixed to the patient's back in a manner that will prevent it kinking as it emerges from the skin. The other end is then fitted with a luer connection and a 0.2 μm bacterial/viral filter.

N.B. The catheter should never be withdrawn through the needle when the latter is still inserted. In this situation, it can be dragged onto the edge of the needle tip causing it to shear, leaving a portion of catheter within the epidural space.

Combined Spinal/Epidural Techniques

Some anaesthetists prefer to perform a spinal anaesthetic initially and to supplement it with an epidural block. This can be performed through a single skin puncture. A Tuohy needle is used first to identify the epidural space and a thinner (and longer than standard) spinal needle then inserted through it and into the dural space. Following injection of anaesthetic, the spinal needle is removed and an epidural catheter inserted. The Huber point should ensure that the catheter does not impinge on the dural puncture site. In any case, if a small-bore pencil point needle is used for the spinal technique, it is unlikely that the catheter could pass through the puncture site.

EQUIPMENT FOR MAJOR NERVE BLOCKS

Most major nerves (including nerve roots and plexuses) lie some distance under the skin, are often covered by muscles and may lie adjacent to substantial arteries and veins. There may be other structures which, if accidentally punctured, can cause significant morbidity (e.g. the pleura). Accurate identification of the nerve (with minimal trauma to the surrounding tissues) is essential to produce a successful block. This requires a sound knowledge of the relevant anatomy, specialized needles and preferably a nerve stimulator to help locate it.

Needles (Fig. 16.6)

Some authorities recommend that nerve-blocking needles should have tips that separate rather than cut the tissue through which they pass. To do this, they should be of the short bevelled type with blunted edges (Fig. 16.1) or have pencil point tips (Fig. 16.2). They should be fitted with a short length of clear flexible tubing with a hub housing, a luer taper and a luer lock. The translucency assists the detection of blood should the needle be accidentally placed in a blood vessel and the flexibility allows the needle to be held in position, usually by one operator, whilst a second injects the anaesthetic solution (the 'immobile needle technique'). This prevents migration of the needle when large volumes of agent are slowly injected. They should have a narrow external diameter (22 or 23 gauge) that is small enough to pass through tissue without excessive force but large enough for blood to pass back easily if accidental vascular puncture occurs. They are supplied in various lengths (30–150 mm) depending on the manufacturer and may have an electrical lead attached for connection to a nerve stimulator. The shaft may be coated in an insulator (Teflon) so that any electrical current passed through the needle comes into contact with the tissues at the tip only (see below).

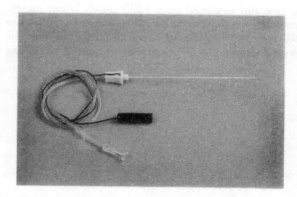

Figure 16.6 An insulated nerve block needle with flexible extension and electrical wire connection.

Nerve Stimulators

These are battery-operated devices that pass a low voltage (up to 9 V) and low current (0.1–5 mA) through the nerve block needle (Fig. 16.7). The current is made to flow in short bursts (1 ms) at a frequency of 1 or 2 Hz (switchable). To use the device, one of its leads is connected to the needle and the other to a self-adhesive electrode (similar to that used for an electrocardiogram) so as to complete an electrical circuit when the needle is passed through the skin. The needle is passed in the

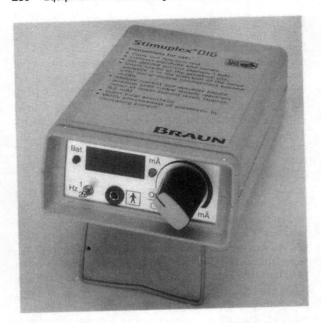

Figure 16.7 The Braun Stimuplex battery-powered nerve stimulator.

general direction of the nerve to be blocked using a current of about 1 mA. This is adjusted by a knob on the device and displayed on a LED panel. When muscle contractions become visible, the current is reduced to 0.2 mA and the needle advanced further. When the needle is 'in close proximity to the nerve, a sudden increase in muscle movement is seen. After an aspiration test to ensure that the needle has not entered a blood vessel, the local anaesthetic may then be injected with the needle held steady ('immobile needle technique').

FURTHER READING

Cesarini MD, Torrieli R, Lahaye F, Mene JM, Cabiro C (1990) Sprotte needle for intrathecal anaesthesia for Caesarean section: incidence of post-dural puncture headache. *Anaesthesia* **45**: 656–658.

Editorial (1994) Peripheral nerve damage and regional anaesthesia. *British Journal of Anaesthesia* **73**: 435–436.

Gerrish SP, Peacock JE (1987) Variations in the flow of cerebrospinal fluid through spinal needles. *British Journal of Anaesthesia* **59**: 1465–1471.

Jones RP, De Jonge M, Smith BE (1992) Voltage fields surrounding needles used in regional anaesthesia. *British Journal of Anaesthesia* **68**: 515–518.

Kopacz DJ, Allen HW (1995) Comparison of needle deviation during regional anesthetic techniques in a laboratory model. *Anesthesia & Analgesia* **81**: 630–633.

Vandermeersch E (1993) Combined spinal–epidural anaesthesia. In: Van Aken H (ed.) *Clinical Anaesthesiology: New Developments in Epidural and Spinal Drugs Administration*. London: Baillière Tindall: 691–708.

—17—

VIGILANCE AND HUMAN ERROR

INTRODUCTION

Operative mortality associated with anaesthesia has been variously quoted as between 1:1000 and 1:10 000 with approximately 1–3 deaths per 10 000 anaesthetics administered.

THE CHANGING PATTERN OF ACCIDENTS ASSOCIATED WITH ANAESTHETIC APPARATUS

Owing to the less frequent use of flammable and explosive anaesthetic agents and the institution of precautions to prevent explosions, particularly in connection with static electricity, accidents caused by fire and explosion have been virtually eliminated. However, as flammable and explosive agents are now hardly ever used in the developed world, many new operating theatre suites are no longer protected against static electricity.

In recent years, deaths from electrocution have been reported, and following the elucidation of the concept of microshock one is left to wonder how many cases of ventricular fibrillation may have been caused in this way in the past.

Other factors that may influence the changing pattern of accidents are increasing complexity of equipment, disparagement of the mundane, and reliance upon assistance (nurse, technician or another anaesthetist).

The major causes for mortality and also of considerable morbidity are:

- insufficient oxygen supply to the brain;
- inadequate carbon dioxide removal;
- administration of excessive amounts of anaesthetic or other associated drugs;
- barotrauma to the lungs;
- obstruction of the airway.

Statistical evidence shows that about 70% of critical incidents can be attributed to human error and only about 13% are due to genuine equipment failure. The scenarios leading to critical incidents are often multifactorial and it must remain the responsibility of designers and manufacturers of anaesthetic equipment, and the users, to minimize the possibility of their occurrence.

The administration and management of general anaesthesia may be depicted as a closed loop as shown in Fig. 17.1. The anaesthetist controls the anaesthetic machine and its accessories. These manipulations have a direct effect upon the patient and are, in turn, observed by the anaesthetist who then further adjusts the machine if necessary.

The anaesthetist's role is vital in that he or she composes the gas mixture, controls the ventilation (be it spontaneous or controlled), observes the response of the patient and must, if possible, anticipate the surgeon and any changes in the patient's condition.

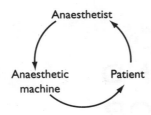

Figure 17.1 Anaesthetic control loop.

Vigilance

Two important attributes of the anaesthetist must be considered for the safe conduct of anaesthetic practice:

- vigilance and
- decision-making ability.

The level of arousal also affects the rate and the quality of both vigilance and the ability to make decisions correctly and rapidly.

Vigilance is defined in the dictionary as watchfulness or caution. Anaesthetic vigilance has been defined by Gravenstein (1986) as a state of clinical awareness whereby dangerous conditions are anticipated. In 1943, research by the Royal Air Force showed that vigilance requiring continuous monitoring and detection of brief, low-intensity and infrequently occurring events over long periods is poor. This is illustrated in Fig. 17.2, which shows rapid fall-off in vigilance after a period as short as half an hour.

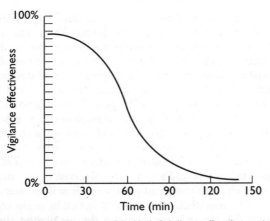

Figure 17.2 An illustration of the kind of vigilance effect that can be expected in the performance of passive tasks with a low signal rate. This shows a notable decline in performance after about 30 min. (Reproduced from Hawkins FH (1987) *Human Factors in Flight*, London: Gower Technical Press.) This would occur over a similar period of uneventful anaesthesia.

Twenty years ago, there were very few aids to vigilance for anaesthetists – just a manually operated non-invasive blood pressure monitor and possibly a pulse plethysmograph; with seriously ill patients an ECG monitor might have been available. With modern anaesthesia there are many vigilance aids, which are described in the next three chapters. Vigilance aids concerned with the performance of the anaesthetic machine itself have already been mentioned in Chapter 7.

Decision-making Ability

The decision-making ability of the anaesthetist is dependent upon training, experience and the feedback of information from the senses of the patient's condition, the anaesthetic machine, the monitoring equipment and the requirements of the surgeon.

Psychological research has shown that the human brain is able to make only a single decision at any one instant. The pathway for human information processing is depicted in a simplified form in Fig. 17.3.

Incoming physical stimuli are received by the sense organs and it is therefore necessary to make sure that stimuli are within the bandwidth of, and are of sufficient amplitude for, those organs. The brain will not necessarily perceive the same message from the stimuli on each occasion, as perception depends upon context and previous experience in handling similar stimuli. The information is filtered and these filters are controlled by feedback loops. At this stage, some of the information may be off-loaded into short-term memory and may be lost if other information bombards the senses simultaneously. The human brain has a single decision channel. All information to be processed must pass sequentially through this one channel. A person can attend only to one thing at a time, although he or she can change from one thing to another extremely rapidly; the danger of preoccupation is obvious. Following a decision during which information from long-term memory may be used, a response is effected via the muscles. This is a grossly simplified description of an extremely complicated process.

Arousal

Both vigilance and the ability to make decisions are affected by the anaesthetist's level of arousal. Arousal is the level of 'wakefulness' and is controlled by the reticular formation in the mid-brain. Arousal ranges from total stupor to hypomania. For any task there is a level of arousal at which one performs most efficiently, as shown in Fig. 17.4. Surprisingly, this optimal level decreases as the difficulty of the task increases, so that overarousal is most likely to occur for difficult tasks. Overarousal often occurs in emergency situations when difficult tasks may

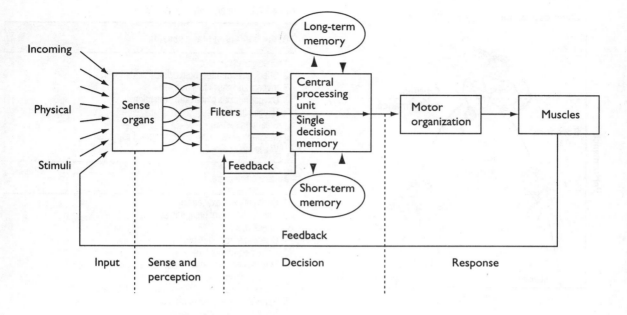

Figure 17.3 Human information processing. A simplified scheme of the pathway followed in decision-making.

need to be carried out rapidly. Underarousal for a particular task slows decision-making and makes it less accurate and also reduces vigilance. Underarousal occurs with boredom and sleep deprivation.

Performance is also adversely affected by physical and mental ill health, and several other stressors are listed in Table 17.1.

Anaesthetist or Pilot?

Much of the aforementioned relates equally well to pilots and their aircraft. The reason is that there are many similarities between administration of anaesthesia and flying. Both skills are carried out by intelligent highly motivated professionals who have undergone many years of expensive training. Both have to carry out many routine but highly skilled procedures and remain vigilant for long periods of time, observing for one of many possible, but hopefully rare, adverse occurrences that may be life-threatening, after which skilled intervention has to be instituted rapidly. Both professions also have to work long and often unsocial hours in imperfect environments and yet have to maintain high standards that are imposed externally as well as self-imposed.

There are two main areas where anaesthetists can learn from the aeronautical world, namely the use of checklists and ergonomic design. Pre-anaesthetic checklists have now become a routine, but pilots use checklists for many routine procedures apart from before take-off.

The design of anaesthetic and monitoring equipment with safety and ergonomics in mind has now become a priority. Until recently the design of anaesthetic and associated equipment has been on a purely

Table 17.1 Stressors contributing to reduction in performance

Environmental stresses	Domestic stresses	Professional stresses
Heat	Marriage	Colleagues
Noise	Divorce	Management
Vibration	Birth	Legal problems
Low humidity	Bereavement	Lack of sleep
	Financial problems	Hunger and thirst
	Health	Lack of rest

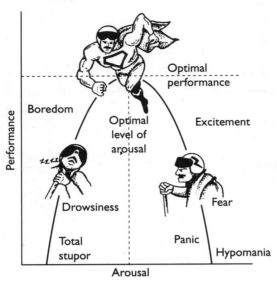

Figure 17.4 The inverted 'U' curve of arousal. Optimum performance for a particular task does *not* occur at maximum arousal. The optimum level varies depending upon the task.

Table 17.2 Pre-anaesthetic checklist

At the beginning of the session
1. Check all controls 'off'
2. Check gas supplies, both cylinder and pipeline
3. Inspect and check function of:
Oxygen/nitrous oxide ratio protection
Oxygen flush
Breathing system
Mechanical ventilator and disconnect alarm
Waste gas scavenging system

Before each case
1. Check reserve oxygen supply
2. Check function of breathing system
3. Check vaporizer
4. Check absorber, if in use
5. Inspect equipment for:
Entotracheal intubation intravenous infusion
Resuscitation
5. Check function of high-vacuum suction apparatus
6. Apply and check monitoring systems
7. Set appropriate alarm levels

functional basis and typical arrangements 'just grew' as new developments occurred and, more probably, as money for purchase became available (see Fig. 7.4).

Pre-anaesthetic Checklist

Many critical incidents could be avoided if another leaf was taken from the pilot's textbook: the pre-flight checklist. This is a written list of checks and measurements that must be made before every flight by every pilot, no matter how experienced or senior. The pre-anaesthetic checklist is now becoming more important with the increasing complexity of the equipment under the anaesthetist's control. A typical checklist is shown in Table 17.2.

A comprehensive checklist that does require the use of an oxygen analyser is reproduced, with references, by kind permission of the Association of Anaesthetists of Great Britain and Ireland and is to be found in Appendix IV.

HUMAN ERROR

Human error is the major cause of anaesthetic mishaps in the same way that 90% of aircraft accidents are due to human error. Taken to the extreme, all mishaps due to failures in anaesthetic and monitoring equipment are also due to human error in the failure to design–out risk of equipment malfunction causing detrimental effects to patients.

Classification of Human Error

Human error may be classified in several ways. One classification is chronological:

- *Active* error is an immediate precursor to an incident or accident with an unfortunate outcome.
- *Latent* errors occur well before the incident or accident and once the latent error has occurred it may go unnoticed for a considerable time before the incident/accident occurs. Examples of latent errors would include design faults and the 'wrong' drug ampoule in the 'right' box.

Another classification differentiates the cognitive level at which the error occurs:

- *Mistakes* occur at a high cognitive level where the intention before an intended action is wrong, leading to an unfortunate outcome.
- *Slips* occur at a much lower cognitive level when the intention is correct but the actual action is wrong.

Runciman *et al* (1993) have summarized a 'psychological' classification of error, as shown in Table 17.3.

Table 17.3 A 'psychological' classification of error. The '**X**' indicates where the error occurs in the chain between intention and planning action (the arrow) and outcome

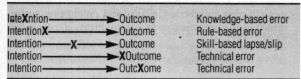

InteXntion ──────▶ Outcome	Knowledge-based error
IntentionX ──────▶ Outcome	Rule-based error
Intention ──X──▶ Outcome	Skill-based lapse/slip
Intention ──────▶ XOutcome	Technical error
Intention ──────▶ OutcXome	Technical error

Reproduced with permission from Runciman et al. (1993).

Knowledge-based errors are the result of forming the wrong intention because of inadequate knowledge, training or experience. Previous experience and familiarity may have a positive or a negative ('jumping to conclusions') effect in this type of error.

Rule-based errors involve failure to apply a rule designed to avoid error, to apply a bad or inadequate rule or to misapply a rule in solving a situation.

Skill-based errors are errors that are the result of 'absent-mindedness'. Most skill-based errors occur in skilled activities. Humans have two control modes for any action: automatic mode and conscious mode. The *automatic* mode of control consists of stored patterns of action which can be executed rapidly with very little attention. These patterns of action are efficient but rigid and may be likened to an 'autopilot'. The *conscious* control system is for novel situations; it is heavily dependent upon cognitive resources. Conscious control is slow, effortful and careful; one of its functions is to monitor automatic control. Skill-based errors may be due to the dissociation between these two modes of control.

Technical errors are those that occur despite correct intention and execution. They may be due to unrecognized abnormal anatomy or physiology or due to technical faults in the equipment concerned.

'STANDARDS' IN ANAESTHESIA

In anaesthesia, the word Standards may refer to standards as written by BSI, ISO, CEN, CENELEC, ASTM, ANSI, etc., which refer to the minimum safety requirements for equipment design, or the word may refer to Standards that have been promulgated by professional bodies regarding the safe conduct of anaesthesia.

A condensation of the recommendations of the internationally recognized professional bodies is given in Table 17.4.

Table 17.4 Recommendations of internationally recognized professional bodies

Essential
- Continuous presence of appropriately qualified anaesthetist
- Oxygen supply failure alarm
- Continuous monitoring of cardiac output
- Observation of reservoir bag and chest excursion
- Ventilator disconnect alarm
- Oxygen analyser of inspired gas
- Electrocardiogram
- Non-invasive arterial blood pressure

Strongly recommended
- Spirometry
- Pulse oximetry
- Temperature
- End-tidal carbon dioxide
- Monitoring of neuromuscular blockade

FURTHER READING

Chappelow J (1994) Psychology and safety in aviation. In Secker-Walker J (ed.) *Quality and Safety in Anaesthesia.* London: BMJ Publishers.

Cooper JB, Newbower RS, Long CD, McPeek B (1978) Preventable anesthesia mishaps: a study of human factors. *Anesthesiology* **49**: 399–406.

Editorial (1990) An International Consensus on Monitoring. *British Journal of Anaesthesia* **64**: 263–266.

Eichorn JH, Cooper JB, Cullen DJ, et al (1988) Anesthesia practice standards at Harvard: a review. *Journal of Clinical Anesthesia* **1**: 55–65.

Gaba DM, Maxwell M, DeAnda A (1987) Anesthetic mishaps: breaking the chain of accident evolution. *Anesthesiology* **66**: 670–676.

Gravenstein JS (1986) Why investigate vigilance? *Journal of Clinical Monitoring* **2**: 145–147.

Green RG, Muir H, James M, Gradwell D, Green RL (1991) *Human Factors for Pilots.* Aldershot, UK: Avebury Technical.

Loed RG (1993) Measurement of intraoperative attention to monitor displays. *Anesthesia and Analgesia* **76**: 337–341.

Parker JBR (1987) The effects of fatigue on physician performance – an underestimated cause of physician impairment and increased risk. *Canadian Journal of Anesthesia* **34**: 489–495.

Reason J (1990) *Human Error.* Cambridge, UK: Cambridge University Press.

Runciman WB, Sellen A, Webb RK, et al. (1993) Errors, incidents and accidents in anaesthetic practice. *Anaesthesia and Intensive Care* **21**: 506–519.

Schreiber P (1985) *Anesthesia Systems – Safety Guidelines.* Telford, Penn, USA: North American Dräger.

Schreiber P, Schreiber J. (1987) *Anesthesia Risk Analysis.* Telford, Penn, USA: North American Dräger.

Thompson PW (1987) Safer design of anaesthetic equipment. *British Journal of Anaesthesia* 59: 913–921.

Utting JE, Gray C, Shelley FC (1979) Human misadventure in anesthesia. *Canadian Journal of Anesthesia* 26: 472–478.

Weinger MB, Englund CE (1990) Ergonomic and human factors affecting anesthetic vigilance and monitoring performance in the operating room environment. *Anesthesiology* 73: 995–1021.

PHYSIOLOGICAL MONITORING: PRINCIPLES AND NON-INVASIVE MONITORING

Contents

INTRODUCTION

Anaesthesia, be it local or general, has a profound effect upon all physiological systems; most of these effects are deleterious and it is therefore important to know how the body is affected. In order to increase patient safety and effect good risk management, all systems affected by anaesthetic drugs must be monitored using equipment that converts physiological variables into visible or audible signals which may then be assessed by the anaesthetist. In this chapter the principles of clinical measurement and clinical monitoring will be discussed. In Chapter 19, the measurement and monitoring of gases is described and in Chapter 20 more invasive monitoring systems relevant to anaesthesia are discussed. The term *monitoring* means the continuous assessment of one or more variables, whereas *measurement* implies the single assessment at a discrete time.

CLASSIFICATION OF MONITORING EQUIPMENT

Patient monitoring equipment may be classified in several ways. *In vitro* equipment usually involves the removal of a sample of blood, urine or gas from a patient and discrete samples are subjected to some form of analysis, for example blood–gas analysis, blood sugar estimation, which may be done at the bedside, or other more complex biochemical or haematological tests done in a pathology laboratory. *In vivo* monitoring refers to the monitoring of physiological variables in real-time usually by the attachment of electrodes or transducers to the body.

In vivo monitoring equipment may be classified according to the principles involved:

- gas monitoring equipment (Chapter 19);
- equipment monitoring electrical signals that are naturally generated by the body (Fig. 18.1a);
- equipment that uses *transducers* to convert non-electrical physiological variables to electrical signals, which may then easily be displayed (Fig. 18.1b);
- equipment that displays the effect that the body has upon some form of energy that has been passed through it (Fig. 18.1c).

Monitoring equipment may also be classified by whether it is:

- Non-invasive (electrocardiography (ECG), electro-encephalography (EEG), non–invasive blood pressure (NIBP), pulse oximetry, capnography);
- minimally invasive (core temperature);
- Invasive (direct arterial blood pressure, central venous pressure (CVP), thermodilution cardiac output).

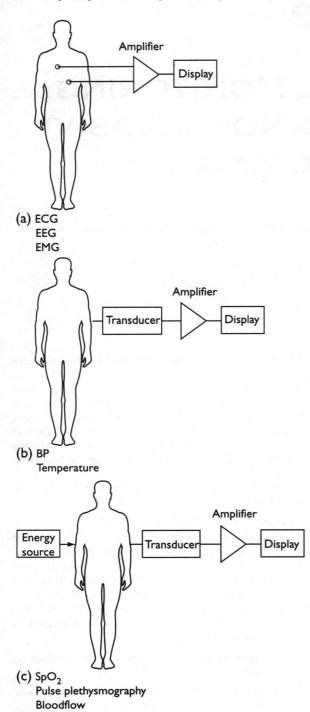

Figure 18.1 Basic classification of monitoring systems.
(a) Monitoring electrical signals generated by the patient.
(b) Conversion of measurand to an electrical signal with a transducer.
(c) Passing energy through the patient and measuring the effect the patient has on it.

The degree of invasiveness affects such things as cost, skills required, and risks such as infection, bleeding and damage to internal organs. Invasive monitoring used in anaesthesia is dealt with in Chapter 20.

GENERALIZED MONITORING SYSTEM

To fulfil requirements of safety, display, recording and alarms, the basic classification of Fig. 18.1 may be enlarged to show other major common components of any physiological monitoring system (Fig. 18.2).

The *measurand* is the physical or chemical property or condition that is to be measured. Except when measuring biological potentials (ECG, EEG, electromyography (EMG), etc.), a *transducer* is necessary to convert the measurand into an electrical signal so that it may be *processed*. The processed signal may then be passed to the following:

- *Display* for immediate real-time assessment by the anaesthetist. This may be a numerical display (liquid crystal display (LCD), light-emitting diodes (LED), cathode ray tube (CRT), analogue meter or bargraph).
- *Alarm system* with upper and lower adjustable thresholds to advise the anaesthetist when the measurand goes outside preset limits.
- *Data storage* to maintain the data for use after anaesthesia is completed for clinical, statistical or medicolegal reasons. Data storage may be *hard copy* directly onto paper or onto magnetic or semiconductor memory for future processing.
- *Data transmission* using standard interface connections so that information gained may be used by other parts of an integrated system.

For most applications, some form of *calibration* will be necessary at regular intervals during its operation.

Almost all monitoring equipment is now *controlled* by microprocessors as this makes it possible to design equipment that requires minimal user calibration and set-up and also provides self-diagnostics in terms of equipment faults.

Other key elements of the design of monitoring equipment that may not be obvious include:

- protection of the patient from faults in the equipment;
- protection of the equipment from damage caused by diathermy, defibrillation, etc.;
- protection of the equipment and also its displayed results from electromagnetic interference (EMI), usually referred to as electromagnetic compatability (EMC);

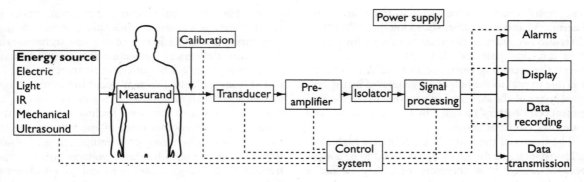

Figure 18.2 Generalized monitoring system showing the major components.

- ergonomics or the ease of use both in its physical design and any necessary training;
- reliability under the conditions in which it might be used.

MONITORING OF PHYSIOLOGICALLY GENERATED ELECTRICAL SIGNALS

All living cells generate minute electrical currents; across every living cell membrane there is a potential difference. When excitable cells, for example muscle cells, act in unison, the generated current is large enough to be detected by electronic means. Commonly measured electrophysiological potentials include the electrocardiogram (ECG), electroencephalogram (EEG) and the electromyogram (EMG). Table 18.1 shows the typical potentials and range of frequencies expected.

With such small potentials, extreme methods have to be used in equipment design to amplify the required signal without amplifying unwanted electrical interference or *noise*. The *signal to noise ratio* is an important parameter in the design of physiological amplifiers. Also, because this is the *only* situation in electronic engineering when deliberate ohmic connection is made with the human body, it is especially important to have *electrical isolation* of very high quality between the components

Table 18.1 Physiologically generated potentials

Measurand	Range of potentials	Signal frequency range
Electrocardiography	0.5–4 mV	0.01–250 Hz
Electroencephalography	5–300 µV	d.c.–150 Hz
Electromyography	0.1–5 mV	d.c.–10 000 Hz

touching the body and any electrical pathway that may lead to electric shock or electrocution.

The Electrocardiograph

Modern ECGs are much more complex than would seem necessary just to display the ECG. This is to fulfil the extra requirements listed above. The electrical signals generated by the beating heart may be detected by placement on the surface of the body, electrodes connected to a high-gain amplifier and may then be displayed on an oscilloscope. As measured at the body surface, typical amplitudes are 1–5 mV with a frequency range of 0.1–100 Hz. This frequency range does not imply that the heart rate is of this range but that the PQRST complex may be broken down by Fourier analysis into components made up from the addition of frequencies in this range. This means that to produce a faithful representation of the electrical events, the ECG amplifier must have a bandwidth covering this range; in other words, it should amplify by a constant amount over the range of 0.1–100 Hz. The greater the bandwidth of an amplifier, the more accurately the output will be a function of the input, but also the greater will be the unwanted interference. This interference may be biological, mainly as a result of noise generated by muscle (EMG) or environmental noise caused by power cables, electrical instruments, transformers or surgical diathermy equipment that becomes electrically or magnetically coupled to the body or monitoring leads. For this reason, the bandwidth is limited to a compromise between the quality of the ECG signal and the acceptable level of interference. For diagnostic purposes, ECG pre-amplifiers usually have a bandwidth of 0.05–100 Hz, but for monitoring in electrically noisy environments, as in the operating theatre, the bandwidth is limited to 0.5–40 Hz. The effect of this narrower bandwidth is to 'round-off' slightly the sharper peaks and troughs of the QRS complex and markedly reduce interference while making it still quite possible to assess arrhythmias and ischaemia. A band-pass rather than a low-pass filter (Fig. 18.3) is also necessary to eliminate the approximately 25 mV of d.c. skin potential that exists at the interface between the recording electrode and the skin. This 25 mV is due in part to the potentials generated by the epidermal layers of the skin, and in part due to the electrochemical cell ('battery') formed by the skin–electrolytic gel–metallic electrode combination.

The tissues of the body have a relatively high electrical resistance and the ECG signal is said to be a *high-impedance source*; it is therefore necessary to use a high-quality amplifier with a high input impedance. Electrical noise is also generated by the components of

the amplifier itself, but careful design can minimize its effect. Safety is a prime consideration, as recording or monitoring the ECG is one of the few techniques in which direct electrical connection is deliberately made to the human body. The patient must therefore be protected from (a) faults that may occur in the monitoring system and (b) an unwanted earth pathway for surgical diathermy or a fault condition leading to an unwanted earth pathway in another piece of apparatus connected to the patient. The monitoring equipment is also protected from damage by high voltages from radio-frequency (RF) surgical diathermy and even defibrillator pulses.

Figure 18.4 shows the components of a modern ECG monitor. A simple amplifier would have a single input terminal and its output would be a function of the potential difference between that input terminal and the ground reference. Any EMI that would be coupled to the input lead, either inductively or capacitively (Fig. 18.5a), would be unlikely to couple to both the input lead and the ground reference to the same extent, and therefore the interference, which may be of much greater amplitude than the ECG signal itself, will also be amplified. Even the simplest of ECG monitors therefore make use of a differential or balanced pre-amplifier (Fig. 18.5b). The reference earth lead is connected to the patient; this lead is often marked 'Right Leg' or 'RL'. However, the ECG is detected as the difference between inverting (−) and non-inverting (+) inputs to the pre-amplifier, which is designed to have a high common mode rejection ratio (CMRR). The CMRR is a measure of the ratio between the wanted and interfering signals; the higher the value of the CMRR the better the quality of the amplifier. Thus any EMI affecting the input leads will be of the same polarity in both leads and will therefore be cancelled out and only the ECG signal will be amplified.

The pre-amplifier is electrically isolated from the rest of the monitor by either transformers with a high degree of insulation between primary and secondary windings or by optical isolators where the amplified signal is converted to light by a light-emitting diode, which is insulated from a photo-detector that converts the signal back into an electrical signal. The very high power of RF surgical diathermy equipment may overwhelm the simple techniques described thus far.

High-quality ECG monitors for use in operating theatres may use adaptive noise filtering, a complex digital electronic technique in which the EMI is detected separately from the ECG signal and then subtracted from the ECG+EMI, thus leaving a clean ECG trace without the EMI.

Early ECG monitors used the so-called 'bouncing dot' type of scan on a cathode-ray tube which had a long-persistence output phosphor. It takes a lot of practice to make a diagnosis from this type of display and it is

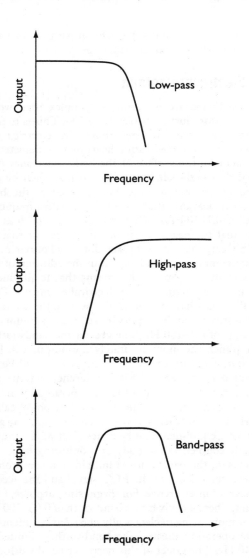

Figure 18.3 Electronic filters – for a constant input amplitude, the output varies as shown.

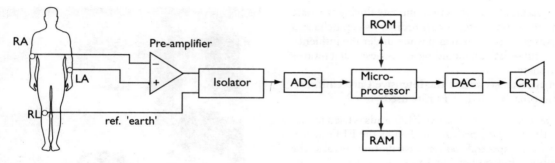

Figure 18.4 Block diagram of a modern ECG monitor.

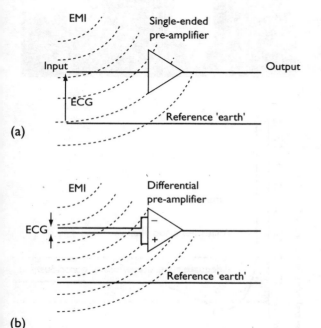

(a)

(b)

Figure 18.5 Effect of electromagnetic interference (EMI) on the ECG signal. (a) Single-input pre-amplifier. Note that the interference to the 'input' and the 'reference earth' is amplified. (b) Identical EMI affecting the positive and negative inputs of a differential amplifier are cancelled out, because the amplifier amplifies the *difference* between the two inputs.

impossible to 'freeze' a frame for further examination as the only 'memory' was the persistence of the phosphor. Today's ECG monitors, and the displays of other analogue traces, make use of a microprocessor memory technique. The analogue signal is converted to a digital signal by an analogue to digital converter (ADC). Sufficient ECG data, now in digital form, is stored in the semiconductor random access memory (RAM) to fill the width of the display screen. As the latest information is stored, so the oldest is erased, thus ensuring that the most up-to-date 5 or 10 s are stored in the RAM. Simultaneously, the entire RAM is read out very rapidly through the microprocessor and a digital to analogue converter (DAC) to a CRT display. Thus a 'rolling' display of the previous 10 s is displayed and may be 'frozen' for closer examination. If an LCD is used it may be driven digitally directly from the microprocessor. ECG monitors for use during anaesthesia may have an alarm that operates when the heart rate goes outside preset limits, but further sophistication is usually not provided unless the machine has been designed for use in intensive care situations.

Before making any decision about the management of a patient from the results of an ECG, it is important that any causes of error or artefacts in the use of the equipment are eliminated. The following may cause erroneous traces:

- wrongly positioned electrodes;
- left-to-right misconnection;
- poor electrode contact with skin;
- electromagnetic interference;
- voluntary or involuntary movement;
- shivering;
- excessive muscle tone.

The Electroencephalograph

The electrical signals generated by the central nervous system are of a much lower amplitude than the ECG and therefore electroencephalography requires even more sensitive amplifiers than the ECG; there is also a greater need for protection from EMI than for the EEG. For diagnostic purposes, a combination of many leads are recorded on paper simultaneously.

The EEG signal is characterized by four frequency bands:

- alpha, 8–13 Hz;
- beta, 13–30 Hz;
- theta, 4–7 Hz;
- delta, <4 Hz.

Alpha and beta waves predominate during the state of conscious awareness, during ordinary sleep delta and theta patterns are formed and when under the influence of powerful sedatives, including anaesthesia, delta waves predominate.

In anaesthesia and in the Intensive Care Unit, different approaches to the EEG are used:

- *Fourier analysis* of one or two EEG leads is used to display the *spectral power distribution* of the EEG in real time. The spectral power distribution breaks the seemingly indecipherable EEG signal down into its component frequencies and displays the 'amount' or power of each frequency at any one time. This form of EEG may be used to indicate the depth of anaesthesia or coma. The *cerebral function analysing monitor* (CFAM) is a much simpler form of EEG analyser, which is said to show depth of anaesthesia or coma.

- *Spectral Edge Frequency* (SEF_{90}) is the frequency below which 90% of the power in the frequency spectrum lies. It is therefore the highest relevant frequency in the EEG signal.

- The *bispectral index* is another method of spectral analysis where not only is the power spectrum displayed but the phase differences between the frequency components are also indicated. This is said to produce an even more sensitive indication in the state of brain function and level of consciousness.

- The *evoked potential EEG* is especially useful during spinal surgery but is also used in intensive care. A stimulus (electrical to the lower limb in the case of spinal surgery, sound or light when the central nervous system is being monitored) is applied to the patient. The effect of the stimulus on the processed EEG is displayed.

An example of an EEG-based depth of anaesthesia monitor, the Dräger pEEG, is shown in Fig. 18.6.

The Electromyograph

The EMG is mainly used in diagnostic neurology but a form of EMG may be used to assess the state of the neuromuscular junction during anaesthesia. An electrical stimulus is applied to a peripheral motor nerve and the resultant muscle contraction is monitored by applying electrodes over the appropriate muscle mass.

MONITORING OF BLOOD PRESSURE

Arterial blood pressure is measured before, during and after every anaesthetic, be it general anaesthesia, sedation or regional conduction anaesthesia. In the seriously

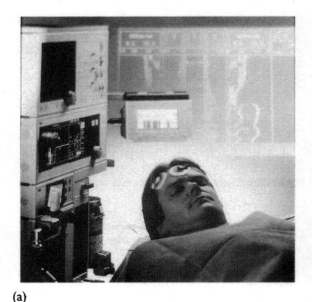

(a)

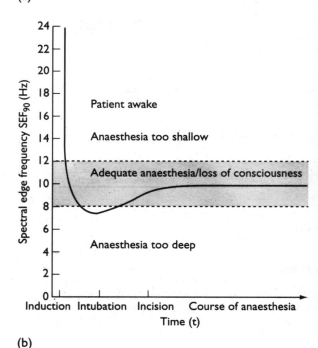

(b)

Figure 18.6 (a) Dräger pEEG monitor for assessing the depth of anaesthesia. (b) Plot from the output of the pEEG monitor.

ill patient or those undergoing major surgery it may be necessary to measure the central venous and pulmonary vascular blood pressure as well.

The measurement and monitoring of arterial blood pressure during anaesthesia has been carried out for many years although, like many physiological variables, it may be measured more because it is possible to do it reasonably easily, than because of its physiological importance.

Historical measurement of blood pressure was originally *direct*, i.e., is by using the *manometer* principle. Direct invasive connection was made to the blood vessel in which it was desired to know the pressure with a vertical narrow-bore glass tube. The pressure caused blood to flow into the vertical tube until such a point when the pressure in the blood vessel was equal to the pressure generated at the base of the tube due to gravity, the density of blood and the height to which the blood had reached. This is shown in Fig. 18.7. Direct invasive blood pressure measurement is described in Chapter 20. The following techniques are available for the measurement of arterial blood pressure:

Non-invasive
- Riva Rocci (auscultation);
- Oscillotonometer (von Recklinghausen);
- Oscillometric;
- Penaz (Finapress).

Invasive
- Aneroid;
- Transducer.

Central venous pressure may be measured by a simple manometer technique whereas pulmonary vascular pressure is always measured using a transducer. It is also important to bear this principle in mind when measuring arterial blood pressure non-invasively. When a patient is supine, the blood pressure measured at the arm will be similar to blood pressure in the head and at the feet. However, if the patient is not supine then the pressure above the level at which it is measured will be lower than that measured at the arm and *vice versa*, as shown in Fig. 18.8. This hydrostatic effect causes the blood pressure to fall by 7.5 mmHg (1 kPa) for every 10 cm in vertical height. If the patient is marginally hypotensive as measured at the arm when in the head-up position he or she may have a very low cerebral perfusion pressure.

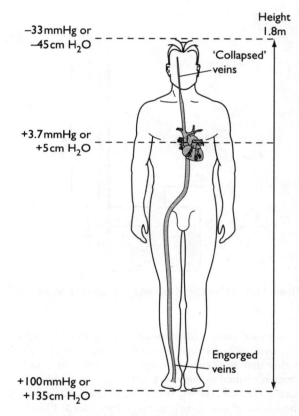

Figure 18.8 Arterial blood pressure is affected by gravity. This effect is shown most dramatically in the venous system.

Methods of Non-invasive Arterial Blood Pressure Measurement

The vast majority of non-invasive arterial-blood pressure measurement are *intermittent* methods in that they measure arterial blood pressure at a discrete moment in time, which is not instantaneous as these methods require a few heart cycles to produce a result. The ideal method of measuring arterial blood pressure would be non-invasively but producing a *continuous* reading. Techniques for continuous measurement are now

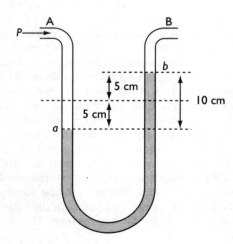

Figure 18.7 A simple manometer. A pressure *P* is applied at A. This causes a depression of the fluid level at *a* and a corresponding rise of the fluid level at *b*. In this case the tube is filled with water and the pressure is 10 cm of water.

becoming available; the most well known, Finapress (Ohmeda), uses 'vascular unloading' and will be described.

Sphygmomanometer

The simplest and cheapest method of measuring arterial blood pressure is with a mercury manometer and cuff system known as a *sphygmomanometer* (Fig. 18.9), using the Riva-Rocci auscultatory technique.

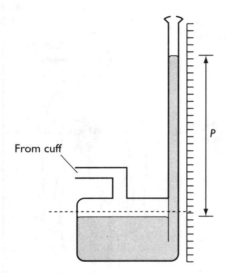

Figure 18.9 The principle of the mercury sphygmomanometer.

An inflatable cuff is placed firmly but not tightly over the brachial artery. The cuff is inflated to a pressure higher than the expected systolic pressure and a stethoscope is applied to the artery distal to the cuff. The pressure in the cuff is slowly reduced and the points at which the *Korotkoff* sounds begin and end are noted. These are said to be equivalent to systolic and diastolic pressures, respectively. The systolic pressure measured in this way is commonly 5–10 mmHg *lower* than when measured directly.

The advantages and disadvantages of sphygmomanometry are shown in Table 18.2.

The size of the cuff has an influence on the accuracy of this technique:

- The width of the inflatable bladder should be 40% of the mid-circumference of the limb; the length should be twice this width.
- A cuff that is too narrow produces erroneously high pressures.
- A cuff that is too loose produces erroneously low pressures.

Table 18.2 The advantages and disadvantages of sphygmomanometry

Advantages	Disadvantages
Low technology	Poor correlation with invasive measurement
No electricity required	Affected by ambient noise
Low cost	Dependent upon observers' hearing
Portable	Dependent upon cuff-size/arm diameter
Rugged	Accuracy affected by vascular disease

The flow of blood under the cuff may be detected by photoplethysmography or by a Doppler ultrasonic flow detector. Arterial blood pressure during anaesthesia is most commonly measured using the oscillometric principle. If one examines carefully the meniscus of the mercury in a mercury sphygmomanometer as the cuff pressure is slowly reduced, small fluctuations, sychronous with heart rhythm, may be seen on the manometer when the cuff is inflated at pressures between systolic and diastolic pressures, with a maximum amplitude at mean arterial blood pressure.

Oscillotonometer

These fluctuations may be detected by a double-cuff device known as an oscillotonometer (Fig. 18.10). A double pneumatic cuff is applied to the upper arm as shown in Fig. 18.10a. The instrument itself consists of two aneroid capsules, one of which is coarse (A) and the other very sensitive (B) inside a sealed case and they are connected by a lever mechanism and a rack-and-pinion to a pointer, as shown in Fig. 18.10b. Capsule A is sealed and responds to changes in pressure in the case. Capsule B is connected to the distal cuff. The valve lever is biased to position 1 where the release valve is occluded and there is free communication between the two sides of capsule B. Manual inflation of the system with the bulb causes an increase in pressure equally in both cuffs and the case of the instrument and this pressure is indicated on the scale as capsule A decreases in volume. When the pressure is in excess of the expected arterial pressure, inflation is ceased and the lever is moved to position 2. A small-bore aperture is now interposed between the inside and outside of capsule B and air is allowed to leak slowly from the system through the pressure release valve. Pulsations occurring in the distal cuff are indicated by fluctuations of capsule B only. As the pressure in the system is released, oscillations will first occur at systolic blood pressure, reach a maximum at the mean pressure, and should finally disappear at the diastolic pressure.

The oscillotonometer gives only a usable clinical accuracy at the systolic pressure. The actual blood pressure is indicated by releasing the lever back to position 1, at which time the scale indicates the cuff pressure.

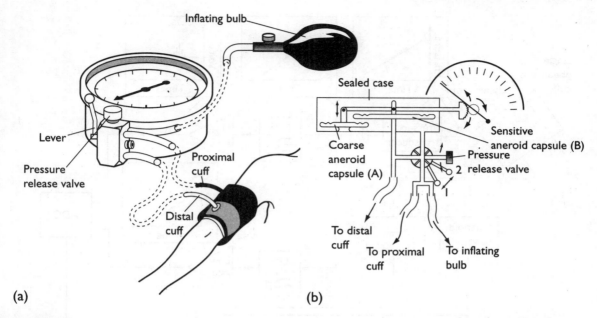

Figure 18.10 The von Recklinghausen oscillotonometer (see text). (Reproduced from Ponte J and Green D (1986) *A New Short Textbook of Anaesthesia.* London: Edward Arnold.)

Automatic Oscillotonometry

It is now common practice to use electronic techniques, again relying on the oscillometric principle. Electronic oscillometric blood pressure monitors make use of a conventional pneumatic cuff surrounding, usually, the upper arm. Some manufacturers use a single tube to connect the cuff to the monitor whilst others use two tubes, separating the pump tube from that along which the pressure in the cuff is sensed. Figure 18.11 shows the principle of the technique. At the centre of the machine is a microprocessor, which controls all the other components. The pump inflates the cuff to above the expected systolic pressure, which is measured by the pressure transducer. The air in the cuff is then allowed to leak slowly out via a solenoid valve, either smoothly or in a series of discrete steps. As the pressure in the cuff falls, the signal from the transducer varies, as shown in the graphs. This signal is amplified in two ways. (1) After passing through a low-pass filter, it is amplified by a comparatively low-gain amplifier, the output of which is then proportional to the cuff pressure at that instant. (2) The signal is also passed through a high-pass filter, which effectively removes the electrical signal due to the slowly changing cuff pressure, and then through a high-gain amplifier so that the comparatively high-frequency oscillations due to the oscillations of the arterial wall alone are amplified. It can be seen that these oscillations

begin at the systolic pressure, are a maximum at the mean pressure, and finally disappear at the diastolic pressure. The signals from both these amplifiers are then passed through an ADC to the microprocessor. The microprocessor, apart from controlling the pump and the solenoid valve, calculates the systolic, diastolic and mean pressures and controls the display and alarms. The microprocessor also compares the results for systolic and diastolic pressures with what would be expected from the mean pressure. This is done because the most accurate measurement made by these machines is the mean pressure, as the maximum oscillations are much more easily detected than the points at which the oscillations just start and disappear.

It is possible that the values of blood pressure obtained with this technique do not exactly correspond to those obtained by direct intra-arterial measurement at the radial artery. This is often due to underdamping of the direct arterial pressure signal, but it has also been shown that pressure measured by the oscillometric technique is comparable to central *aortic* blood pressure. The heart rate is always displayed at the same time since it is so easy for the microprocessor to calculate this from the period between each oscillation.

Oscillometric non-invasive blood pressure monitors may also have integral printers that record the blood pressure, heart rate and time at preset intervals. It most accurately displays *mean* blood pressure.

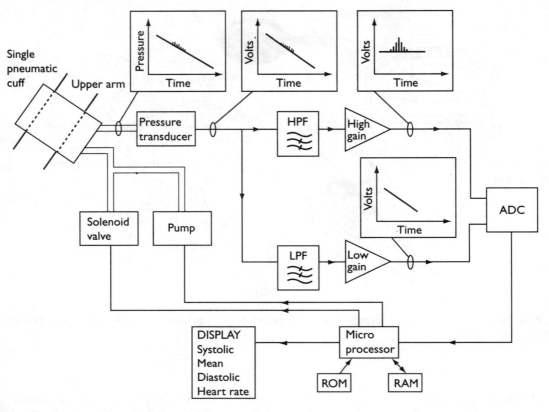

Figure 18.11 Schematic diagram of the automatic non-invasive arterial blood pressure monitor using the oscillometric principle.

The disadvantages of conventional oscillometric blood pressure monitoring are:

- it can make only discrete blood pressure measurements, at best, once every 2 minutes or so;
- there is a small risk of nerve damage owing to repeated compression.

A recent development is a non-invasive blood pressure monitor using a very small pneumatically inflated cuff applied to a finger (Fig. 18.12). The cuff also contains an infrared photoplethysmograph. The technique is based on the concept that if an externally applied pressure is equal to the arterial wall pressure at all times, the artery will not change in size. If the arteries under the cuff are therefore kept at the same size, the blood volume contained within them will remain constant as will the absorption of the infrared light and therefore the photoplethysmograph signal will remain constant. A microprocessor-controlled servo-system maintains the cuff pressure so that the light absorption remains constant. The pressure in the cuff is therefore instantaneously the same as that in the artery and a continuous blood pressure reading is therefore available.

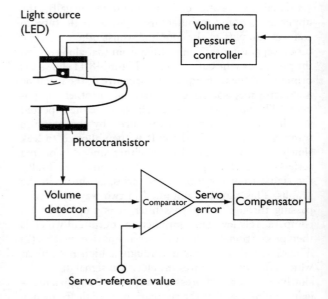

Figure 18.12 Principle of the Finapress continuous non-invasive blood pressure monitor.

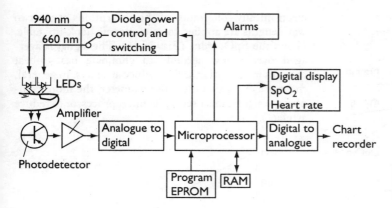

Figure 18.13 Electronic components of the pulse oximeter. (LED, light emitting diode).

PULSE MONITORING

The character of the arterial pulse, its rate and its rhythm have always been important, not only to the mystique of medicine but also to scientific diagnosis, and no more so than in the practice of anaesthesia. Although the greatest amount of information may be gained by palpation of the radial pulse, it is usually inconvenient to do this throughout a long surgical procedure. For this reason several non-invasive methods have been developed for electronic monitoring of the arterial pulse. Pulse plethysmography, as the technique is called, also forms the basis of two modern monitoring techniques: pulse oximetry described below and continuous non-invasive blood pressure monitoring.

Pulse plethysmography is based upon the measurement of the increase in the volume of an extremity, usually a finger or an ear lobe, during or shortly after systole.

All pulse plethysmograph devices now use the technique of photoplethysmography. A low level of electromagnetic energy (light or near-infrared) is passed through the extremity. Most of the energy, which must be at a wavelength to which the part is translucent, is detected by a semiconductor sensor or photodetector suitable for that wavelength. An increase in volume of the part is then detected as an increase in the absorption of the incident light during systole. The signal from the photodetector is then amplified and may be displayed on a cathode-ray oscilloscope. This technique may be so sensitive that the dichrotic notch is easily visible. The 'light' used is usually not at visible wavelengths as it is customary to use near-infrared, because it is then possible to use a detector that is sensitive only to these wavelengths, thus eliminating artefacts caused by ambient light.

PULSE OXIMETRY

It is extraordinarily difficult to guess the state of a patient's arterial oxygenation subjectively. The ability to detect decreased haemoglobin oxygen saturation depends on many factors including circulatory state, skin pigmentation, haemoglobin concentration, ambient light colour and intensity. The introduction in the early 1980s of pulse oximetry allows reasonably accurate objective assessment of haemoglobin oxygen saturation of arterial blood (SpO_2), cheaply, non-invasively and with a very low morbidity.

Apart from the objective indication of SpO_2, pulse oximetry may be described as 'fail-safe' in that the technique fails and therefore alarms if the pulsatility of the pulse waveform decreases to below a critical level. Further information may be gained by the display of a plethysmograph trace, which enables the differentiation between the pulse waveform and artefacts. No pulse oximeter should be used unless a plethysmograph trace is displayed.

Knowledge of the principles of the technique allows one to understand the limitations and use the information displayed safely. The absorption spectra of normal adult haemoglobin in its saturated and desaturated states are shown in Fig. 18.14. Also shown are the absorption spectra of two common dyshaemoglobins, carboxyhaemoglobin and methaemoglobin, which lead to erroneous oxygen saturation values being indicated by conventional pulse oximetry, as described later. It can be seen from the spectra of oxygenated and deoxygenated haemoglobin that there is a change in absorption dependent upon the amount of oxygen being carried by the haemoglobin molecule. In living tissue it is necessary to separate the change in energy absorption resulting from any change in oxygen saturation from all other energy

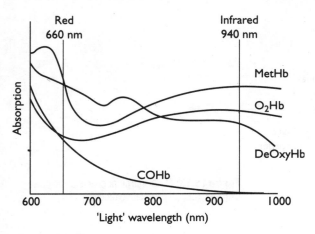

Figure 18.14 Absorption spectra of whole blood and two common interfering dyshaemoglobins between 600 nm and 1000 nm showing the two commonly used wavelengths of pulse oximetry.

absorbants at those wavelengths. This separation is done by assuming that, over short periods of time, in peripheral tissue, absorption of the energy will be constant by all tissue components except that resulting from the pulsation of arterial blood.

Energy from LEDs of wavelengths 660 nm and 940 nm is projected through peripheral tissue (finger, toe, ear-lobe, bridge of nose). The emerging energy, after absorption by all the tissue layers including arteries and arterioles, is detected by a semiconductor sensor. To allow a single site for the transducer, the LEDs are energized alternately at a rate of around 1 kHz. The signal from the sensor is electronically separated into plethysmograph signals for each of the wavelengths. These signals are pulsatile owing to the variability of the arteriolar cross-sectional area and the change in axis of erythrocytes with cardiac cycle. In simple terms the absorption due to tissues other than the arterial system are constant (Fig. 18.15) and therefore can easily be eliminated

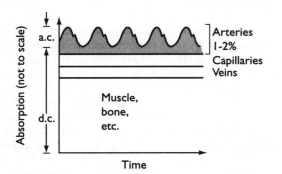

Figure 18.15 Composition of the absorption signal as detected by photoplethysmography (not to scale).

electronically. The ratios of the absorptions at the two wavelengths are applied to an electronic 'look-up' table, giving the SpO_2 value (Fig. 18.16). The signal is averaged over a few seconds to eliminate beat-to-beat changes in saturation and to reduce artefacts. In general, the more expensive the pulse oximeter, the more complex the algorithms used by its microprocessor to reduce artefacts.

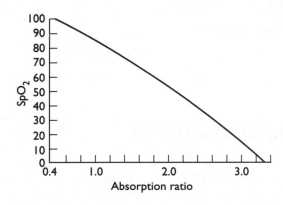

Figure 18.16 Theoretical ratio of absorption of red (660 nm) and infrared (940 nm) light energy related to haemoglobin oxygen saturation.

The Limitations of Pulse Oximetry

The advantage of pulse oximetry is that it is easily applied and has a much more robust probe than transcutaneous blood gas monitoring. However, it must be remembered that it is indicating *percentage haemoglobin oxygen saturation in arterial blood* and not partial pressure of dissolved oxygen, although these are related by the *oxygen dissociation curve* (ODC). The ODC is changed by several other variables as shown in Fig. 18.17 and also varies with other types of haemoglobin. *P50* is an abbreviation for the partial pressure of oxygen at which the haemoglobin is 50% saturated and is a useful shorthand term for quantifying shifts in the ODC.

Safety in the use of pulse oximetry depends upon a knowledge of the *limitations* of the technique. These limitations (Table 18.3) may be classified in two ways, namely as to whether they are *technical* or *physiological* limitations and whether they are *safe* or potentially *dangerous*. Safe limitations may be defined as conditions when the pulse oximeter is not indicating the correct value of arterial haemoglobin oxygen saturation but the user is warned that the value may be inaccurate. Dangerous limitations are those where the device appears to be operating satisfactorily but is indicating the wrong value of saturation.

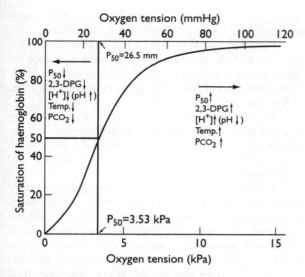

Figure 18.17 Oxyhaemoglobin dissociation curve.

Table 18.3 Limitations of pulse oximetry

	SAFE	DANGEROUS
Technical	Mechanical artefacts Electromagnetic interference Magnetic resonance imaging	Accuracy Calibration Delay 'Flooding' 'Penumbra'
Physiological	Pulse dependence Pulse volume Pulse rhythm	Abnormal haemoglobins Other absorbents Dyes Delay Pulsatile veins (pigmentation)

Mechanical artefacts are caused by any movement of the probe on the extremity. The technique is especially sensitive to this problem as the energy absorption resulting from arterial pulsation is only 1–2% of the total absorption. Most pulse oximeters are able to detect excessive movement and indicate malfunction unless it is rhythmic and approximately at the heart rate. Mechanical artefacts are obvious when the oximeter displays a plethysmograph trace. *Electromagnetic interference* (EMI) may also cause malfunction that is obvious if a trace is displayed and always leads to an alarm situation. The most common source of EMI in hospital practice is radiofrequency surgical diathermy. However, a recent problem is the susceptibility of all electromedical equipment to the electromagnetic radiation from cellular telephones. Although the emissions from cellular telephones are of low power, when they are in close proximity the electric field emitted is often strong

enough to disrupt microprocessor function. A special class of EMI is the intense magnetic field in the vicinity of magnetic resonance imaging or nuclear magnetic spectroscopy equipment. With such equipment, nothing metallic should be in the high field area. Special pulse oximeters have been developed in which both the LEDs and the photodetector are housed in the case of the apparatus and the energy is led to the patient and back to the photodetector by optical fibres.

Pulse oximetry is *pulse dependent*; the technique requires an adequate pulse volume and may be said to be fail-safe as all devices warn of an inadequate pulsatile signal. With ever advancing computer software, modern pulse oximeters are better able to function with irregular *rhythms*.

It is essential that the dangerous limitations of the technique are understood. Pulse oximeters are *type-calibrated* by the designers and manufacturers using fit, healthy young adults with normal adult haemoglobin (HbA) levels who are desaturated by stages from 100% down to a minimum of 80%. It would be unethical to desaturate below 80% and therefore any values of SpO_2 are less likely to be as accurate as those above 80% as calibration <80% is by extrapolation.

The calibration of pulse oximeters is performed against *in vitro* arterial blood samples tested in a co-oximeter, which is a spectrophotometer dedicated to assessing haemoglobin oxygen saturation. SpO_2 should never be compared with saturation values indicated by blood–gas analysis as saturation in this case is derived from the measurement of pH, pCO_2 and pO_2.

Accuracy is quoted by most manufacturers as being of the order of ± 2%. *In vitro* methods of calibration are under development (see further reading). There is much argument as to whether pulse oximeters are calibrated to measure *functional* or *fractional* oxygen saturation. Strictly, pulse oximeters indicate neither functional nor fractional but 'the value of oxygen saturation as indicated by pulse oximetry using the wavelengths of 660 nm and 940 nm' and for this reason the abbreviation SpO_2 should always be used.

There may be *delays* between a change in oxygen saturation and its indication by a pulse oximeter. These technical delays may be due to an irregular pulse volume or rhythm slowing the computation of SpO_2 or due to averaging algorithms, which produce more accurate but slower results. When relying upon pulse oximetry to indicate hypoxia, it must be remembered that the technique gives a comparatively late warning of, for example, failure of oxygen supply of mechanical ventilation. For this reason it is important that there are separate measurement systems and alarms for inspired oxygen concentration and failure or disconnection of mechanical ventilation. Placement of the probe centrally (tongue, cheek) rather than peripherally (finger, toe) may halve the delay in indication of desaturation.

Extraneous energy sources, especially bright visible or infrared light, may *flood* or overload the semiconductor detector. If the pulse oximeter does not alarm to indicate flooding, it may display a value of 85%. This is because a ratio of red/infrared of 1 is equivalent to an SpO_2 of 85%. A similar problem, which has been called the *penumbra effect*, often occurs with small infants and children. In this case the pulse oximeter may over-read or under-read because of a different path-length of tissue for each of the wavelengths. This occurs with very small fingers or when the LEDs are projecting tangentially through the tip of a digit. For this reason, probes especially designed for use with babies and children have been produced and should always be used.

The most serious limitations of pulse oximetry are related to the fact that because currently available devices only use two wavelengths, the displayed value is always based on a calibration curve for normal HbA. Current pulse oximeters are unable to detect dyshaemoglobins and will therefore produce erroneous results without warning. Co-oximeters are safe to use in the presence of abnormal haemoglobins because they use more than two wavelengths; one machine uses as many as 17. Multi-wavelength co-oximeters actually indicate the proportions of the common dyshaemoglobins.

Of the dyshaemoglobins, carboxyhaemoglobin is the most dangerous as it is fairly common and makes the pulse oximeter *over*-read. The absorption spectrum of carboxyhaemoglobin is shown in Fig. 18.14. Carboxyhaemoglobin is caused by the inhalation of even very small quantities of carbon monoxide. Common sources of carbon monoxide are the internal combustion engine, conflagrations, barbecues, tobacco smoke and inadequately ventilated combustion of coal or gas in heating systems. **It must now be considered negligent to use pulse oximetry on patients who have been at risk of carbon monoxide inhalation.** For every 1% of carboxyhaemoglobin circulating, the pulse oximeter over-reads by approximately 1%. Fifty per cent of cigarette smokers have carboxyhaemoglobin concentrations of >6%; those involved in accidental inhalation may have much higher concentrations.

Methaemoglobinaemia, whose absorption spectrum is also shown in Fig. 18.14, may be congenital or, more commonly, acquired. This dyshaemoglobin may be considered 'safer' as the greater the concentration of methaemoglobin, the more the indicated SpO_2 tends toward the value of 85%. Acquired methaemoglobinaemia occurs when the iron of haemoglobin is oxidized from the ferrous Fe^{2+} to the ferric Fe^{3+} form. There are a large number of drugs and other chemicals that may induce methaemaglobinaemia, including several antimalarials, dapsone, EDTA, local anaesthetic agents, methylene blue, nitrates, nitrites, nitric oxide, para-aminosalicylic acid (PAS) and the sulphonamides.

Fetal haemoglobin (HbF) has similar absorption spectra to HbA and therefore pulse oximeters indicate SpO_2 within the same limits of accuracy as with HbA. This is also true of HbS although in both cases the ODC will be shifted.

Certain *dyes* such as methylene blue and indocyanine green, which may be administered for diagnostic purposes, have a drastic effect upon the accuracy of pulse oximeters. The accuracy recovers rapidly after bolus injection as the dye dilutes.

Bilirubin was reported to render pulse oximetry inaccurate when compared with co-oximetry. Examination of the absorption spectrum of bilirubin shows no absorption at 660 nm and 940 nm. The discrepancy between pulse oximetry and co-oximetry was due to the fact that co-oximeters operate over different wavelengths, normally visible, where bilirubin does absorb. This demonstrates how important it is to compare like-with-like. The latest multi-wavelength co-oximeters can distinguish bilirubin and also HbF. The accuracy of pulse oximetry is not effected by jaundice although the ODC will be shifted.

Pulsatile veins may cause pulse oximeters to *under*-read as the technique cannot tell the difference between pulsating veins and arterioles. This was first noted in cases of tricuspid incompetence but recently there has been some suggestion that venules in neonates and children with hyperdynamic circulation may be more pulsatile than in adults owing to the shorter length of the arterio-venous anastomoses in the microcirculation.

Skin *pigmentation* and opaque nail varnish usually make pulse oximeters fail safely but there have been some conflicting reports of inaccuracies.

MONITORING OF BODY TEMPERATURE

It is important to monitor body temperature during anaesthesia to avoid excessive deviation from 37°C. The causes of deviation from normal body temperature are listed in Table 18.4.

The body temperature may be monitored by several different devices:

- mercury thermometer (intermittent)
- liquid crystal thermometer (intermittent)
- thermocouple
- thermistor
- infrared tympanic thermometer.

Table 18.4 Causes of deviation from normal body temperature

Body temperature may decrease due to:	Body temperature may increase due to:
Preoperative hypothermia	Sepsis
Exposure peroperatively	Malignant hyperpyrexia
Evaporation from open body cavities	Malignant neurolept syndrome
Contact with cooler environment	Excessive insulation from environment
Infusion of cool fluids (IV and bladder)	Excessive heat input from environment
Vasodilatation caused by anaesthetic drugs	
Inhalation of cold, dry gases	

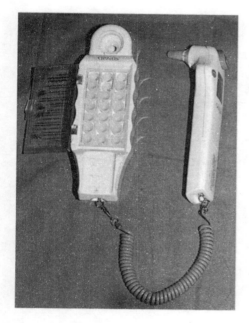

Figure 18.18 Tympanic thermometer.

The clinical *mercury thermometer* is a conventional thermometer relying upon the expansion of a liquid with increase of temperature. There is a small constriction introduced just above the mercury bulb so that when the temperature of the mercury in the bulb reduces as the thermometer is removed from the body cavity, the mercury column is broken thus retaining the reading. Low-reading clinical thermometers are available for assessing the hypothermic patient. Used orally or rectally, the reading approximates to the core temperature; used in the axilla the reading is approximately 1°C below core temperature.

Liquid crystal thermometers have the advantage of being less delicate than mercury thermometers; however, they will only indicate surface temperature.

Thermocouples rely on the Seebeck effect; a potential difference is generated at the junction of two dissimilar metals proportional to the temperature difference between one junction at the point of measurement and a similar junction at a reference temperature. At clinical temperatures, thermocouples are therefore more difficult to use than thermistors. *Thermistors* are electrical resistors usually made from a semiconductor material chosen for its large change in resistance with change in temperature; thus the electronics involved are much simpler and the calibration much easier.

A recent introduction in temperature measurement, which is almost non-contact, is the *infrared tympanic thermometer*. A small probe, which consists of a series of thermocouples forming a 'thermopile', is aimed at (but not in contact with) the tympanic membrane, radiation from which is detected by the thermopile. The voltage generated is proportional to the tympanic temperature (Fig. 18.18).

FURTHER READING

Hutton P, Prys-Roberts C (eds) (1994) *Monitoring in Anaesthesia and Intensive Care*. London: WB Saunders.

Moyle JTB (1994) *Principles & Practice of Pulse Oximetry*. London: BMJ Publishing Group.

Webster JG (ed.) (1992) *Medical Instrumentation – Applications & Design*. Boston: Houghton Mifflin.

PHYSIOLOGICAL MONITORING: GASES

Contents ━━━

INTRODUCTION

Unlike other specialities involving clinical measurement, safety and quality in the practice of anaesthesia are intimately related to the measurement of the concentration of both inhaled and exhaled gases. This chapter describes the methods used to measure these gases both in the gaseous form and, in the case of oxygen and carbon dioxide, in their dissolved state.

INSPIRED OXYGEN CONCENTRATION

Inspired oxygen concentration is most commonly measured by one of three methods. Two of these are electrochemical: the galvanic cell, more commonly referred to as a fuel cell, and the polarographic cell. The third method is physical, relying on the paramagnetic property of oxygen.

Galvanic and Polarographic Cells

The galvanic or fuel cell (Fig. 19.1a) is similar to the cell of a primary battery but the potential difference between the anode and cathode is proportional to the oxygen tension to which it is exposed. A typical fuel cell consists of a goldmesh cathode separated from the gas under test by a gas-permeable plastic membrane. The anode is made of lead and the electrolyte is potassium hydroxide.

Oxygen is consumed at the cathode, the reaction being:

$$O_2 + 4e^- + 2H_2O \rightarrow 4(OH^-)$$

At the anode, electrons are released by a combination of hydroxyl ions, from the potassium hydroxide electrolyte, with lead:

$$Pb + 2(OH^-) \rightarrow PbO + H_2O + 2e^-$$

As the fuel cell is temperature sensitive, compensation has to be provided, usually by a thermistor. The oxygen concentration may be displayed by a simple voltmeter calibrated in percentage of oxygen.

The polarographic oxygen cell is of the same type as is used for the analysis of oxygen in blood. The construction is shown in Fig. 19.1b. A fine platinum cathode is separated from the gas under test by a thin layer of electrolyte and contained by a Teflon membrane which is permeable to oxygen gas. A polarizing voltage of about 0.6 V is applied between the cathode and a platinum anode, which is also immersed in the electrolyte solution. Oxygen diffuses through the membrane into the electrolyte solution at the cathode. Electrons combine with the oxygen at the cathode and reduce them to hydroxyl ions. A current thus flows that is proportional to the oxygen concentration. The current is very small

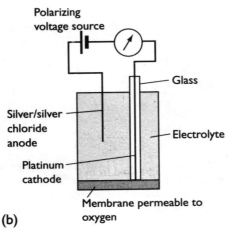

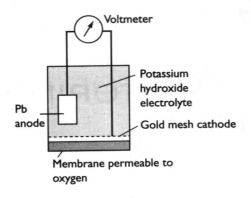

(a)

(b)

Figure 19.1 Working principles of (a) a galvanic oxygen fuel cell and (b) a polarographic oxygen analyser.

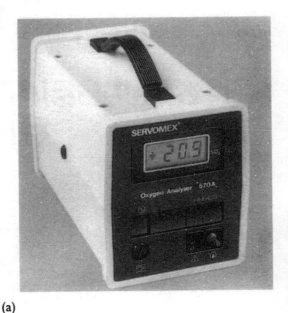

(a)

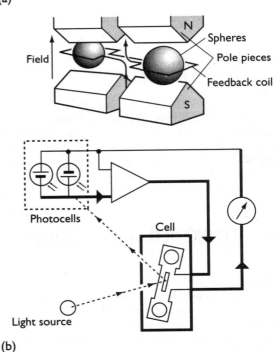

(b)

Figure 19.2 (a) Servomex paramagnetic oxygen analyser; (b) working principles.

and therefore requires amplification. Unfortunately, the polarographic analyser is sensitive, sometimes very sensitive, to nitrous oxide. Both galvanic and polarographic oxygen cells have a limited life.

Paramagnetic Oxygen Analysers

Paramagnetic oxygen analysers rely on the unusual magnetic property of the oxygen molecule called paramagnetism, whereby it is attracted by a magnetic field, in contrast to most other gases, including nitrous oxide, which are weakly diamagnetic and are therefore repelled. Conventional paramagnetic oxygen analysers, for example the Servomex (Fig. 19.2), consist of a small chamber into which is drawn the gas mixture under test. In the chamber are a pair of nitrogen-filled non-magnetic spheres, in a dumbbell arrangement, supported in a non-uniform powerful magnetic field by a hair-spring balance. A gas mixture containing oxygen in the chamber will be attracted to the magnetic field thus displacing

the spheres. The amount of displacement will be dependent upon the concentration of oxygen. Movement of the dumbbell arrangement about its axis is detected by directing a small beam of light onto a mirror on the dumbbells and thence to photocells. Any deflection of the beam causes an increase or decrease in current through a feedback coil that is part of the dumbbell assembly. The current is varied until the dumbbells return to the null position. The current required to do this is also directed through a meter that is calibrated in percentage of oxygen. The Servomex oxygen analyser is commonly used to check oxygen pipelines and air–oxygen mixers, to test the output of anaesthetic machines and to check the calibration of fuel cells.

Another oxygen analyser based on this principle has been developed by Datex (Fig. 19.3). A small sample of gas mixture is continuously drawn through a capillary tube at the same rate as a gas of known constant oxygen concentration (air). A powerful pulsed magnetic field is arranged over the junction of the two capillary tubes. This causes a pulsed pressure difference to occur between the two tubes if there is a difference in the oxygen concentration between the two tubes. The pressure difference is measured with a semiconductor transducer, and the resultant electrical signal is displayed as oxygen concentration and used for controlling alarms and even gas mixing valves.

been developed for the measurement of individual anaesthetic agents, although most of them are not agent-specific. Techniques include:

- interferometry;
- surface absorption;
- ultraviolet;
- infrared absorption spectroscopy;
- photo-acoustic spectroscopy.

The Riken Gas Indicator

The Riken gas indicator (Fig. 19.4) is an interferometer (interference-refractometer). It depends for its operation on the fact that there is a difference between the refractive index of clean air and that of air containing another gas. Light from a small lamp bulb is condensed

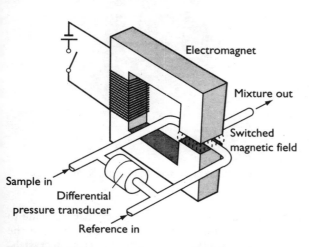

Figure 19.3 Datex paramagnetic oxygen analyser.

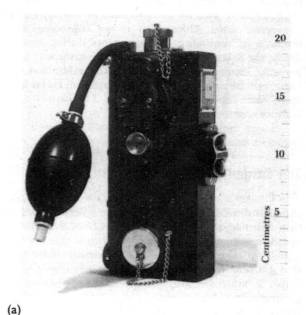

(a)

CARBON DIOXIDE, NITROUS OXIDE AND THE VOLATILE ANAESTHETIC AGENTS

Until recently, the only measurement technique capable of measuring oxygen, nitrous oxide, the volatile anaesthetic agents and any other gas was mass spectrometry; a technique new to anaesthesia, Raman spectroscopy, is almost as versatile. Many other physical techniques have

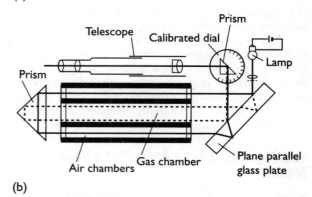

(b)

Figure 19.4 (a) The Riken gas indicator; (b) working principles.

into a beam, which is split into two parallel beams by prisms. Each parallel beam then passes through a chamber, one of which contains clean air and the other the sample of gas to be analysed. There is a difference in the effective length of the paths taken by the two beams, which, when they are brought together again, causes the appearance of an interference fringe that includes two characteristic dark lines, one of which is taken as the reference. The position of the reference line may be moved by a control knob until it falls on a reference point on the scale when the sampling chamber is filled with air. By means of a small manual aspirator, the sample of gas is then drawn into the sampling chamber and this causes a change in the position of the reference line on the scale. The displacement is proportional to the concentration of the gas. There is a vernier scale for more precise reading.

The interferometer may be calibrated for any required gas or vapour; one calibrated for halothane in oxygen may be used for other vapours by reference to a conversion table. Although it is not convenient for repeated or continuous measurements during anaesthesia, the Riken gas indicator is a most satisfactory and portable instrument for checking the calibration of vaporizers for any known anaesthetic agent and is far less costly than most other instruments. The battery and bulb are easy to replace.

Large bench-type interferometers are used by vaporizer manufacturers for calibration purposes.

The Dräger Narcotest Halothane Indicator

The Dräger Narcotest halothane indicator (Fig. 19.5), although obsolete, illustrates a relatively simple technique that depends on the effect that the volatile anaesthetic agents have on silicone rubber. The gases containing the vapour circulate around strands of the rubber under tension and alter its length by changing its modulus of elasticity. A bimetallic strip compensates for changes in environmental temperature. A clamp may be used to secure the pointer during transit. The Narcotest has the advantage that it requires no electrical power and may be kept continuously in-line during anaesthesia.

The disadvantages include its maximum span of up to 3% halothane; its non-specificity, although calibration factors enable it to be used for other agents; and the fact that it is markedly affected by nitrous oxide in the carrier gas. Since the operation of this device is dependent upon rubber/gas and oil/gas solubility coefficients, it has been suggested that it approximates to an 'MAC meter'.

The Engström Emma Anaesthetic Vapour Monitor

Several materials exhibit a marked piezoelectric effect. When quartz crystals are mounted between electrodes

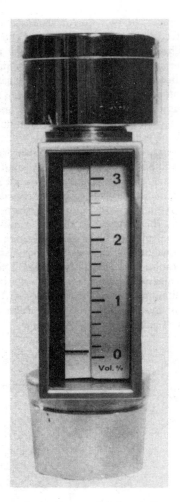

Figure 19.5 The Dräger Narcotest halothane indicator.

and are accurately cut to shape, they may be made to oscillate at a specific frequency. The transducer of the Engström Emma (Fig. 19.6) contains two such crystals, one of which is coated with a layer of silicone oil that can absorb or release halogenated anaesthetic molecules. When a carrier gas containing halogenated vapours passes through the transducer, molecules of the agent are absorbed onto the silicone oil, changing the mass of the oil-coated crystal and hence its fundamental frequency with respect to the uncoated reference crystal. The measurement of vapour concentration is made by comparison of the frequencies of the two crystals.

Nitrous oxide produces a small change in calibration, at worst less than 0.2% on the meter scale. If one is using nitrous oxide mixtures, the device can be re-zeroed for the proportion of nitrous oxide in use. Carbon dioxide has no appreciable effect in clinical concentrations. The response time of the instrument is 0.1 s.

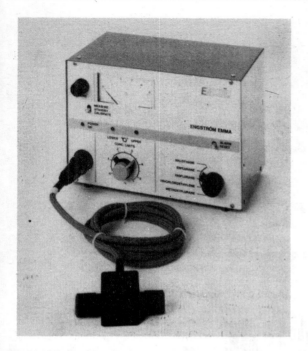

Figure 19.6 The Engström Emma anaesthetic vapour analyser.

If the transducer is installed in the expiratory limb of a breathing attachment, water vapour may be absorbed by the non-oily crystal and produce a low reading.

The Engström Emma measures the concentration of any substance that is absorbed by the silicone oil and since all volatile anaesthetic agents are oil-soluble, they can be detected. However, it is incapable of distinguishing one agent from another.

Infrared Absorption Spectroscopy

Asymmetric polyatomic molecules absorb infrared (IR) radiation. Carbon dioxide, nitrous oxide and water vapour absorb strongly, whereas helium, argon, hydrogen, oxygen and nitrogen do not.

Molecules that absorb IR radiation convert the IR energy into vibrations at frequencies dependent on molecular mass and atomic bond strength. Hence different compounds absorb IR radiation at different frequencies. Thus, it is possible to determine what a compound is and also its concentration. Even fairly simple molecules such as CO_2 may absorb at more than one wavelength; the absorption is caused by the molecule being caused to vibrate and thus take up energy; this vibration may be in several planes or modes each absorbing at a different wavelength.

The Beer–Lambert law shows the relationship between the absorption of energy and the concentration of gas under test:

$$A = \log \frac{I_0}{I_1} = \varepsilon dC$$

where A = absorption, I_0 = incident intensity, I_1 = exit intensity, ε = molar extinction coefficient, d = path length of cell and C = concentration of sample.

At IR wavelengths, absorption may also be affected by the so-called 'pressure broadening' of the molecular frequencies by certain carrier gases, especially helium, argon or hydrogen.

The principles of a typical IR analyser are shown in Fig. 19.7. IR radiation from a nichrome wire filament is directed through a test cell via a chopper wheel, which has several windows. The windows in the chopper wheel are composed of narrow-bandwidth filters of the wavelength of the absorption peaks of the gas or gases of interest. In the case of the capnograph, the filter passes only energy of wavelength 4.26 μm. In the multigas analyser, 3.3 μm is the common absorption peak for enflurane, isoflurane and halothane as they all absorb at this wavelength, and 4.5 μm for nitrous oxide. Thus, discrete pulses of IR energy at a series of different wavelengths, appropriate to the gases under test, pass through the test cell. The IR detector receives the IR signals which, after amplification and processing, are displayed as the concentrations of each of the component gases or vapours under test.

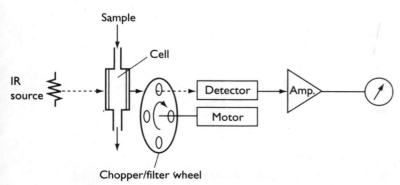

Figure 19.7 Components of a typical infrared analyser.

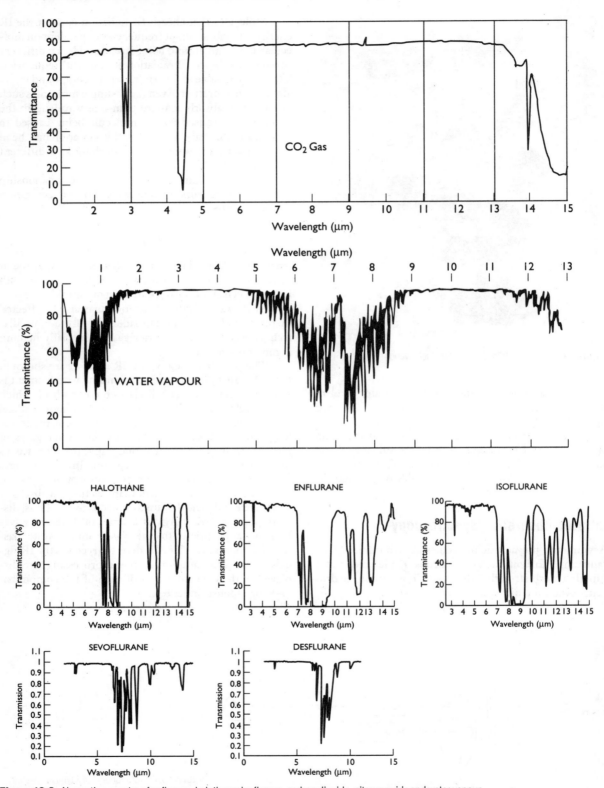

Figure 19.8 Absorption spectra of enflurane, halothane, isoflurane, carbon dioxide, nitrous oxide and water vapour.

The main advantages of this system are that it rapidly measures the concentration of nitrous oxide, end-tidal and inspired carbon dioxide, and the volatile agents. However, in the near-IR range, as the absorption peaks of most of the volatile anaesthetic agents are identical at 3.3 μm (Fig. 19.8), it is impossible to distinguish between them. It is necessary to select the correct calibration for the expected vapour and mixtures, or the wrong vapour concentration will be displayed. It is also necessary to remove water vapour, as it is a strong absorber at this wavelength.

A similar problem may occur with interference between carbon dioxide and nitrous oxide. It has recently been observed that high levels of blood alcohol may interfere with the calibration when exhaled gas is sampled (or analysed). Most IR multigas analysers also include either a fuel cell or a paramagnetic oxygen analyser.

Infrared gas monitors capable of distinguishing between different volatile anaesthetic agents need to analyse at longer wavelengths as well, where there are more differences in the absorption spectra.

The Miran Infrared Spectrophotometer

The Miran (Fig. 19.9) is a high-quality IR spectrophotometer that is often used for testing the calibration of vaporizers, and also in the assessment of environmental pollution in the operating theatre by anaesthetic agents. A heated nichrome wire IR source is directed through a variable interference filter, which is calibrated in wavelength. This filter may either be set at a wavelength that is a known absorption peak of an agent, or may be continuously varied to scan through the near-IR spectrum, in order to analyse gas samples. The beam of IR energy then passes through a chamber, of known path length, to the detection system. Two chambers are

provided, one with a very short path length, for the measurement of gases and vapours at anaesthetic concentrations, and the other with a long path length, for analysing environmental gases in the parts-per-million range.

Brüel and Kjaer Anaesthetic Gas Monitor

Acoustic techniques for the analysis and measurement of gas and vapour concentrations may be based on the physical property that, if energy is applied to a gas or vapour, it will expand, causing an increase in pressure.

The Brüel and Kjaer anaesthetic gas monitor (Fig. 19.10) utilizes photo-acoustic spectroscopy. Nitrous oxide, carbon dioxide and the halogenated anaesthetic vapours absorb specific wavelengths in the IR region. If these gases and vapours are irradiated with pulsatile IR energy, of a suitable wavelength, then a sound wave is produced that can be detected by a microphone.

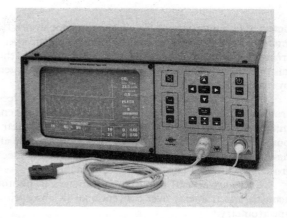

Figure 19.10 Brüel and Kjaer's anaesthetic gas monitor type 1304.

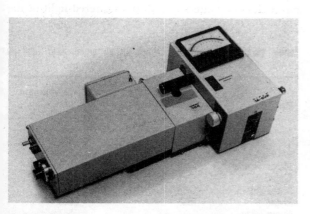

Figure 19.9 Miran variable-wavelength variable-path length infrared spectrophotometer, capable of measuring gas concentrations in the percentage range or the parts-per-million range.

The schematic representation in Fig. 19.11 shows the principle of the measurement system. The gases under test are drawn through a small measurement chamber which is irradiated by an IR source. The radiation is 'chopped' by a rapidly rotating wheel. In order to differentiate between nitrous oxide, carbon dioxide and the volatile agents, the IR beam is chopped at three different frequencies. To do this, the chopper wheel has three concentric bands of holes, and this causes the IR energy to pulsate at three different audio frequencies. Each part of the now divided beam passes through a narrow-band filter appropriate to the absorption of carbon dioxide, nitrous oxide or the halogenated hydrocarbon anaesthetic vapours. The absorption of the IR energy causes each gas to expand and contract at its relevant audio frequency.

This periodic expansion and contraction produces a pressure fluctuation of audible frequency that can be

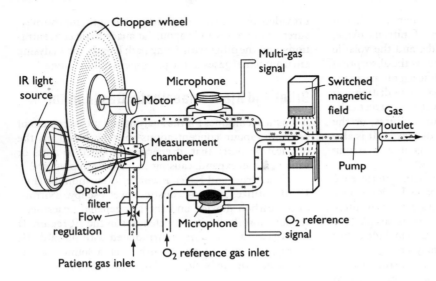

Figure 19.11 Working principles of the Brüel and Kjaer anaesthetic gas monitor.

detected by a microphone. As oxygen does not absorb IR energy, it cannot be measured by photo–acoustic spectroscopy, but an alternating magnetic field applied to the gas mixture will induce an audible signal in the oxygen by making use of its paramagnetic property.

The multigas signal from the microphone is electronically filtered into its four component parts: oxygen, nitrous oxide, carbon dioxide and halogenated hydrocarbons. As the halogenated anaesthetic vapours in use all have similar IR absorption spectra, photo–acoustic spectroscopy is unable to distinguish between them.

There are several important advantages in photo-acoustic spectrometry over conventional IR absorption spectrometry:

- The photo–acoustic technique appears to be extremely stable, with virtually no zero drift, and its calibration remains constant over much longer periods of time.
- The very fast rise and fall times give a much truer representation of any change in gas concentrations.

When reading the specification of a gas analyser, it is important to note the conditions under which such things as the rise time are measured. Rise time is usually quoted from the input to the measuring device. However, Brüel and Kjaer quote the rise time when a step change in concentration is made at the patient end of the monitoring catheter.

Hook and Tucker Halothane Meter

This analyser exploits the fact that halothane absorbs energy in the ultraviolet (UV) part of the spectrum. A mercury discharge lamp is used to create UV energy which is passed through an absorption chamber contain-

ing the gas under test. The energy absorbed is measured by comparing the output from photocells before and after the measuring chamber.

Raman Scattering

This new technique for gas monitoring makes use of a property similar to fluorescence. When gas molecules are bombarded with energy of a discrete wavelength, they may scatter energy at very low levels at a different wavelength. The difference or 'shift' is characteristic of the species of molecule (Table 19.1).

Intense monochromatic energy from an argon laser (plasma tube) of wavelength 488 nm irradiates a cell that forms part of the laser (Fig. 19.12). The gas under test is aspirated through the cell. Energy is scattered by the gas molecules. The filters absorb the scattered light of the

Table 19.1 Raman frequency shifts for an argon laser (488 nm 20 492 cm⁻¹)

Gas	Frequency shift Wave number (cm⁻¹)	Wavelength (nm)
Halothane	717	505.7
Enflurane	817	508.3
Isoflurane	995	512.9
Carbon dioxide	1285	520.6
Nitrous oxide	1285	520.6
Carbon dioxide	1388	523.4
Oxygen	1555	528.1
Nitrous oxide	2224	547.4
Nitrogen	2331	550.6
Water	3650	593.8

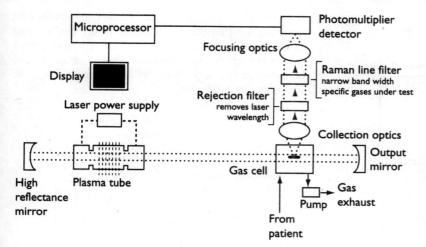

Figure 19.12 Working principles of the Raman anaesthetic gas monitor.

same wavelength as the laser, that is the 'unshifted' laser wavelength. Any 'shifted' wavelengths pass on through a rapidly rotating filter wheel with narrow-band pass filters appropriate to each of the gases and vapours of interest. The very low levels of light are then detected with a photomultiplier tube.

Raman scattering is a new technique in gas analysis with exciting possibilities for multigas analysis, and with the advantages that it is cheaper and more reliable than mass spectroscopy and more versatile than IR absorption spectroscopy.

Mass Spectrometry

Mass spectrometry has the advantage that it can be used to monitor continuously the full range of gases encountered in anaesthesia and intensive care. Its disadvantages include its complexity and cost. Mass spectrometry relies on the different molecular weights of the gases to be monitored.

The basic principle of the technique is shown in Fig. 19.13. The gas mixture to be monitored is drawn into a sampling chamber by a vacuum pump. The pressure in the sampling chamber is about 1 mmHg or 133 Pa. A very small amount of this gas is slowly drawn through a molecular leak into the *dispersion chamber*, which is highly evacuated to around 10^{-6} mmHg by a high-vacuum pump. The ions of the various species are attracted towards a collector electrode or electrodes. On their passage through the dispersion chamber they are deflected by either a strong *magnetic field* in the case of the magnetic sector mass spectrometer or by powerful *electromagnetic forces* in the case of the more common quadrupole mass spectrometer. The various species are separated by the fact that they have different masses and their trajectories are therefore different, as shown in Fig. 19.14.

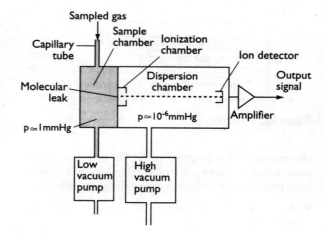

Figure 19.13 Mass spectrometry.

However, CO_2 and N_2O both have a mass of 44 and CO and N_2 both have a mass of 28 and would therefore not be distinguishable. During the process of ionization and dispersion many of the ions are broken down into sub-species. Mass spectrometry can distinguish between gases with equal molecular masses by measuring the mass of the whole molecule and comparing this value with the current produced by the sub-species.

Position of Sampling

The sampling of respiratory gas may be done in one of two ways, namely sidestream and mainstream. Because of their methods of analysis, mass spectrometers and Raman spectrometers use sidestream sampling, as do most IR instruments. Only the precise tubing recommended by the manufacturer should be used, and only of

Magnetic Sector Mass Spectrometer

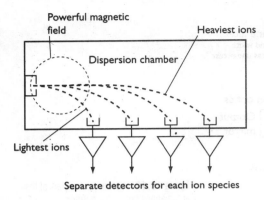

Quadrupole Mass Spectrometer

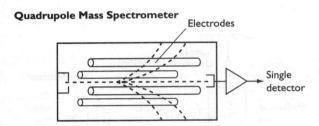

Figure 19.14 Magnetic sector vs quadrupole mass spectrometers.

the recommended length. Typical IR instruments sample at a flow rate between 50 and 150 ml/min. The problems encountered with sidestream sampling include:

- water-vapour condensation; only the specified type of tubing should be used;
- distortion of the respiratory waveform by too high a flow rate, the capillary tube being too long, or the capillary tube diameter being too large.

It is also important that the tip of the sampling tube should always be as near as possible to the patient's trachea, but the sampled gas mixture must not be contaminated by inspired gas during the expiratory phase. This is a definite risk if the sample is extracted near the patient end of a co-axial Mapleson D breathing system and may give rise to erroneously low end-tidal readings. With sidestream sampling, sometimes the gases should not be returned to the breathing system, because sometimes they are denatured by the measuring technique.

Mainstream sampling, although more cumbersome, does have advantages over sidestream monitoring. The gas to be analysed never leaves the respiratory attachment. Windows that are transparent to the IR wavelengths in use form part of an adaptor or even the catheter mount, and a miniature IR source, filter-wheel, motor and detector are attached over the

windows (Fig. 19.15). The advantages of mainstream sampling are that there is no delay in the rise and fall times of gas composition changes, no gas is lost from the attachment, no mixing occurs along a capillary tube before analysis, and there are fewer problems with water vapour condensation.

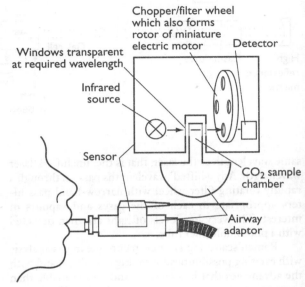

Figure 19.15 The principle of the Hewlett-Packard mainstream carbon dioxide gas analyser.

Response Time

There is always a delay between any change in gas concentration and its indication on the display of the gas analysis system. This delay has two main components: the delay in the gas sample reaching the analysis element as it travels along the sampling tube and the delay in the analysis itself. Mainstream analysers do not suffer from the time taken for the gas to flow along the capillary tubing but with the sidestream analyser this is dependent upon the length of the tubing, which should be kept as short as possible, and the rate at which gas is aspirated along the tube. The delay in actual measurement of the gas concentration is known as the *rise time*; the measurement *time constant* is the time it takes for the indication of concentration to rise from 0% to 63% of the final reading (Fig. 19.16).

Breathing Attachment Disconnect Alarms

Breathing disconnect alarms use one of two principles: detection of exhaled tidal volumes, or pressure changes

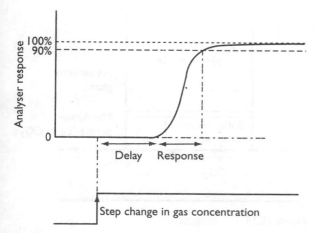

Figure 19.16 Response time of gas analysers to a change in gas concentration.

in the breathing attachment. Both of these methods are related to time. With the tidal volume method, a preset exhaled tidal volume must recur at greater than a minimum preset frequency whereas with the pressure method the airway pressure must exceed a certain preset level and then reduce to below that level rhythmically at greater than a minimum preset rate. The tidal volume method is applicable to both spontaneously breathing and ventilated patients and usually forms part of a respirometer. The pressure method is applicable only to ventilated patients. It usually incorporates an alarm for excessive inspiratory pressure due, for example, to kinking of the endotracheal tube, but gives no indication of decreased tidal volume with, say, deteriorating compliance.

MEASUREMENT OF RESPIRATORY VOLUMES

The measurement of inhaled and, more importantly, exhaled respiratory volumes during anaesthesia is normally carried out by one of the following techniques:

- turbine respirometer (Wright's);
- positive displacement (Dräger);
- calibrated bellows;
- hot-wire anemometry (not with flammable agents);
- vortex shedding.

Hot-wire anemometry and vortex shedding are flow measurements; flow is integrated with respect to time (giving volume.) The principles of these techniques are discussed in Chapter 4.

THE MEASUREMENT OF NITRIC OXIDE

The use of inhaled nitric oxide as a therapeutic agent has led to the urgent requirement of a method of measurement (Etches *et al.*, 1995). However, there are currently only industrial and laboratory methods available. It is important that nitric oxide be measured accurately, as it can cause methaemoglobinaemia and excessive concentrations are fatal. It is critically important to be able to detect nitrogen *dioxide* in the inhaled gas as it is a decomposition product of nitric oxide and causes pulmonary oedema.

All industrial analysers designed for the measurement of the oxides of nitrogen are environmental instruments intended to measure low concentrations in the presence of atmospheric oxygen at 21% or less. The accuracy of these devices cannot be guaranteed when the carrier gas has a high concentration of oxygen. The two types of analyser in common use are:

- The *chemiluminescence* analyser is based on the reaction of NO with ozone (O_3) in a chamber to produce energized NO_2 molecules. These energized NO_2 molecules emit photons of light in the range 590–2600 nm; the amount of light emitted is proportional to the original concentration of nitric oxide. In a parallel system there is a catalytic converter before the reaction chamber to reduce NO_2 present in the sample to NO. The total oxides of nitrogen are then measured at NO. The difference between the two readings is the NO_2 concentration.
- *Electrochemical* analysers generate a potential difference proportional to the nitrogen oxide concentration. This is due to the migration of ions generated from the reaction between NO or NO_2 and the electrolyte. A separate cell is used for NO and NO_2.

It is important that any industrial method of the measurement of these gases be tested and calibrated with the concentrations of oxygen that they will be used with in any clinical application.

MEASUREMENT OF GASES IN BLOOD

Although it is now possible to continuously monitor oxygen saturation with pulse oximetry (Chapter 18), mixed venous oxygen saturation (Chapter 20) and even the partial pressure of oxygen, carbon dioxide and pH by means of intravascular electrodes, these measurands are more commonly measured by *in vitro* blood gas analysis.

The Blood Gas Analyser

Bench blood gas analysers need a very small, heparinized sample of blood (100–300 µl) to make the analysis. This blood is passed across four electrodes simultaneously in a temperature-stabilized cuvette, as shown in Fig. 19.17. The electrodes measure the partial pressure of dissolved oxygen using a Clarke electrode, carbon dioxide using a Severinghaus electrode and pH with a conventional 'glass' pH electrode; the fourth electrode is a reference electrode.

The Clarke polarographic electrode has already been briefly described (see p. 279) as a method of measuring gaseous oxygen, in this case, with a membrane that passes oxygen but not blood.

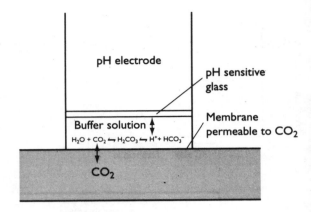

Figure 19.18 P_{CO_2} electrode.

The Severinghaus Carbon Dioxide Electrode

The Severinghaus electrode relies on the fact that the relationship between the logarithm of the partial pressure of carbon dioxide and pH is linear over the range 1.3–12 kPa (10–90 mmHg). The electrode consists of two components: a buffer solution and a glass pH electrode (Fig. 19.18). The blood is separated from the buffer solution by a semipermeable membrane usually made of Teflon or silicone rubber, which allows the CO_2 dissolved in the blood to equilibrate with CO_2 in the buffer solution. The pH of the buffer solution is measured with the pH electrode. The pH or 'glass' electrode

is used in the Severinghaus electrode also independently to measure the plasma pH. The glass electrode is an *ion-specific electrode*, which is an electrode that responds only to a specific ion in aqueous solution. A solution, usually of hydrochloric acid, of known pH is separated from the solution under test by a membrane made of special glass. A reference electrode, usually silver–silver chloride, is placed in the hydrochloric acid. An electrochemical cell is formed between the glass electrode and a reference electrode (Fig. 19.19); the output of the cell is proportional to the pH or in the case of the Severinghaus electrode to P_{CO_2}.

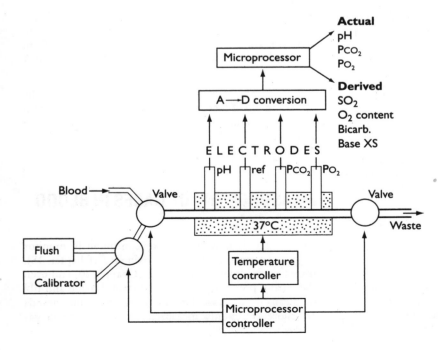

Figure 19.17 Blood gas analyser.

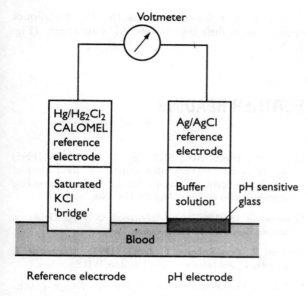

Figure 19.19 pH electrode.

Table 19.2 Composition of glass ion-selective membranes of clinical use

	Composition (%)						
Analyte	**SiO$_2$**	**Al$_2$O$_3$**	**Na$_2$O**	**Li$_2$O**	**CaO**	**Fe$_2$O$_3$**	**P$_2$O$_5$**
pH	72		22		6		
Li$^+$	60	25		15			
Na$^+$	71	18	11				
K$^+$	69	4	27				
Ca^{2+}	3	6	6		<1	16	67

Other Ion-Selective Electrodes

Glass ion-selective electrodes may also be made for other ions useful in clinical practice by carefully selecting the proportions of the constituents of the glass (Table 19.2).

All blood gas analysers display values of serum bicarbonate, base excess, oxygen saturation and oxygen content. However, it must always be remembered that the only actual values are pH, P$_{O_2}$ and P$_{CO_2}$; all other displayed values are derived making assumptions of haemoglobin concentration, type and quality. The cuvette is temperature controlled at 37°C. If the patient's temperature is not 37°C, then the corrected values may be obtained automatically so long as the patient's temperature is dialled into the blood gas analyser.

The Co-oximeter

Although not strictly a method of measuring oxygen in blood, the co-oximeter is usually associated with the blood gas analyser. The co-oximeter measures the percentage oxygen saturation of haemoglobin *in vitro* in discrete blood samples. In some ways it is much simpler than the pulse oximeter (Chapter 18). The co-oximeter

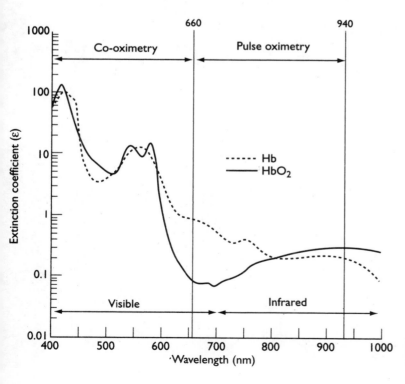

Figure 19.20 Spectrum: Co-oximetry vs pulse oximetry.

bears more resemblance to a bench spectrophotometer and the Bere Lambert law is more closely adhered to than in pulse oximetry.

A small sample (200–400 µl) of heparinized blood is injected into a cuvette of known fixed width or *path length*. The erythrocytes are disrupted either by subjecting them to a soap solution or ultrasonic energy; thus a solution of free haemoglobin in plasma is produced. Conventional spectrophotometry then takes place at several wavelengths, usually in the visible range. Early oximeters used in cardiac catheter laboratories used two wavelengths but modern devices use between five and 17. The advantage of using multiple wavelengths is that abnormal haemoglobins can be detected and quantified. The multiple wavelengths are produced either by a filter wheel with multiple narrowband filters or by scanning with a diffraction grating or prism (Fig. 19.20). The result is usually available within 30 s and includes: $SO_2\%$, total Hb concentration, oxygen content, methaemoglobin%, carboxyhaemoglobin%; some devices being capable of distinguishing fetal haemoglobin (HbF). In strictly scientific terms, SpO_2 should not be directly compared with the SO_2 derived from a Co-oximeter as the two techniques operate over different ranges of wavelength (Fig. 19.20).

FURTHER READING

Etches PC, Harris ML, McLinley R, Finer NM (1995) Clinical monitoring of inhaled nitric oxide: comparison of chemiluminescent and electrochemical sensors. *Biomedical Instrumentation & Technology* 29: 134–140.

Gravenstein JS (1990) *Gas Monitoring & Pulse Oximetry*. Boston: Butterworth-Heinemann.

Hutton P, Prys-Roberts C (eds) (1994) *Monitoring in Anaesthesia and Intensive Care*. London: WB Saunders.

O'Flaherty D (1994) *Principles & Practice of Capnography*. London: BMJ Publishing Group.

Webster JG (ed.) (1992) *Medical Instrumentation – Applications & Design*. Boston: Houghton Mifflin.

— 20 —

PHYSIOLOGICAL MONITORING: ADVANCED MONITORING SYSTEMS

Contents

INTRODUCTION

This chapter describes aspects of more advanced monitoring that would only be employed for patients who are either very ill or undergoing major surgery. Some of these techniques are *invasive* or *minimally invasive*. Invasive monitoring includes techniques that breach the skin or mucous membrane such as direct blood pressure monitoring, both arterial and central venous, and intravascular blood gas monitoring. Minimally invasive monitoring includes those techniques in which probes are inserted into body cavities but there is no breach of the mucous membrane, for example, core temperature measurement and oesophageal Doppler ultrasound monitoring.

BLOOD PRESSURE MEASUREMENT

With currently available technology, direct invasive pressure monitoring is the only method available for the measurement of central venous, intracardiac and pulmonary artery pressures. Invasive pressure measurement is still often used for monitoring peripheral arterial blood pressure when a continuous read-out is required, despite the introduction of non-invasive continuous methods (see Chapter 18).

The advantages of invasive arterial pressure monitoring are:

- continuous reading;
- instantaneous reading;
- pressure waveform displayed;
- easy blood sampling.

The disadvantages of invasive arterial pressure monitoring are:

- difficulty of insertion of cannula;
- risk of haemorrhage;
- risk of infection;
- risk of distal ischaemia;
- risk of emboli (air, clots);
- difficulties with calibration;
- inaccuracy due to manometer effect;
- inaccuracy due to overdamping or underdamping of the system;
- greater expense than non-invasive blood pressure monitoring.

In order to obtain accurate readings it is necessary to understand the physical principles. The first principle is the *manometer effect* already described in Chapter 18. An equilibrium is reached between the blood pressure and the force of a column of liquid which is related to the density of the liquid and the acceleration due to gravity.

Simple manometers are used for estimation of *central venous pressure* (CVP). Connection with a central great vein is made via cannulation of the internal jugular or subclavian veins, or by the use of a catheter extending from a peripheral vein centrally. The manometer system contains heparinized normal saline, maintaining the blood/saline interface at the tip of the cannula or catheter. The CVP is measured as the height of the saline column measured vertically from the mid-axillary line at the level of the right atrium, as shown in Fig. 20.1. The zero point must be chosen carefully each time as small changes in its selection induce a comparatively large error in CVP. CVP measurement in the intensive care situation is now commonly done with a transducer.

Arterial blood pressure is too high to make use of a simple manometer and although it is possible to measure mean arterial blood pressure with a simple aneroid pressure gauge, a transducer is usually used. Even with a transduced system it is important to remember that errors may still be induced by forgetting the manometer effect caused by the height of the liquid connection between the artery and the transducer.

The Pressure Transducer

Pressure transducers convert the variable pressure to a varying electrical signal. Although catheter-tip pressure transducers have been used experimentally, the conventional method of invasive pressure measurement is to connect the blood in a vessel to a pressure transducer via a saline-filled catheter which is made of a hard plastic so that changes in pressure are minimally distorted by any change in diameter of the tubing with changes in pressure. Most pressure transducers are *resistive* in that a change in pressure produces a change in electrical resistance, often in the form of a bridge circuit. Traditionally blood pressure transducers were reusable devices, the blood/saline pathway having to be cleaned and sterilized after each use. These were soon surplanted by transducers with a sterile disposable 'dome' with a diaphragm which was held in contact with the flexible surface of the transducer. The set-up for invasive arterial blood pressure measurement is shown in Fig. 20.2.

A small bore cannula is inserted in an artery and as short a length as possible of 'manometer' tubing connects the cannula to the transducer dome. An automatic flushing system maintains a constant flow of heparinized saline at about 5 ml/h through the system to reduce the risk of blockage by clot formation. It is important that the transducer, once zeroed, is maintained at the same level as the cannula in the case of arterial pressure measurement, otherwise there will be a manometer effect either increasing or decreasing the indicated value of pressure. In the case of venous or pulmonary artery pressure measurements, the transducer should be zeroed and kept at the level of the right atrium.

Both the forms of transducer so far described are

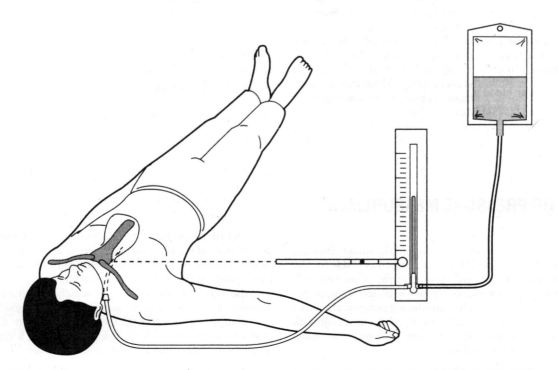

Figure 20.1 Central venous pressure measurement using a manometer system. The reading must be referred to the level of the right atrium.

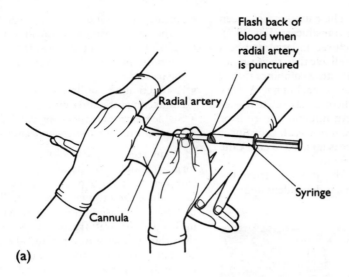

(a)

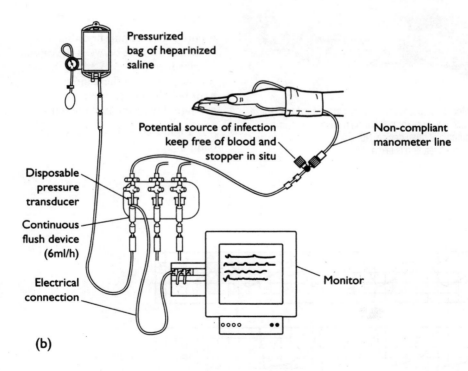

(b)

Figure 20.2 Invasive arterial blood pressure measurement. An air-tight, fluid-filled system connects the artery to the transducer. A pressurized bag of fluid is used to flush the system continuously at about 6 ml/h through an automatic flush device.

expensive and easily damaged. Their use has now been replaced by disposable pressure transducers (Fig. 20.3). These may be cheaply manufactured in large numbers and tend to be more robust and reliable than their predecessors. The technique of manufacture combines that of integrated electronics with micro-machining. A very small diaphragm, usually of silicone, has resistive elements etched on its dry side. An internal film resistor network is etched by laser to calibrate each transducer during manufacture so that there is no need to check the calibration between changes of device.

Accurate transmission of the pressure from the blood vessel to the indicated value is dependent upon:

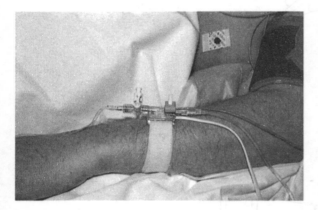

Figure 20.3 Modern disposable blood pressure transducer. These transducers are accurately calibrated during manufacture and incorporate an automatic flush device. NB. It is still necessary to 'zero' the system each time a reading is taken.

- Accurate calibration of the transducer (at manufacture in the case of disposable transducers).
- Careful zeroing initially, regularly and especially when the position of the transducer is moved in relation to the patient.
- A functioning continuous flush system to keep the connecting tube and cannula clear of obstruction.
- Stable electronic processing of the transducer signal.
- Careful attention to *resonance* and *damping*.

Any recording system that is to reproduce a waveform accurately must be able to reproduce the amplitude and phase difference of all the harmonics that summate to produce the original waveform. To achieve this it is necessary to design the system with a much higher undamped natural frequency or resonant frequency than the original waveform and then apply the correct amount of damping until the displayed waveform corresponds with the waveform under test. The resonant frequency and the damping of both the hydro-mechanical components and the electronics must be considered; the electronic component is determined by the designer of the monitoring equipment but there are several factors that can affect the hydro-mechanical part:

- bore of the cannula or catheter;
- bore of the tube between the cannula/catheter and the transducer;
- distensibility of the tubing;
- air bubbles in the system;
- range of movement of the transducer diaphragm.

Figure 20.4 shows the effects of over- and under-damping.

(a)

(b)

(c)

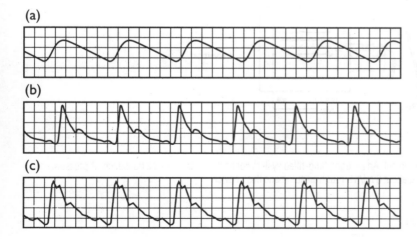

Figure 20.4 Intra-arterial pressure recordings: (a) excessively damped; (b) 'critically' damped to provide accurate readings; (c) 'underdamped'.

Risks of Direct Arterial Blood Pressure Monitoring

The risks are as follows:

- haemorrhage;
- infection;
- peripheral ischaemia (Allen's test);
- air embolism;
- clot embolism;
- damage to vessel;
- arteriovenous fistula formation.

MEASUREMENT OF CARDIAC OUTPUT

Thermodilution

Currently the most common but most invasive method of measuring cardiac output is by *thermodilution*. The advantage of the thermodilution technique is that central pressures may be monitored via the same flow-directed catheter and mixed venous samples of blood may be withdrawn for estimation of oxygen saturation. The disadvantages of thermodilution are those risks associated with flow-directed pulmonary artery catheters already stated above plus:

- risk of damage by injectate under pressure;
- significant extra fluid input;
- possibility of lowering of body temperature;
- intermittent readings of cardiac output;
- variation in indicated cardiac output with variation in rate of injection;
- high cost of catheters.

The principle of thermodilution is similar to dye dilution but instead of a coloured dye, a bolus of cold normal saline is used. A flow-directed pulmonary artery catheter is placed with its tip in a branch of a pulmonary artery. This catheter has four lumens: (1) directly to the tip to measure the pressure at the tip and for mixed venous blood sampling; (2) connected to the latex balloon around the distal end of the catheter proximal to the tip orifice (Fig. 20.5); (3) containing two electrical conductors connected to a

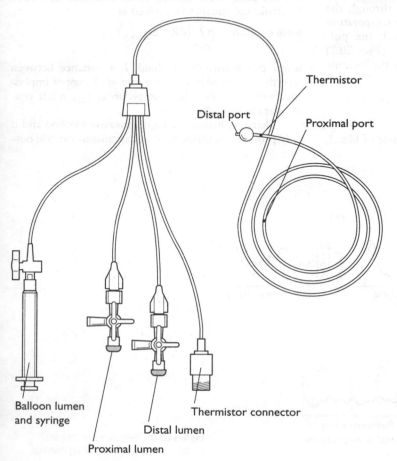

Balloon lumen
and syringe

Proximal lumen

Distal lumen

Thermistor connector

Distal port

Proximal port

Thermistor

Figure 20.5 Flow-directed pulmonary artery catheter (see text).

temperature-sensing thermistor near the distal end of the catheter; and (4) terminating in a port some way back from the tip such that it may be used to measure CVP and used for injecting the cold saline bolus. This catheter is usually also used to measure right-sided cardiac, pulmonary artery and capillary wedge pressures. It is inserted via a peripheral vein with a pressure transducer connected to the port of the lumen from the tip of the catheter. The catheter is advanced until a CVP trace is observed. The latex balloon is then inflated with air and the catheter slowly advanced, the flow of blood directing the tip through the right atrium, tricuspid valve, right ventricle, pulmonary valve and into either of the main pulmonary arteries (Fig. 20.6). The catheter is then slowly advanced until the balloon is just occluding a smaller branch of a pulmonary artery and the pulmonary capillary wedge pressure is measured. **The balloon is then immediately deflated** to avoid ischaemia of that lung segment. Once the pressures have been estimated, the cardiac output can be measured. A bolus of saline of known temperature and volume is **rapidly** injected via the proximal port of the catheter. This bolus mixes with the blood as it passes through the right side of the heart. The curve of the temperature change in the blood as it passes through the pulmonary arteries is plotted automatically (Fig. 20.7) and the cardiac output is calculated using the formula below.

$$Q = \frac{V D_i S_i (T_B \times T_i) \times 60}{dT.t.D_B S_B \times 1000} \qquad \text{litres/min}$$

where Q = cardiac output, S_B = specific heat of blood,

S_i = specific heat of injectate, T_B = temperature of blood, T_i = temperature of injectate, dT = mean temperature change, D_i = density of injectate, D_B density of blood, V = volume of cold saline, t = time in seconds.

It is usual to repeat the measurement three or four times over the course of a few minutes and then take an average value.

Impedance Plethysmography

Cardiac output may also be estimated completely non-invasively by measuring the electrical impedance of the thorax. The impedance changes with changes in the distribution of blood in the thoracic cavity. The most accurate way is by placing self-adhesive electrodes circumferentially, as shown in Fig. 20.8. A *constant current generator* producing a few milliamperes at around 100 kHz is applied and the changes in impedance are estimated by measuring the voltage change across the thorax as shown. Impedance changes to a certain extent with respiration but this signal is of a much lower frequency than changes due to cardiac function and therefore are easily electronically eliminated. An expression for stroke volume may be derived as:

$$\text{Stroke volume} = \rho \frac{L^2}{Zo^2} (dZ / dt)_{min} \cdot T_{LVE}$$

where ρ = resistivity of blood, L = distance between recording electrodes, dZ/dt = rate of change of impedance with time, Zo = basic impedance, T_{LVE} = left ventricular ejection time.

Thermodilution is a highly invasive method and it only provides an estimate of instantaneous cardiac out-

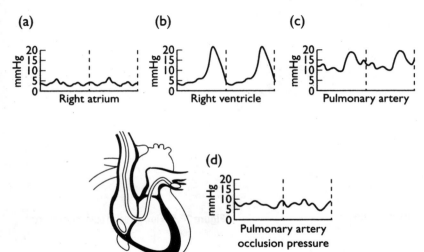

(a)
Right atrium

(b)
Right ventricle

(c)
Pulmonary artery

(d)
Pulmonary artery
occlusion pressure

Figure 20.6 Pressure waveforms with pulmonary artery catheter during insertion.

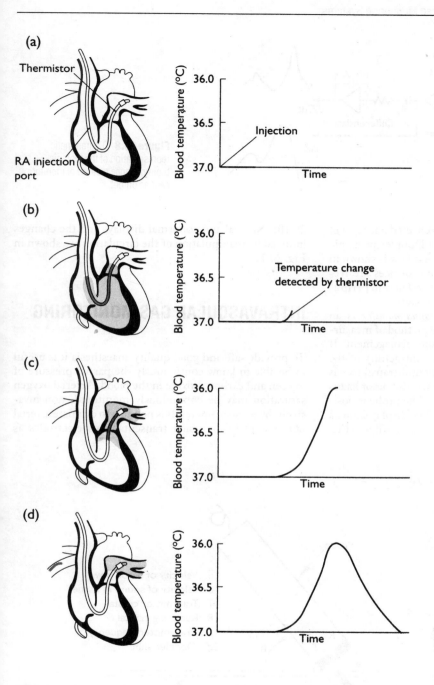

Figure 20.7 Thermodilution method for measuring cardiac output. The cold saline is rapidly injected via the right atrium injection port and the change in temperature is sensed by the thermistor. Note the absence of a recirculation peak and that there is no elevation of the baseline.

put; impedance plethysmography requires good electrical contact with the patient and is easily interfered with by electromagnetic interference. It would be very useful to have an easily applied measure of cardiac output and fluid balance during all major surgery. Poor perfusion of vital organs may occur during surgery for several reasons, including trauma, sepsis, preoperative dehydration, vasodilatation, insensible loss and myocardial depression.

Doppler Ultrasound

Ultrasound (1–10 MHz) energy travels at an almost constant velocity of 1500 m/s. If it is directed at a surface, a proportion of the energy is reflected. If the surface is stationary with respect to the emitter, then the reflected energy will be of the same frequency as the source. If the reflector is moving away from the source then the reflected energy will have a lower frequency; if it is

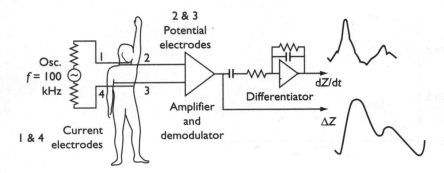

Figure 20.8 Diagrammatic representation of the thoracic bioimpedance method of monitoring cardiac output.

moving towards the source then the reflected energy will be of a higher frequency. This is the Doppler principle and its use in the measurement of blood flow is shown in Fig. 20.9. Simple Doppler ultrasound devices are frequently used to detect and measure blood flow in peripheral vessels and to assess cerebral perfusion.

The *oesophageal Doppler ultrasound monitor* is an easily applied and minimally invasive method of measuring cardiac output and assessing fluid management. It gives a continuous indication of the contractility of the heart and of fluid balance. An ultrasound transducer is inserted through the mouth and down the oesophagus and directed at the descending aorta. The probe is positioned to produce an optimal signal. The display shows a Doppler flow-velocity waveform against time (Fig. 20.10). Normal and abnormal displays and the changes induced by manipulation of the circulation are shown in Fig. 20.11.

INTRAVASCULAR GAS MONITORING

To provide safe and good quality anaesthesia it is useful to be able to know continuously the partial pressure of oxygen and carbon dioxide in the blood. Arterial oxygen saturation may be continuously monitored, non-invasively, by pulse oximetry. It is possible to estimate arterial pO_2 and pCO_2 by using transcutaneous electrodes as

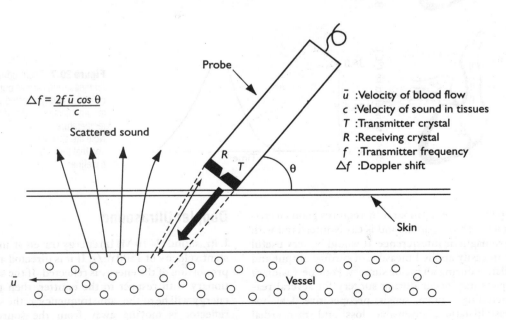

$$\Delta f = \frac{2f\bar{u}\cos\theta}{c}$$

$\bar{u}$: Velocity of blood flow
c : Velocity of sound in tissues
T : Transmitter crystal
R : Receiving crystal
f : Transmitter frequency
Δf : Doppler shift

Figure 20.9 Doppler ultrasound measurement of blood flow.

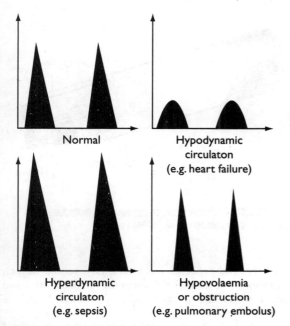

Figure 20.10 Stylized appearances of normal hypodynamic and hypovolaemic waveforms as displayed by the oesophageal Doppler ultrasound monitor. (Reproduced with permission from Singer M (1994) Using the waveform shape. *International Proceedings Journal* **1**(1): 22–34.)

described in Chapter 19 but although these are useful with neonates they are not successful with adults. To monitor pO_2, pCO_2 and pH continuously it is necessary to use *intra-arterial* transducers.

Intra-arterial Subminiature Gas Electrodes

Subminiature Clarke, Severinghaus and pH electrodes at the tips of catheters have been developed but are difficult to calibrate and insert.

Fibreoptic Photoluminescence

A more successful technique that is now commercially available is the use of photoluminescence at the tip of a fibreoptic catheter. The technique relies upon the choice of dyes that have the property of *fluorescence*; when a high-energy photon of monochromatic light source is subjected to the dye, a lower energy photon is emitted from the dye. Different dyes are selected such that the amount of energy emitted indicates the concentration of a particular analyte that is surrounding the dye (Fig. 20.12).

The dye is coated on the tip of an optical fibre along which high-energy light is directed; the emitted energy is transmitted back to the optical unit of the monitor along the same fibre. Figure 20.13 shows the tip of the intravascular catheter containing fibres for measuring pO_2, pCO_2 and pH; there is also a thermistor at the tip to measure the blood temperature as the response of the dyes is temperature sensitive.

Mixed Venous Oxygen Saturation

With the critically ill patient, a great deal of useful information about the circulation and gas exchange can be obtained by comparing arterial oxygen saturation with mixed venous oxygen saturation. Arterial saturation may be monitored non-invasively by pulse oximetry whereas mixed venous saturation requires samples from a pulmonary artery catheter or may be monitored continuously with a fibreoptic oximeter. The principle of the SvO_2 monitor is similar to the pulse oximeter but is much simpler as the light energy is directly reflected by the erythrocytes in the pulmonary artery. The energy from a broad-spectrum incandescent light source is filtered to produce rapidly cycling energy in two or three narrow bands. This energy is directed along an optical fibre in a flow-directed pulmonary artery catheter to be reflected directly by erythrocytes in the pulmonary

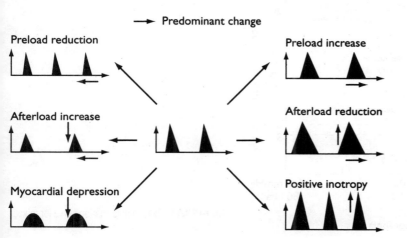

Figure 20.11 Changes in waveform shape following inotropic, preload and afterload manoeuvres. (Reproduced with permission from Singer M (1994) Using the waveform shape. *International Proceedings Journal* **1**(1): 22–34.)

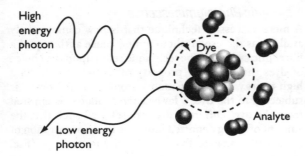

Figure 20.12 In a fluorescence-based system, the dye molecules absorb the excitation light and then emit light that indicates the concentration of the analyte. (Reproduced with permission from Lumsden et al. (1994).)

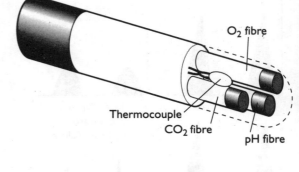

Figure 20.13 Photofluorescence catheter tip. (Reproduced with permission from Lumsden et al. (1994).)

artery. A second fibre carries the reflected light back to the optical unit. A calculation of haemoglobin oxygen saturation is made in a similar way to the co-oximeter. Because so few wavelengths are used, the calibration of this device can be adversely affected by carboxyhaemoglobin and methaemoglobin in the same way as with pulse oximetry. Assuming normal haemoglobin, HbA, the following inter-related variables can affect the SvO_2:

- arterial oxygen saturation, SaO_2, SpO_2
- cardiac output
- haemoglobin
- oxygen consumption.

The graph in Fig. 20.14 shows the oxygen dissocia-

tion curve and expected values of mixed venous oxygen saturation. The normal SvO_2 is in the range 60–80% and occurs when the oxygen delivery and demand are normal.

A *high SvO_2 of > 80%* may indicate increased delivery caused by raised inspired oxygen concentration (FiO_2) or a decreased demand caused by anaesthesia, hypothermia, sepsis or skeletal muscle paralysis. A *low SvO_2 of < 60%* may be of much more serious import:

- Reduced oxygen delivery
  Hb: anaemia, haemodilution, haemorrhage
  SaO_2: arterial hypoxaemia

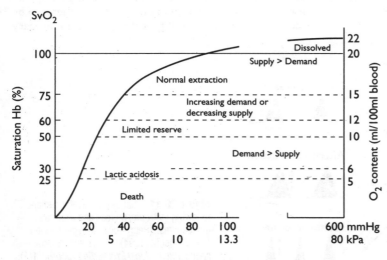

Assuming: pH is 7.4 and normocapnia

Figure 20.14 Oxygen dissociation curve for mixed venous blood.

CO: cardiogenic shock, arrhythmias, hypovolaemia, hypotension
- Increased oxygen demand
  hyperthermia
  pain
  convulsions
  shivering.

The advantages of continuous SvO_2 monitoring are:

- early indication of changes in the cardiovascular, respiratory and general condition of the patient;
- optimization of cardiovascular drug regimens;
- optimization of fluid loading;
- optimization of ventilator management;
- warning of the detrimental effects of procedures such as turning and tracheal suction.

FURTHER READING

Hutton P, Prys–Roberts C (1994) *Monitoring in Anaesthesia and Intensive Care*. London: WB Saunders.

Lumsden T, Marshall WR, Divers GA, Riccitelli SD (1994) The PB3300 intra-arterial blood gas monitoring system. *Journal of Clinical Monitoring* 10: 59–66.

Sykes MK, Vickers MD, Hull CJ (1991) *Principles of Measurement and Monitoring in Anaesthesia and Intensive Care*. Oxford: Blackwell Scientific.

Webster JG (ed.) (1992) *Medical Instrumentation – Applications & Design*. Boston: Houghton Mifflin.

Norfleet EA, Watson CB (1985) Continuous mixed venous oxygen saturation measurement: a significant advance in hemodynamic monitoring. *Journal of Clinical Monitoring* 1: 245–258.

— 21 —

AUTOMATIC
RECORD KEEPING

Contents

INTRODUCTION

The first anaesthetic records were allegedly written in 1894 in order to settle a wager about patient's intraoperative stability (Beecher 1940)! The most important reason for keeping a contemporary record of the progress of an anaesthetic is to allow the anaesthetist to keep track, in real-time, of what has happened and what medications have been given to help guide the immediate intraoperative and postoperative management of the patient (Eichhorn 1993).

FUNCTIONS OF THE ANAESTHESIA RECORD

The functions of the anaesthesia record (Friesdorf et al 1993) include:

- treatment control and decision making;
- information transfer to colleagues managing the patient postoperatively and in the future;
- medico-legal documentation;
- audit and quality control;
- cost calculation;
- departmental administration;
- research;
- training and medical education.

Hand-written anaesthesia records do have certain advantages, namely:

- Information from the patient and the monitoring and anaesthetic equipment has to pass through the brain, consciously or subconsciously, before it is committed to paper, whereas trends in measured values may not become apparent until an automatic alarm is sounded.
- The human brain acts as a 'filter' eliminating artefacts which may well be otherwise recorded faithfully by an automatic system. Lawyers may well pick on these artefactual and inaccurate recordings erroneously. One currently available integrated anaesthetic apparatus consistently alarms and records 'Asystole!' when there is poor connection of an ECG lead, rather than alarming 'ECG lead off'; this is despite the fact that the same integrated monitoring system is recording a regular plethysmograph tracing. The capture of inaccurate data may have a more serious effect on the management of the patient if these results are included in any automatic trend analysis system.
- Many automatic record keeping systems require familiarization with software and also require time to be spent recording data such as administered drugs via a keyboard.
- Presently there is no common data-bus amongst manufacturers. A data-bus is the multiwire electrical connection between pieces of equipment. The International Standards Organization has, for many years, been trying to get agreement for a common data-bus system but has not yet succeeded.

- A further advantage may be seen by some anaesthetists in that the data may be 'smoothed', removing genuine extremes of vital signs.

ADVANTAGES OF AUTOMATIC RECORD KEEPING

The advantages of automatic recording of anaesthetic data are:

- Increased legibility (many anaesthetists cannot read their own writing when it has been photocopied and produced in court).
- Accuracy, but this is only so if any artefacts are accurately removed.
- Time-saving, making more time available for the anaesthetist to actually observe the patient and the procedure.
- Automatic trend analysis, which may alert the anaesthetist sooner than by manual methods if this form of analysis is available.
- Central alarm functions rather than having to scan many pieces of equipment when an alarm sounds.

- Theoretically, it would be possible for a senior anaesthetist to be able to observe the progress in several operating theatres simultaneously whilst supervising junior anaesthetists.
- Automatic recording also can generate a huge database of standardized information for research and audit.
- Standardized legible data are available for non-medical personnel for the purposes of billing, cost-control and administration.

EQUIPMENT FOR AUTOMATIC ANAESTHESIA RECORD KEEPING

There are several commercially available automatic anaesthesia record keepers. They are of the format shown in Fig. 21.1. Digitized information is received at frequent intervals from the monitoring devices and this forms the main input. Manual input from the anaesthetist is from a keyboard or a touch-screen. Real-time information appears on a CRT screen and hard-copy is available from a conventional printer. Information is also stored using conventional information technology methods; this information is then available for audit, administration and research.

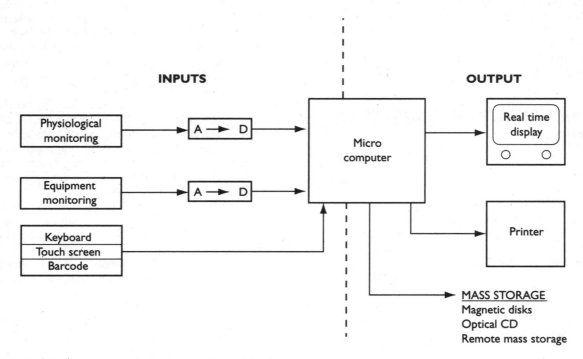

Figure 21.1 Basic components of a simple automatic record-keeping system.

FURTHER READING

Beecher HK (1940) The first anesthesia records. *Surgery, Gynecology and Obstetrics* 71: 689–693.

Eichhorn JH (1993) Anesthesia record keeping. *International Journal of Clinical Monitoring and Computing* 10: 109–115.

Friesdorf W, Schwilk B (1992) Patient-related data management. *Journal of Clinical Monitoring* 8: 308–314.

Friesdorf W, Konichzeky S, Grob-Alltag F, Schwilk B (1993) Ergonomics applied to anaesthesia record keeping. *International Journal of Clinical Monitoring and Computing* 10: 251–259.

Gravenstein JS (1989) The uses of the anesthesia record. *Journal of Clinical Monitoring* 5: 256–265.

— 22 —

ATMOSPHERIC POLLUTION

Contents

INTRODUCTION

There have been many epidemiological studies on the alleged adverse effect of chronic exposure to trace concentrations of anaesthetic gases and vapours in operating theatres and recovery rooms. The evidence is somewhat conflicting and inconclusive. The most frequently quoted references suggest that:

- There is a tendency to increased incidence of spontaneous abortion in female anaesthetists, anaesthetic nurses, and also the wives of men working in theatres.
- There is an increased incidence of minor congenital abnormalities amongst children of anaesthetic personnel.
- There appears to be a higher incidence of females among babies born to anaesthetists.
- There is a reduced fertility in female dental assistants exposed to unscavenged nitrous oxide for more than 5 hours a week.
- There is an increased incidence of subjective complaints (headaches, fatigue, sleep loss, nervousness, pruritis).
- There is a higher rate of cancer (leukaemia and lymphoma) amongst exposed females.
- There is a higher incidence of liver disease in anaesthetists.
- There is an increased incidence of renal disease in exposed females.

- Dentists exposed to chronically high levels of nitrous oxide have developed neurological symptoms suggestive of a vitamin B_{12} deficiency. This finding has been confirmed in rats chronically exposed to nitrous oxide.
- Animal studies (in rats) also show that chronic exposure to nitrous oxide has resulted in litters that are reduced in number and size compared with control animals.

It must be stressed, however, that some epidemiological studies did not confirm some of these claims. For example, a major 10-year prospective study in the UK of 13 500 pregnancies in 11 000 women doctors showed no relation between the number of hours spent in the operating theatre or medical speciality, and reported miscarriages after confirmed pregnancy. Neither was there any increase in congenital malformations observed.

It would seem prudent, however, to reduce levels of anaesthetic agents in the environment where they are used. This would include the operating theatre, recovery rooms, dental suites and the maternity unit. Various organizations in different parts of the world have introduced recommendations for maximum acceptable levels of pollution to protect staff working in these areas. In the USA, for example, this is done through the National Institute of Occupational Safety (NIOSH) and the American Conference of Industrial Hygienists (ACIGH) and in the UK by the British Health and Safety Commission (HSC). There is also a proposal (in draft form at present (prEN 740)) covering countries in the European Community.

In the UK there is a legal requirement on employers to control industrial and medical pollution with the introduction of a government approved code of practice entitled 'Control of Substances Hazardous to Health' (COSHH), which was introduced in October 1989 and updated in 1994. This code of practice has been drawn up by the HSC's Advisory Committee on Toxic Substances under section 16 of the Health and Safety at Work Act (1974) for the purpose of providing practical guidance on the control of substances hazardous to health in the workplace. However, it is a separate organization, the Health and Safety Executive (HSE), that has the power to enforce the code of practice.

This code came into force on 1 October 1989 (although defined exposure limits were only introduced in 1996 (EH40/96)) and covers a wide variety of substances including anaesthetic gases and vapours. COSHH regulations require an employer to protect employees by:

1. assessment of risk;
2. prevention or control of exposure;
3. installation and maintenance of control measures as well as regular examination and testing of the control measures;
4. monitoring of exposure at the workplace;
5. provision of health surveillance;
6. provision of information and training.

Under item 2, COSHH recommends that 'Exposure should be controlled to a level to which nearly all the population can be exposed day after day without adverse effect on health'. This reference exposure is usually expressed as the upper acceptable limit for an agent averaged out in any 8 h period of potential exposure (8 h TWA (time-weighted average)).

Recommended exposure limits for anaesthetic gases and vapours in some countries are set out in Table 22.1 based on the 8 h TWA. The levels are expressed as parts per million (ppm) or as millilitres per cubic metre (ml/m³).

Surveys have shown that when no steps are taken to avoid pollution, these limits may be exceeded. For instance, two studies reported in the published code (COSHH) showed from a 20-hospital survey that the levels of halothane varied between 0.1 and 60 ppm and for nitrous oxide between 200 and 300 ppm when no steps were taken. However, a 27-hospital survey showed the mean TWA exposures to halothane were 1.7 ppm and to nitrous oxide 94 ppm.

THE EXTENT OF POLLUTION

This depends on five factors:

- the quantity of anaesthetic gases and vapours employed;
- the employment of a scavenging system and its efficiency;
- the amount of leakage from the anaesthetic equipment;
- the efficiency of the air-conditioning and ventilation system in an operating theatre or anaesthetic room;
- the size and layout of the operating theatre and any other place where anaesthetic vapours are used.

Anaesthetic Gases and Vapours

The quantity of gases and vapours used may vary considerably depending on the breathing system used. At one extreme is the Mapleson D system, where there is a fresh gas flow of about 8 litres/min, of which 70% may be nitrous oxide, and to which other volatile anaesthetic agents may be added. At the other extreme is the low-flow circle system, where flows may be reduced to less than 1 litre/min. Also, there is substantial pollution from unscavenged 'Entonox' demand valves used in maternity units.

Table 22.1 Exposure limits to anaesthetic gases and vapours measured in parts per million (ppm) or as millilitres per cubic metre (mg/m³) and expressed as 8-h time-weighted averages (8-h TWA)

Country		N₂O		Halothane		Ethrane		Isoflurane	
		ppm	ml/m³	ppm	ml/m³	ppm	ml/m³	ppm	ml/m³
UK	1996	100	180	10	80	50	380	50	380
USA	1994	50		50		75			
Switzerland	1994	100		5		10		10	
Sweden	1994	100		5		10		10	
Italy	1994	50		2		2		2	

The Employment of a Scavenging System and its Efficiency

Surplus anaesthetic gases and vapours are vented from a breathing system or ventilator, via an expiratory valve and, if allowed to escape into the immediate environment, would pollute it. However, the valve is normally adapted to discharge into a scavenging system which collects the escaping gas and vents it to the atmosphere remote from a populated area. The efficiency of the scavenging system depends on its rate of extraction and the gas-tight fit of its components. The former must be greater than the discharge of pollutant gases in order to be effective. These systems are discussed in greater detail later in the chapter.

Leakage

However efficient a scavenging system may be, its purposes will be defeated if gases and vapours are permitted to escape from the apparatus. Overt leaks from the high-pressure and regulated-pressure parts of the anaesthetic machine may be easily detected. Leaks from the breathing system may be less obvious, however, and may even be due to diffusion through the rubber or neoprene parts. The latter often absorb significant quantities of some of the volatile agents during the administration of one anaesthetic, only to release them during the next anaesthetic. For this reason new and unused breathing attachments should be used for the administration of an anaesthetic to a patient who exhibits sensitivity to a particular anaesthetic agent, for instance in the case of malignant hyperpyrexia.

Leakage may also result from carelessness when certain vaporizers are refilled.

The Efficiency of the Air-conditioning System

The frequency of air changes is often quoted as a measure of the efficiency of an air-conditioning system. A figure of 20 per hour is usually considered satisfactory. However, the circulation of air throughout the theatre is often uneven, and frequently the recovery area, where the patient exhales anaesthetic agents, is poorly ventilated and there may be no arrangements for scavenging. The nurse attending the patient is often in direct line with the exhaled gases.

There are two further considerations:

. Some air-conditioning systems are wholly or partially recirculating, and may result in the vapours from one location polluting another.
. Thought must be given to the siting of the external outlet of the extract system, which again may pollute other areas in which people work.

The Size of the Premises

'Dental chair' anaesthetics for dental extractions are frequently administered in small rooms. This, in itself, is probably of little importance, since the anaesthesia is of only short duration and most dentists employ general anaesthetics only occasionally, so exposure of the personnel (except the travelling anaesthetist!) is limited. However, the advent of inhalational methods for relative analgesia and sedation has resulted in much more prolonged exposure. In these techniques high flow rates of nitrous oxide may be used.

CONTROL OF POLLUTION

The control of pollution should be tackled along the guidelines recommended in COSHH in the UK and NIOSH in the USA, namely:

- Instilling an awareness in personnel working in the potentially affected environment.
- Installation of effective scavenging equipment (see below).
- Ensuring good working practices by:
  (a) always using the devices provided;
  (b) daily inspection of these devices to establish that they are functioning;
  (c) considering the use of low-flow systems where appropriate;
  (d) checking for leaks in the breathing system;
  (e) flushing out the breathing system (including the reservoir bag) through the scavenging device provided, at the end of an anaesthetic;
  (f) considering capping off the breathing system at the end of an anaesthetic so as to prevent anaesthetic vapours that have impregnated the breathing hoses from polluting the environment;
  (g) the filling of anaesthetic vaporizers in a fume cupboard that includes a spill tray;
  (h) amending workplace practice by reviewing rotas so that the same personnel are not always working in those areas of highest pollution.
- Efficient room air-conditioning so as to remove any pollutant that may have inadvertently escaped. (A minimum of 15 changes per hour with a balanced supply and extraction process.)
- Regular monitoring of the theatre environment.

That which constitutes regular monitoring appears to be the most difficult issue to resolve. Monthly or fortnightly checks might miss a week in which the levels could, due to a fault, contravene COSHH/NIOSH guidelines. An employer (the hospital), if sued by an employee, could well find the case difficult to defend.

MEASUREMENT OF POLLUTION

The extent of pollution in the theatre environment is now quantifiable. It may be measured by various methods, some of which are described below.

Operating theatres. With the introduction of low-cost, non-dispersive infrared analysers, trace quantities of anaesthetic agents can be measured continuously. A single analyser (e.g. the Ollair Gas Handling Unit) can be set to measure 12–24 sampling sites and record the extent of pollution (for nitrous oxide) at the sites on a continuous basis, logging the results on a chart recorder and producing an alarm when excessive levels are recorded.

Theatre personnel. Individuals can be issued with sampling badges (for volatile anaesthetics) and sampling tubes (for nitrous oxide) that are worn for approximately 8 h. They are placed at shoulder height (to measure respirable exposure). The pollutants are adsorbed onto the material in the sampler in proportion to their concentration in the ambient atmosphere. For volatile agents, the material is based on activated charcoal, whereas for nitrous oxide a molecular sieve is used. At the end of the sampling period the samplers are sent to a specialist laboratory where the pollutants are measured using a gas chromatograph linked to an infrared detector.

SCAVENGING SYSTEMS

A scavenging system transports waste gases and vapours from a ventilator or breathing system and discharges them at some safe remote location. It includes several components, namely:

- a *collecting system*, which conveys waste gases from the breathing system to a transfer system;
- a *transfer system*, which consists of a section of flexible wide-bore hose linking the collecting system to the receiving system;
- a *receiving system*, which behaves as a reservoir to store surges in the flow of waste gas. From here these gases have to pass via disposal tubing to
- a *disposal system*. This transports the waste gases to a site on the outside of a building, away from populated areas.

Two or more of these items may be embodied in a single item of equipment.

Waste gas normally passes through the collecting and receiving system to the disposal system, using only the power generated in exhalation by the elastic recoil of a patient's lungs. At this stage there is little difference between the various systems employed. It may then pass through the disposal system using this same power (*passive scavenging*). However, it may be assisted by some form of gas or electrically powered apparatus which generates a subatmospheric pressure (*active scavenging*). Only systems that employ active scavenging are able to deal with the wide range of expiratory flow rates (30–120 litres/min) seen in anaesthetic practice, especially when certain ventilator systems are used. These systems (as opposed to passive systems) are, therefore, the only ones that can be recommended, and this is provided that they meet the specification and performance criteria approved by those countries in which they are in use (e.g. BS 6384: 1987 UK).

The Collecting System

This has two components:

- A 30 mm male conical connection (Fig. 22.1a) that is fitted either to the expiratory port of a ventilator, the demand valve (for Entonox) or to the APL valve of a breathing system. The version that fits the APL valve shrouds all the exit apertures on the body of the valve enclosing them in a gas-tight fit. (The latter is often called a banjo fitting because of its shape.)
- A 30 mm female conical connection (Fig. 22.1b) that fits over the first to form a gas-tight fit. Its other end remains attached to the patient end of the transfer system.

Having two components in the collecting system allows the female part to be detached and reattached to different breathing systems as required. The selection of a unique 30 mm taper for this connection is intended to prevent other breathing system components from being attached to it in error.

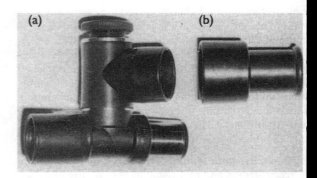

Figure 22.1 A collection system showing (a) a shrouded APL valve encased in a gas scavenging collector system and terminating in a 30 mm conical male taper; (b) 30 mm female conical taper linking the former to a transfer system.

The collecting system may also house an overpressure relief valve (Ohmeda AGS system), which is normally set to blow off at 1 kPa (10 cmH₂O). This device (Fig. 22.2) prevents excessive pressure building up in the breathing system should the scavenging system become obstructed (for instance if the transfer tubing was kinked or blocked).

The Transfer System

This consists of a length of wide-bore, kink-resistant tubing that joins the collecting system to the receiving system.

The exhaled gases emerge intermittently from the breathing system, their volume and flow pattern varying according to the type of apparatus in use. For example, with spontaneous respiration there may be a fresh gas flow of, say, 8 litres/min, and therefore that is the volume of gases to be scavenged per minute; however, the peak flow rate, during the period when the APL valve is open, may be much higher (up to 45 litres/min). Furthermore, some ventilators that have gas-driven bellows discharge the driving gas as well as exhaled gas into the scavenging system. This may well produce intermittent flow rates of in excess of 100 litres/min. It is important therefore to match the performance of the rest of the system to that of the anaesthetic equipment.

However, it would be dangerous to attach the collecting apparatus directly to a scavenging system that was actively extracting gas in excess of 120 litres/min as this would suck gas out of both patient and breathing system!

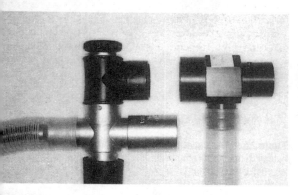

Figure 22.2 A collection and transfer system incorporating an overpressure relief valve (set at 1 kPa) in the female component.

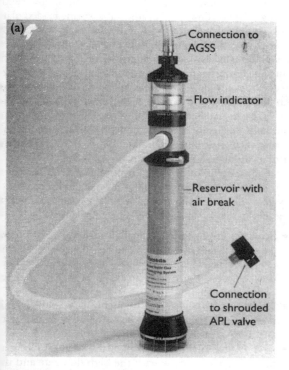

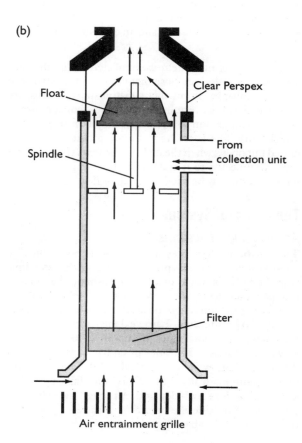

Figure 22.3 (a) An Ohmeda receiving system for use with active gas scavenging (AGS). (b) Internal arrangement of a receiving system.

The solution is to install a safety device (*receiving system*).

The Receiving System

The receiving system (Fig. 22.3) consists of:

- A reservoir (normally a rigid material cylinder) for the expired and driving gases, from which they are passed to the disposal system. It may also temporarily store this gas if the extraction rate falls below the recommended level.
- An air break. The reservoir is open-ended at its base to allow entrainment of air when there is insufficient expired gas. This prevents the transmission of subatmospheric pressure from the scavenging system to the patient. It also provides an emergency escape route for the gas should the scavenging system fail.
- A flow indicator to show that the unit is working when connected to an active disposal system. There is normally a clear Perspex window sited near the top of the reservoir in which a coloured float appears when the extraction rate is normal (i.e. 120 litres/min). When the flow drops below 80 litres/min this disappears from view.
- A filter sited in the base of the unit to prevent fluff entering and blocking the system.
- An entry port on the side and an exit port on the top of the container.

The receiving system is connected to the disposal system via a wide-bore hose that is sufficiently strong to prevent collapse from the subatmospheric pressure within it. The hose terminates in a probe which houses a screw-fit connection to the disposal system socket (terminal unit). The latter houses a valve that is normally closed but opens when the male probe from the receiving unit is connected to it and screwed on (Fig. 22.4). The terminal unit may be sited on a wall or flexible pendant.

The Disposal System

Active Disposal Systems

The subatmospheric pressure required to power the disposal system is usually provided by an exhauster unit (Fig. 22.5). This works in a similar fashion to a fan and requires a low level of maintenance and no lubrication. The size of the unit depends on the number of scavenging sites to be supplied. Large exhauster units can provide waste gas flow rates of up to 2400 litres/min, servicing 20 sites. Large sites often have a 'Duty' and a 'Standby' unit, which are linked. The 'Standby' unit operates automatically if the 'Duty' unit fails, as well as during periods of high demand. Although the exhauster unit is sited outside the operating theatre suite (sometimes a considerable distance away), the operating

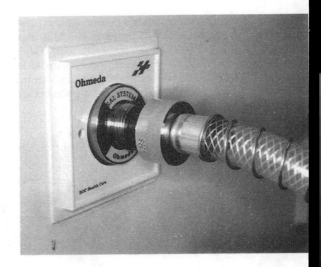

Figure 22.4 The probe from the receiver unit inserted into the wall-mounted terminal unit prior to the attachment of the screw-threaded securing connector (nut).

control switch is sited at a convenient location within the theatre suite.

Pressure fluctuations within the disposal system are controlled within precise limits by a vacuum/flow-regulating valve. It consists of an adjustable spring loaded plate covering the valve aperture and behaves as an air-entrainment valve should the vacuum exceed a predetermined level. This level is set, by adjusting the spring tension, during commissioning of the system, to provide the correct flow rates. Several valves may be fitted to large scavenging systems so as to protect and control specific areas.

The exhauster unit discharges the waste gas to a suitable outside location via rigid pipework. A water trap, with an isolating tap, is included in this pathway to drain any accumulated condensation.

The use of an existing hospital piped vacuum system has often been advocated in the past. However, these systems cannot be recommended as they may be unsatisfactory in design and may well be dangerous as:

- Scavenging requires a high-flow system with a small pressure gradient between the terminal unit and the exhaust unit, whereas the piped vacuum in a hospital uses a lower flow with a larger pressure gradient between the vacuum pump and the terminal unit.
- The extra demand upon the medical vacuum for this purpose may result in other users being deprived of an adequate medical vacuum in an emergency.
- The displacement (flow rate) of the vacuum line may be inadequate to cope with the high flow rate and the pulsating nature of the output of some ventilators.
- The outlet of the vacuum system may be so located that the expired gases would pollute areas where other personnel are working.

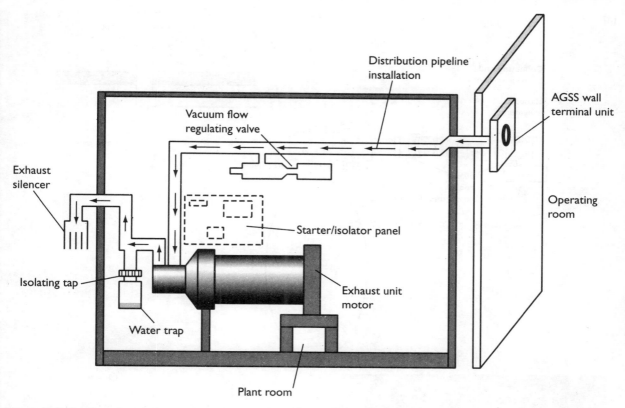

Figure 22.5 The disposal unit (exhauster) in an active gas scavenging unit.

- More importantly, as vacuum lines do not contain safety valves (vacuum/flow-regulating valves, see above), there is a danger that an excessive 'vacuum' may be applied to a patient.

Collecting systems for scavenging in paediatric breathing systems are discussed in Chapter 14.

Passive Disposal Systems

Although these systems are not now recommended, a brief description is included so as to contrast the differences between passive and active systems.

In a passive system (Fig. 22.6), the receiver may house a 2 litre neoprene reservoir bag, an inlet and outlet and two relief valves. One of these valves opens at 1 kPa (10 cmH$_2$O) to prevent pressure build-up resulting from an obstruction in the scavenging system. The other valve can be opened if there is a subatmospheric pressure within the system greater than 50 Pa (0.5 cmH$_2$O) caused by excessive suction from the ventile (see below).

The outlet from the receiver is connected to a wide-bore tube, which passes through one of the walls or the roof of the building and terminates in a ventile. A ventile is a device that uses the wind to entrain the exhaust gases

or air. Unfortunately, the passive system can be relied upon to operate satisfactorily only when the outlet is installed in a suitable position and when the wind is blowing from the desired quarter. It may be affected by the proximity of other buildings. Under adverse conditions the flow may be in the opposite direction, and, because it would be possible for the scavenged gases from one operating theatre to be expelled into another, each point must have its individual ventile. Branching of the pipework is unsatisfactory. Usually the system terminates on the roof. As the waste gases pass to the cooler areas above the ceiling of the operating theatre, they become denser, thus tending to slow their flow, and water vapour may condense and run back down to the theatre, possibly carrying infection. A water trap is therefore essential.

Absorption Systems

Although these systems can remove the vapours of volatile anaesthetic agents from waste gases, they do not absorb nitrous oxide and therefore cannot be recommended as a scavenging system that meets current standards. They are included out of interest as

(a)

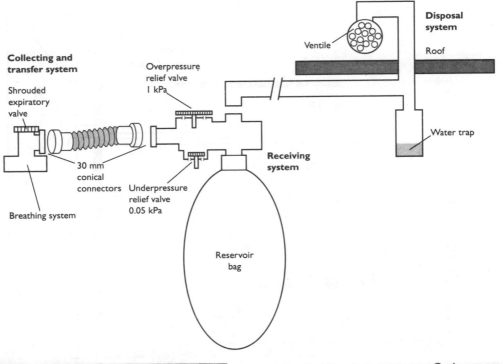

Disposal system

Ventile

Roof

Collecting and transfer system

Shrouded expiratory valve

Overpressure relief valve 1 kPa

Water trap

30 mm conical connectors

Underpressure relief valve 0.05 kPa

Receiving system

Breathing system

Reservoir bag

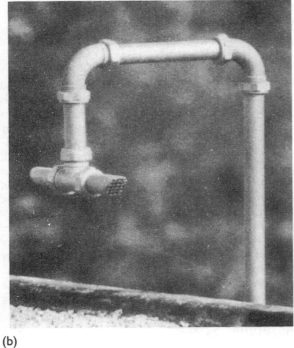

(b)

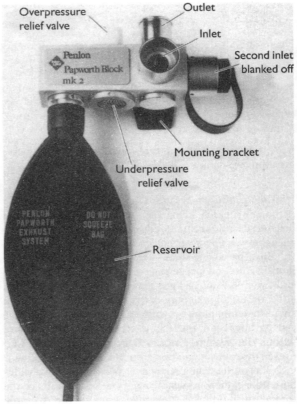

Overpressure relief valve

Outlet

Inlet

Second inlet blanked off

Penlon Papworth Block mk 2

Mounting bracket

Underpressure relief valve

Reservoir

PENLON PAPWORTH EXHAUST SYSTEM

DO NOT SQUEEZE BAG

(c)

Figure 22.6 (a) A passive scavenging system. (b) A ventile for passive waste gas disposal. (c) A receiving system for passive scavenging.

there may be occasions where they could be used with a low-flow breathing system where nitrous oxide was not employed and where scavenging was unavailable.

Most systems employ activated charcoal, in canisters of 1 kg, to absorb the volatile anaesthetic vapour efficiently. They have a low resistance and may be incorporated in the expiratory limb of a breathing system (Fig. 22.7). The canister increases in weight as the vapour is absorbed, and this may be monitored by a spring balance on which it is mounted. When the weight reaches the level stated, it should be discarded.

Care must be taken to ensure that it is disposed of in a safe location, where it will not permit the vapour to be released and pollute the atmosphere breathed by other people. Used canisters should not be allowed to fall into the hands of drug addicts, who have been known to heat them in order to gain the release of vapour. Indeed, the use of heat to release this has been employed in one type

of canister, which being made of suitable metal, may be placed in the autoclave in order to discharge it. If this system is employed, one must again ensure that the discharge of vapour-laden steam from the autoclave is to a safe location.

Unfortunately, recent research incriminating nitrous oxide rather than the volatile anaesthetic agents has rendered the employment of the relatively simple Aldasorber less appropriate.

Other Devices

All the devices described are intended for use with adult breathing systems. Paediatric scavenging devices are described in Chapter 14. However, there are other situations where gaseous anaesthetic pollution can occur, notably in recovery rooms. Here, patients may continue to exhale anaesthetic agents postoperatively in close proximity to recovery room staff. The collecting systems described above cannot scavenge gas from many of the oxygen delivery devices often used on patients in these sites. Devices such as that shown in Fig. 22.8 are more

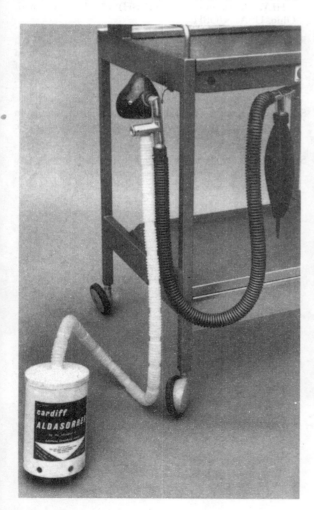

Figure 22.7 The Aldasorber.

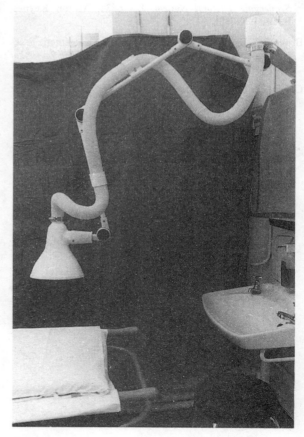

Figure 22.8 A collection system for use in recovery rooms.

suitable. A funnel attached to wide-bore hose (which is then attached to a special active gas scavenging system) can be sited close to a patient's face to remove pollutants. The funnel is supported by a series of levers. The efficiency of the device requires a calm patient! A restless one may constantly move away from the optimal extraction zone of the device. In view of this, a greater interest in efficient air conditioning would be appreciated by many of the medical and nursing staff when the design of theatres is being considered.

FURTHER READING

Askrog V, Harvard B (1970) Teratogenic effects of inhalation anaesthesia. *Nordisk Medicine* 3: 490.

Austin IC, Shaw R, Crichton R, Cleaton-Jones PE, Moyes D (1978) Comparison of sampling techniques for studies of nitrous oxide pollution. *British Journal of Anaesthesia* 50: 1109–1112.

British Standards Institution (1987) *Anaesthetic Gas Scavenging Disposal System*, BS 6834. Milton Keynes, Bucks, UK: BSI.

Bruce DL, Bach MI (1976) Effects of trace anaesthetic gases on behavioural performance of volunteers. *British Journal of Anaesthesia* 48: 871.

Cohen EN (1980) *Exposure in the Workplace*. Littleton, MA: PSG Publishing Company.

Deacon R, Perry J, Lumb M, et al (1978) Selective inactivation of vitamin B12 in rats by nitrous oxide. *Lancet* ii: 1023.

Hatch DI, Miles R, Wagstaff M (1980) An anaesthetic scavenging system for paediatric and adult use. *Anaesthesia* 35: 496–499.

Health and Safety Commission (1988) *Control of Substances Hazardous to Health Regulations 1988. Approved Code of Practice*.

Health and Safety Executive (1996) *Occupational Exposure Limits*. Guidance Note EH 40/96. Sudbury: HSE Books.

Knill-Jones RP, Moir DD, Rodrigues LV, Spence AA (1972) Anaesthesia practice and pregnancy: controlled survey of women anaesthetists in the United Kingdom. *Lancet* ii: 1326.

National Institute for Occupational Safety and Health (1977) *Criteria for a Recommended Standard: Occupational Exposure to Waste Gases and Vapours*, DHEW Publication No. (NIOSH) 77–140. Cincinnati, Ohio, USA: NIOSH.

Rowland AS, Baird DD, Weinberg CR, Shore DL, Shy CM, Wilcox AJ (1992) Reduced fertility amongst women employed as dental assistants exposed to high levels of nitrous oxide. *New England Journal of Medicine* 327: 993–997.

Spence AA, Knill-Jones RP (1978) Is there health hazard in anaesthetic practice? *British Journal of Anaesthesia* 50: 713.

Symington I (1994) Controlling occupational exposure to anaesthetic gases. *British Medical Journal* 309: 968–969.

—23—

INFUSION
EQUIPMENT

Contents

BASIC COMPONENTS OF AN INFUSION SYSTEM

The majority of intravenous infusions are administered by gravity from flexible plastic bags and plastic bottles using pre-sterilized, disposable giving (administration) sets. These giving sets are of several types:

- simple fluid administration – no filter, approximately 15 drops/ml;
- blood and fluid administration with clot filter, approximately 15 drops/ml;
- fluid administration with micro-dropper, no filter, approximately 60 drops/ml;
- burette, 100–150 ml in volume, with or without micro-dropper;
- platelet giving sets.

Simple fluid administration sets must not be used to administer blood without a filter.

The rate of infusion depends upon:

- the height of the fluid container above the infusion site;
- the resistance to flow caused by the giving set;
- occlusion of the tubing by a rate-controlling device;
- the physical properties of the fluid to be administered;
- the bore of the administration cannula;
- the back-pressure in the veins of the patient.

The manufacturers of giving sets quote the size of drops, which may be 15–20 drops/ml, but it must be realized that the actual volume of the drops depends upon the physical properties of the fluid being administered. For more accurate control of fluid administration, such as is required in paediatric practice, giving sets with micro-droppers may be used. Most micro-droppers, when using normal clear fluids, have a drop size of 60 drops/ml. With a burette, increased safety is ensured as only volume for 1 h can be administered. Platelet transfusions require special platelet giving sets in order to reduce the risk of platelet aggregation occurring in the giving set, as would occur with conventional blood giving sets.

Rapid Infusion

When rapid infusion of blood or other fluids is required, the rate of administration may be increased by the use of a Martin's pump (Fig. 23.1), which is used when the infusion solution comes from a rigid bottle, or by a pressure infusing device (Fig. 23.2) when it is in a plastic bag. This may consist of an inflatable pressure bag, which may even be contained in a rigid box to increase the speed at which pressure may be applied.

Whenever fluids are administered intravenously at a rapid rate, provision should be made for warming them to body temperature, otherwise serious cooling of the body may ensue (Fig. 23.3).

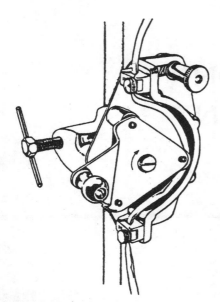

Figure 23.1 A Martin's infusion pump.

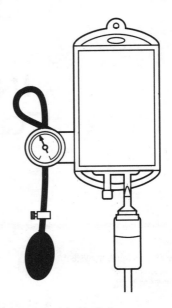

Figure 23.2 Pressure infusion device.

Accurate Infusion Control

It is often necessary in anaesthesia, in intensive care and in the management of pain to be able to infuse drugs accurately and safely at a continuous rate over long periods of time. Large-volume infusions may be administered accurately by using an infusion pump, whereas infusions at very slow rates may be given using a syringe pump or driver. A classification of so-called infusion pumps is shown in Fig. 23.4.

Electronic Drop Counters

Electronic drop counters do not control the rate of infusion, but they accurately inform the user of the rate thereof. A small beam of light, which may be infrared and thus invisible, is passed through the drop chamber of the giving set and interruptions of this beam are detected by a photoelectric cell. From a measure of the time between drops, the rate of infusion is electronically calculated and displayed. These devices are only as accu-

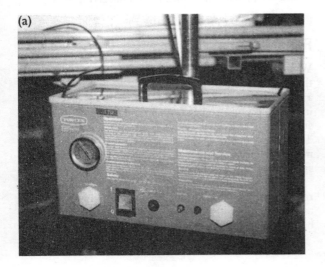

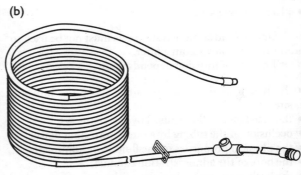

Figure 23.3 (a) Hot water blood warming system. (b) Coil through which the blood passes.

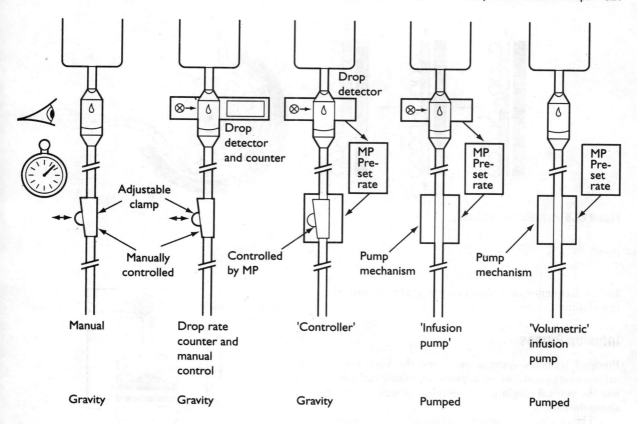

Figure 23.4 Types of infusion pumps. MP, microprocessor.

rate as a knowledge of the size of individual drops, and this size must be programmed into the device each time it is used. Obviously the rate of infusion may not remain constant between estimations with these devices.

PRINCIPLES OF INFUSION PUMPS

Most of the so-called infusion pumps are similar in appearance but may be very different in principle and in the accuracy of infusion rate. Some do not actually pump the liquid but use gravity as the source of energy. It is therefore necessary when using infusion pumps to ascertain the mechanism by which they work.

Infusion Controllers The infusion controller (Fig. 23.4) usually uses a photoelectric drop-counting system in conjunction with some form of adjustable occlusion of the infusion tubing controlled by a microprocessor. The infusion is by no power other than gravity, but is controlled by the microprocessor, which adjusts the clamp

mechanism to compensate for changes in resistance to flow in the cannula or the patient's vein. This method of infusion is more accurate than by simple manually controlled giving sets and always includes alarms that are activated if the desired infusion rate is not maintained.

The Stepper Motor

The driving force in the majority of infusion pumps and electronic syringe drivers is an electrical machine called a stepper motor. The stepper motor may be directly controlled from a digital microprocessor system. The speed of a conventional electric motor driven from either an a.c. supply or a d.c. supply may vary with voltage, mechanical load or the frequency of the supply. It is difficult without electronic feedback to control such a motor accurately. The stepper motor is designed so that a series of pulses applied to the stator windings of the motor cause the shaft to rotate by a fixed amount for each pulse, typically 1.8°, 2.5°, 3.75° or 7.5°, irrespective of the load, within certain limits. Infusion systems may be designed so that a pulse generator, whose frequency may be varied, can produce accurate control of an infusion

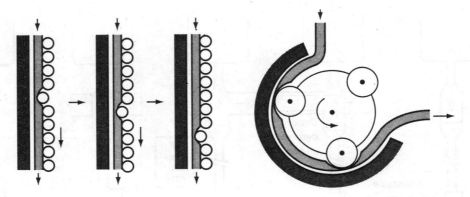

Figure 23.5 Peristaltic mechanisms.

and the frequency adjustment may be calibrated directly in millilitres per hour.

Infusion Pumps

Pumped infusion systems overcome the variation in infusion rate caused by back-pressure, tubing resistance and the vertical height of the reservoir container or bag above the patient.

The driving mechanism of infusion pumps may be a peristaltic arrangement or may use a small syringe with associated valve in the manner of a conventional piston pump. A decade ago, the most accurate (and expensive) infusion pumps used syringes and were referred to as volumetric infusion pumps; the peristaltic pumps were less accurate as they depended on the quality of the infusion tubing and the constancy of the droplet size for the accuracy of their infusion rate. Most modern infusion pumps use the peristaltic principle and are as accurate as the syringe-type owing to the use of precision silicone tubing and not relying upon drop counters to judge the infusion rate.

The principle of the peristaltic infusion pump is shown in Fig. 23.5. The tubing of a giving set is rhythmically compressed by a series of rotating rollers or by a ripple with a series of mechanical 'fingers' as shown. The stepper motor driving either of these two mechanisms is controlled by a microprocessor.

Figure 23.6 shows a typical syringe-type infusion pump mechanism. This is also driven by a stepper motor controlled directly by a microprocessor. The volume of the syringe is usually about 5 ml. The syringe 'cassette' is supplied sterile and disposable. Fluid is drawn rapidly from the reservoir bag into the syringe in less than 1 s. The valve is then actuated so that the syringe contents are expelled at the required rate into the patient, and then the

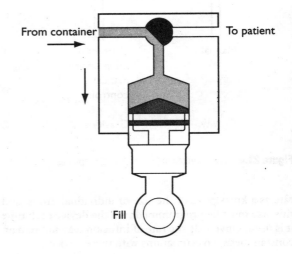

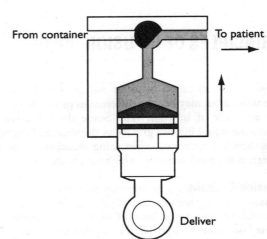

Figure 23.6 Principle of a syringe-type volumetric infusion pump.

process is repeated. Although, in theory, this produces an intermittent flow, it also produces a very accurate overall infusion rate with only 1 s interruptions infrequently.

The low-budget infusion systems rely upon drop counting to control the infusion rate. The required infusion rate is dialled-in on the control panel and the 'dedicated' microprocessor in the pump compares the required rate with the rate of drops passing the photo-detector, and thus maintains the stepper motor at the desired speed. The rate of infusion is once again dependent upon the drop size and the rate selector will have been calibrated for a specific giving set and for a specific fluid. The size of the drops will be dependent upon the physical properties of the fluid being infused and its temperature.

Most infusion pumps (Fig. 23.7) still make use of a photo-electric drop detector as a means of detecting when the fluid reservoir is empty.

Modern infusion pumps are able to detect air-in-line and line blockage, which sound alarms.

Safety

There are several potential hazards with infusion pumps, most of which are automatically protected against, but the user must still be aware of the following:

- too rapid rate of infusion (administration set not properly clamped when pump not in operation);
- failure of power source, be it mains or battery;
- infusion of air;
- continued infusion after cannula has become extravascular;
- rate of infusion upset by more than one infusion through the same cannula or catheter;
- fault condition occurring in the pump device caused by allowing intravenous liquids to spill on the pump.

Syringe Drivers

The simplest mechanical syringe driver is driven by a clockwork mechanism. However, these are only obtainable at a single fixed rate of infusion and therefore find little use in anaesthesia and intensive care. Clockwork syringe drivers are mainly used for narcotic infusions for pain control in terminal care or occasionally for heparin infusions. There is a range of small battery-operated syringe drivers (Fig. 23.8). These pumps are mainly used for insulin infusion and the relief of cancer pain with narcotic infusions. They may have a variable rate that is adjusted with a small screwdriver. The driving mechanism is a miniature d.c. motor that is switched on and off intermittently and drives a screw-threaded rod (or a screw) which is linked to the syringe plunger, causing its advancement. These syringe pumps are small

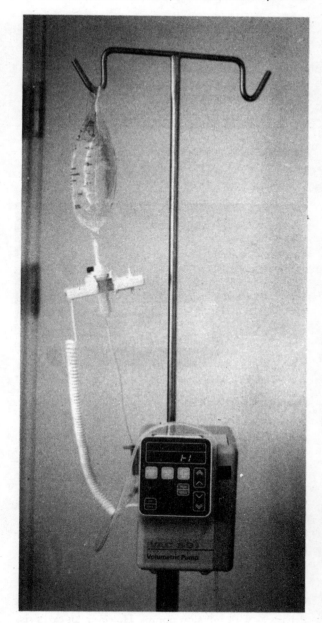

Figure 23.7 Volumetric infusion pump.

and light enough to be worn in a holster by an ambulant patient.

Syringe drivers used in intensive care and anaesthesia usually make use of stepper motors, again connected to the syringe plunger by a lead screw. Thus each pulse applied to the stepper motor causes the advancement of the syringe plunger by a known amount. The pulse generator driving the stepper motor may be calibrated from 0.1 ml/h to 99.9 ml/h in steps of 0.1 ml/h. It is

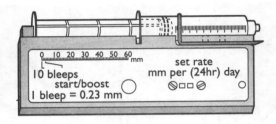

Figure 23.8 Graseby syringe driver.

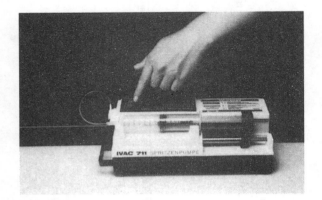

Figure 23.9 A syringe driver.

important that only syringes recommended by the manufacturer are used, otherwise the calibration will be adversely affected. These syringe drivers (Fig. 23.9) may be free-standing or pole-mounted, and are mains driven, but may have a rechargeable battery option for the transport of patients. Electronic syringe drivers have alarms for occlusion and empty syringe.

Safety

The same safety problems may occur with syringe drivers as with infusion pumps. However, an extra risk factor may be apparent. If the syringe pump is physically higher than the vascular access to the patient there is a risk of *syphoning*, whereby the weight of liquid in the catheter between the syringe and the patient may draw more from the syringe than has been programmed, resulting in overdose. Syringe drivers should have protection against the syringe plunger moving faster than its motor-drive.

If syringe pumps are mounted with the syringe in the vertical position, the outlet of the syringe should be *downwards* so that bubbles formed by gas coming out of solution are not driven into the patient.

Target Controlled Infusion

The infusion devices used for total intravenous anaesthesia (TIA) are usually conventional digitally controlled infusion pumps and syringe drivers as already described. Although the drugs used for TIA are short-acting and have short half-lives, it is necessary with the currently available intravenous anaesthetic agents to reduce progressively the infusion rate during the operative procedure to avoid undue accumulation. A new infusion pump is now available that, although not actually measuring the plasma concentration of the infused agent, automatically adjusts its own infusion rate using an algorithm which maintains a constant plasma concentration. The selected plasma concentration may be adjusted at any time by the anaesthetist and the pump alters the infusion rate such that the new level is acquired in the minimum time. The inputs to the pump are: target plasma concentration, patient weight, patient height and drug concentration. This target controlled infusion (TCI) pump is currently available only for the infusion of propofol.

PATIENT-CONTROLLED ANALGESIA

The quality of postoperative pain relief and patient autonomy have improved with the use of patient-controlled analgesia (PCA). The quality of postoperative analgesia, until the introduction of PCA, was actually decreasing owing to the decreasing number of qualified nursing staff, in the name of 'efficiency'. Intramuscular bolusing with opioids at 3–4 hourly intervals may produce good analgesia although smaller boluses at more frequent intervals produces less swings in analgesia and in the side-effects of the analgesic drugs. The disadvantages of intramuscular injections 'when required' are:

- wide swings in plasma concentration of drug;
- delay between onset of pain and pain relief;
- patients not willing to call hard-pressed nursing staff;
- wide variation in patient dose requirement.

The delay between the onset of pain and relief is caused by a summation of:

- too few qualified nursing staff and therefore patients' needs not attended to immediately;
- strong analgesic drugs are drugs of abuse and are therefore 'controlled' and require *two* qualified staff to administer them.

The advantages of PCA are:

- patient autonomy;
- immediate relief of pain;
- analgesia tailored to patients' requirements.

The key points in any PCA system are:

- route of administration;
- type of administration (bolus, background infusion);
- ease of programmability (dose, lock-out);
- ease of priming;
- power source;
- safety;
- security;
- portability;
- display;
- printout.

PCA is most commonly by the intravenous route but may also be into the epidural space. The simplest method of administration is by bolus-dosing; here a pre-set bolus, which may be programmed either by volume of injectate or in more complex systems by weight of drug in milligrams, is injected on demand. There is a pre-programmed lock-out time during which a further bolus is not permitted, thus allowing for the time of onset of action of the previous bolus and protecting against overdosage.

A background continuous infusion may also be available with some devices. The advantages of a background infusion are that smaller boluses are required and if the patient sleeps for a period he or she is unlikely to awake in severe pain owing to the long period since the last bolus dose.

PCA devices may be mains or battery powered (Fig. 23.10) but all electrically powered devices must have a battery capability in case of mains failure or the need to move the patient around the hospital. A further feature of some battery-powered PCA devices is that they are designed for ambulant use and are therefore miniature; these devices are especially useful in labour.

PCA devices may have complex memories and displays showing not only the selected program but also giving a 'history' of their usage on a particular patient. The history may then be used to reprogram the PCA more closely to the patient's requirements. There may also be the facility for connecting the PCA to a printer to down-load the history.

Although it is advantageous to have all of these facilities on PCA devices, it must be borne in mind that:

- the capital cost of each device will be considerable;
- at least one PCA device is necessary for each major (and minor?) case each day;
- the complexity of setting-up and programming for each patient will be considerable and lead to errors;
- maintenance of staff training is costly in time and money.

There is much to be said for the use of simple disposable PCA devices, as shown in Fig. 23.11. This device is powered by the pressure induced in the drug solution by the latex balloon surrounding it. The bolus is 0.5 ml and the lock-out is approximately 5 min.

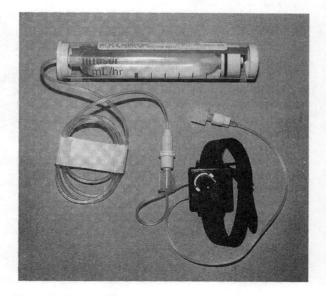

Figure 23.11 A disposable PCA device.

Of prime importance with PCA is safety and security. All devices must be safe against overdosage either caused by fault conditions or drug syphoning. There must also be security against tampering and adjustment of parameters by unauthorized staff, patients or visitors.

FILTRATION

Intravenous fluids should be filtered to protect the patient from microscopic foreign material. Blood for transfusion that is more than 24 h old should be filtered

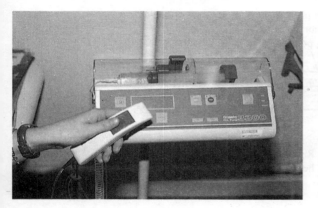

Figure 23.10 A Graseby PCA.

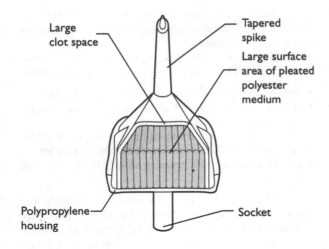

Figure 23.12 A blood filter.

(Fig. 23.12) to remove micro–aggregates that form from the breakdown products of the cellular components and platelets. Blood filters are of two basic types: screen filters and depth filters. Screen filters function as 'sieves' and are usually constructed from a woven mesh. They have a regular pore size, often of 40 μm. The efficiency of a screen-type filter at removing foreign matter increases progressively with each unit of blood passed as the pore size tends to decrease progressively down to 20 μm. Screen-type filters are said to be less damaging to the red cells than are depth filters. Depth filters consist of a pack of synthetic fibre, often Dacron, not formed into a mesh. The mechanism of 'filtration' is actually by adsorption of unwanted material, down to a size of about 10 μm, onto the surface of the fibres. This adsorption is probably due to electrical charge differences between the particles and the fibres. With the depth filter, the efficiency at removal of unwanted material decreases with each unit of blood, probably as a result of channelling in the pack of fibres.

Intravenous crystalloids may be filtered with much finer sieve-type filters to remove foreign particulate matter including bacteria. The Pall intravenous 'Site Saver' extends the life of the giving set, which should normally be replaced every 24 h, to up to 96 h. The construction of the 'Site Saver' is shown in Fig. 23.13. All particulate matter larger than 0.2 μm is removed by a 0.2 μm filter membrane. Air is also continuously vented through a hydrophobic membrane, which has 0.02 μm pores, thus protecting the patient from air embolism. Use of the 'Site Saver' also protects against microbiological contamination.

AUTOTRANSFUSION

When a large blood loss may be expected during surgery, it may be possible to reuse the patient's own blood, provided that is uncontaminated and free from clots. Uncontaminated blood is aspirated by the machine, anticoagulant is added and it is stored temporarily in a reservoir. It may then be transfused back into the patient via a filter.

FURTHER READING

Gambling DR, White PF (1995) Role of patient-controlled epidural analgesia in obstetrics. *European Journal of Obstetrics, Gynecology & Reproductive Biology* 59: (Suppl): S39–46.

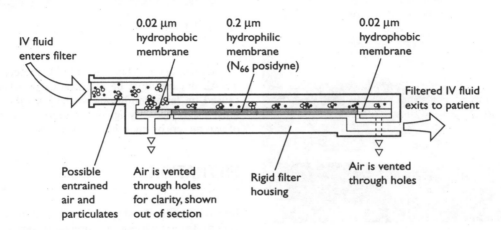

Figure 23.13 Pall intravenous 'Site Saver'.

Jastremski M, Jastremski C, Shepherd M, et al (1995) A model for technology assessment as applied to closed loop infusion systems. Technology Assessment Task Force of the Society of Critical Care Medicine. *Critical Care Medicine* 23: 1745–1755.

Lehmann KA (1995) New developments in patient-controlled postoperative analgesia. *Annals of Medicine* 27: 271–282.

Lindley C (1994) Overview of current development in patient-controlled analgesia. *Supportive Care in Cancer* 2: 319–326.

Shaw HL (1993) Treatment of intractable cancer pain by electronically controlled parenteral infusion of analgesic drugs. *Cancer* 72: (Suppl 11): 3416–3425.

Sherry E, Auty B (1992) Controlled infusion devices: applications in anaesthetic practice. *European Journal of Anaesthesiology* 9: 273–285.

—24—

MEDICAL SUCTION APPARATUS

Contents

INTRODUCTION

Suction apparatus is vital to the safe practice of anaesthesia and intensive care. It is used for clearance of mucus, blood and debris from the pharynx, trachea and main bronchi and during surgery for providing a clear field for the surgeon. Special suction apparatus is also used for other purposes, for example gastrointestinal, wound and pleural drainage.

COMPONENTS

The apparatus has several components, including:

1. A *power source*, which generates the subatmospheric pressure necessary for the removal of the debris. It may take the form of a large power plant that services a whole hospital or a small single unit that services a single patient.
2. *Transfer tubing*. This may be a rigid pipeline, where the power source is large and remote (such as in a central hospital supply), which connects the power source to the items below. In a small unit, it may be a suitable length of flexible tubing.
3. A *collection vessel*, which may use the subatmospheric pressure supplied to entrain and store the debris prior to its disposal. The vessel is, in turn, connected to:

4. A suitable length of *suction tubing*, the other end of which is usually fitted with a detachable, rigid suction tip (sucker). With portable hand-held apparatus, the latter may be connected directly to the collection vessel for ease of use.

Power Source

Suction apparatus requires a power source that generates a subatmospheric pressure. The most powerful will produce a high vacuum. However, this pressure can only be a maximum of 1 atm (100 kPa) less than the normal environment (i.e. sea level), which is not as powerful as other medical gas services (i.e. 400 kPa for respirable gas and 700 kPa for surgical power tools). Therefore, it has to be used efficiently.

The subatmospheric pressure required may be created by:

- An electric motor or other source of rotational energy that may be used to drive a mechanical pump, various forms of which are shown in Fig. 24.1a–e.
- Pneumatically driven pumps that usually work on the venturi injector principle (Fig. 24.1f). They may be driven by compressed air, oxygen, steam or water.
- A manually operated spring-loaded bellows arrangement with unidirectional valves (Fig. 24.1g) (small suction units only).

Pump Types

Figure 24.1a shows a piston pump, which is capable of creating a high vacuum but, in transportable models, has a comparatively low displacement. Figure 24.1b shows a diaphragm pump, which is a variation of the piston pump; it is mechanically much simpler but often has the disadvantage of being much noisier than the conventional piston pump. Figure 24.1c shows a form of rotary pump that can produce a high vacuum. Figure 24.1d shows a rotary pump, which may be designed to produce a very high displacement as would be required in the high-volume aspirator used in dental surgery. It works in the same way as a vacuum cleaner and does not produce a very high degree of vacuum; it is also comparatively noisy. Figure 24.1e shows a pump that works on the principle of the Archimedean wheel. This can be made quite small but produces a high vacuum and high displacement. Many hospitals now use this type of pump as the main source of pipeline medical vacuum. Figure 24.1f shows compressed gas passing through a narrow orifice and entraining gas using a venturi principle. Finally, Fig. 24.1g shows a spring-loaded bellows, which

sucks in gas via a one-way valve and then blows it out via the other.

A large power source may be:

- permanently sited, supplying the other components of the suction apparatus via a vacuum or gas pipeline; or
- transportable, usually powered by mains electricity and supported on castor wheels; or
- truly portable, powered by a battery or cylinder of gas or by human energy (hand- or foot-operated).

Efficiency

The efficiency of the suction apparatus depends upon:

- the degree of negative (*subatmospheric*) pressure that can be produced by the pump, with particular regard to the time taken to achieve it;
- the *displacement*, i.e. the volume of air at atmospheric pressure that the pump is able to move per unit time;
- the *internal resistance* of the suction apparatus and the length and diameter of the transfer pipeline and suction tubing;
- the *viscosity* of the matter to be aspirated.

A pump that is able, through better engineering and design, to produce a high vacuum (*subatmospheric pressure*) in a faster time will be more efficient. However, if the pump has a small *displacement* this will limit the volume of air that the pump is able to move per unit time and so will reduce its efficiency. Different pump designs may have differing displacement and high-vacuum capabilities and therefore may be selected for specific tasks. For example, liposuction requires a *high vacuum* to dislodge fat globules (*high viscosity*) but a small displacement as a relatively small amount of this (and no air) is removed. Dental suction, on the other hand, requires *high displacement* to remove the large amounts of water spray, air and dental debris but does not require a high vacuum. This pump must also have a *low internal resistance* and be connected to a relatively wide-bore sucker and suction tubing to maximize the flow of debris.

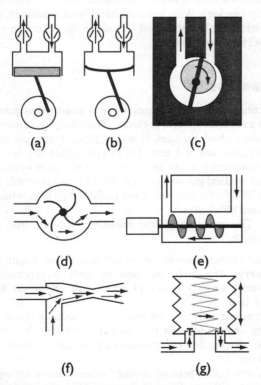

Figure 24.1 Vacuum pumps. (a) Piston pump; (b) diaphragm pump; (c) high vacuum rotary pump; (d) low vacuum rotary vane pump; (e) rotary pump using an Archimedean wheel; (f) gas-powered pump using the Venturi principle; (g) a bellows pump.

Examples of Types of Suction Apparatus

Figure 24.2 shows a portable, electrically driven piston pump attached to a sucker jar; Fig. 24.3 shows a high-volume aspirator using an electrically driven rotor; and Fig. 25.4 shows the working principles of a pneumatically driven pump working on the injector or venturi principle. When driven from an oxygen cylinder, these pumps are very wasteful of oxygen, but they have the virtue of being portable. Figure 24.5 shows a foot-operated bellows-type pump attached to a sucker jar.

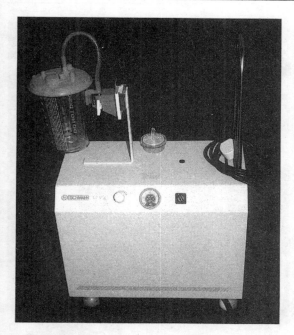

Figure 24.2 A transportable electrical suction device.

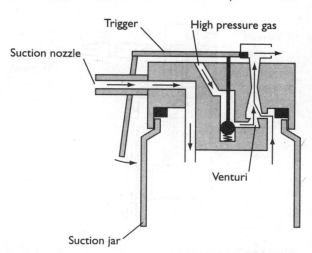

Figure 24.4 Working principles of a suction device using a Venturi injector.

Labels: Trigger, High pressure gas, Suction nozzle, Venturi, Suction jar

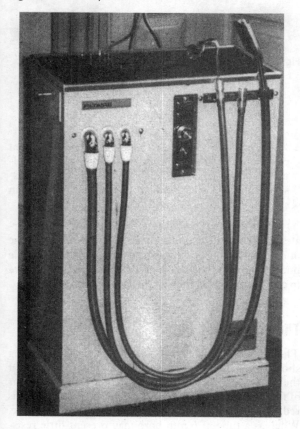

Figure 24.3 A high-volume aspirator, which is used particularly in the dental operatory.

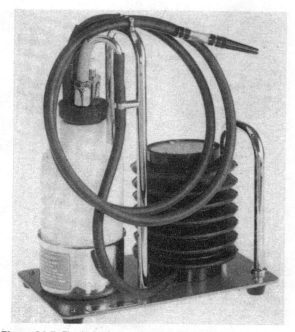

Figure 24.5 The Ambu foot-operated suction pump.

The Collection Vessel Assembly

This has two components:

- *The suction controller* (Fig. 24.6), which is a device with a variable orifice that can be adjusted manually to regulate the force of vacuum applied to the patient. It may include a float assembly and a back-up filter to prevent liquid material entering the system. It is normally connected via flexible tubing to a collection vessel (Fig. 24.7), which is attached to:

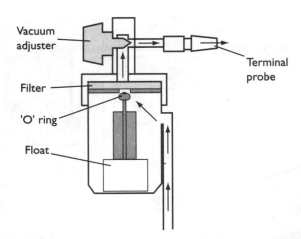

Figure 24.6 A suction controller.

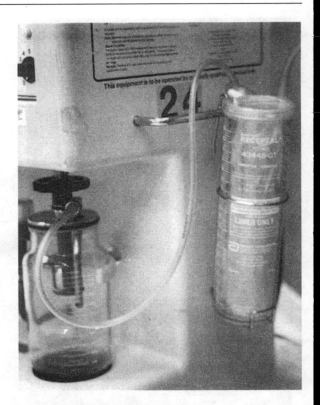

Figure 24.8 Receptal disposable collection vessel system.

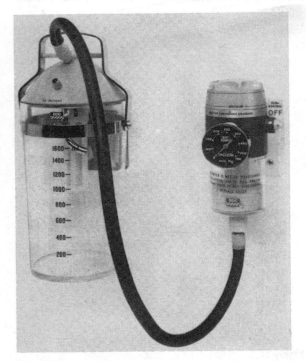

Figure 24.7 A pipeline vacuum unit. On the right is the controller, which is plugged directly into a flush-fitting outlet (obscured in this picture). On the left is the reservoir jar.

- *The collection vessel (or reservoir jar)*. Whatever the source of the vacuum, the size of the collection vessel is important. Sufficient capacity should be allowed for all the matter to be aspirated. Too large a capacity, however, will not only be cumbersome but will also increase the time taken for the vacuum to build up in it, even if the inlet from the patient is completely occluded. The connection between the collection

vessel and the rest of the apparatus should be kept clean and free from damage. A common cause of failure in suction apparatus is a leak at this point. The vessel should be graduated so that the volume of an aspirate such as blood can be estimated.

With the increased danger of infection from aspirates, as with hepatitis and other serious infections, the use of disposable collection vessels or those with disposable liners (Fig. 24.8) should be used so that staff never have to come into contact with the aspirate when cleaning.

The Suction Tubing

The internal diameter and length of the suction tubing should allow the greatest possible amount of suction at the patient end. As discussed in Chapter 1, the behaviour of fluids shows that the resistance of the delivery tube is reduced by keeping it as short and as wide as possible. Whereas a tube of 6 mm bore may present little resistance to air, it will considerably impede the passage of blood, mucus and vomit.

The flow of air alone through the tubing may be laminar, but when it is mixed with liquids or solid matter it is likely to become turbulent, increasing the resistance. The wall of the suction tubing must be of sufficient firmness and thickness to prevent collapse under the vacuum or kinking.

The Suction Nozzle or Catheter

It may be necessary to use a long, narrow catheter, as, for example, in bronchial suction, but otherwise excessive length should be avoided. Suction 'ends' should taper to the nozzle so that as much of the length as possible may be of the wide diameter. The shape of the tip should be smooth so as to prevent damage to delicate surfaces, and it is sometimes desirable to have two or more holes (Fig.24.9a), so that if one is blocked, possibly by mucous membrane being sucked into it, the other will continue the suction. This type of blockage is more common when the vacuum is too high, in which case provision may be made to admit air into the delivery tube or collection vessel by means of a bleed valve or hole. If there is a hole in the proximal end of the suction catheter or Yankauer hand piece, it may be occluded when required by a finger (Fig. 24.9b). The advantage of placing the bleed valve or finger-hole at this point is that it does not reduce the flow along the suction tubing.

REFINEMENTS OF MEDICAL SUCTION APPARATUS

The following refinements are added to a suction apparatus (see Figs 24.6 and 24.7):

Cut-off valve This is fitted inside the collection vessel or controller or both, and usually consists of a float which, being lifted by the rising level of aspirate, operates a valve to shut off the connection with the vacuum source. Its purpose is to prevent liquid from a full collection vessel entering the pump mechanism and causing failure, or entering the pipes of a pipeline system.

Occasionally, a cut-off valve, having been closed, is held closed by the vacuum acting upon it. It is then necessary, after emptying the reservoir, to either stop the vacuum source or pull the float down again and so reopen the valve.

Bacterial filter This should be fitted to prevent air that has been contaminated during its passage through the apparatus from infecting the atmosphere when it is blown out of the pump. It is best placed between the collection vessel and the pump so as to protect the latter. If it becomes wet, it will become ineffective and may also obstruct the air flow. Filters should be changed at regular intervals, depending on their size, lest they themselves become a source of infection.

Vacuum control valve or regulator This may be fitted between the pump and the collection vessel. A vacuum control valve is a bleed valve that, when opened, admits air, thereby reducing the degree of vacuum. A vacuum regulator, on the other hand, operates on a similar principle to a pressure regulator and so no energy is wasted by allowing air into the system. It is usual to use a vacuum regulator to control the degree of vacuum in a pipeline system terminal unit.

Vacuum gauge These gauges, which are normally calibrated in mmHg or kPa, are fitted to the tubing between the vacuum control valve and the collection vessel, or immediately above the collection vessel itself. Note that modern vacuum gauges operate so that the needle goes counter-clockwise as the vacuum increases. However, there are still many in use that work clockwise with increasing vacuum.

Foam prevention Foaming may be a problem in the collection vessel, since it causes closure of the cut-off valve when the vessel is far from full. Foam may even pass the valve and contaminate the filter or the pump, causing

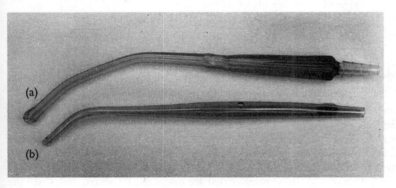

Figure 24.9 Two examples of hand-held suction nozzles.

failure. Foam may be suppressed by the addition of methylated spirits (highly flammable) or, more effectively, by silicone-based emulsions.

Stop valve This valve may be used to occlude the delivery tubing to close the nozzle. It allows the build-up of a vacuum in the reservoir during a standby period and is particularly useful when the pump gives a low displacement.

Two collection vessels There are two ways in which two vessels rather than one might be used:

- In one arrangement a selector enables the second vessel to be used and the first one to be isolated either when the latter is full, or leaking when there is a fault in a washer or a split in the collection vessel. It is of particular importance when large volumes of fluid, as in ascites or major haemorrhage, are being aspirated.
- In the second arrangement the collection vessels are in series, so that if the first is overfilled, the overflow goes harmlessly into the second without contaminating the pump or pipeline. Unfortunately the mechanical principles, though simple, are not always appreciated by the theatre staff, and misconnections are common.

PIPELINE VACUUM UNITS

Piped vacuum systems are now installed in most major hospitals. The 'behind the wall' equipment and terminal outlets are described in Chapter 3. Medical suction apparatus may be plugged into this system wherever there is a terminal outlet.

There are two types of local vacuum unit:

- Free-standing floor units, often with two large collection vessels, used for surgical purposes in the operating theatre (Fig. 24.10).
- Wall-mounted units. These have a single collection vessel that may often plug straight into the pipeline outlet, as shown in Fig. 24.7. There are several types of these controllers available for specific purposes. The most common type has a high-suction capability, which can be adjusted to provide up to the full vacuum pressure available from the wall outlet. Low-suction controllers are especially limited to provide safe suction for intrapleural drainage or nasogastric suction.

NB. It is worth noting that the pressure gradient between the pump and the terminal outlet can be no more than 1 atm (i.e. the difference between atmospheric pressure and a vacuum). Therefore, the efficiency of the system depends on the displacement of the pump and the internal volume of the transfer pipelines. A scenario

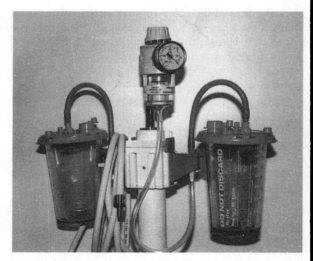

Figure 24.10 Free-standing medical suction unit.

might arise when, if all the suction equipment in a hospital were turned on simultaneously, the displacement would be exceeded and the pressure gradient could drop to levels insufficient to provide adequate suction. It would be wise, therefore, to use the apparatus only when necessary so as not to jeopardize the efficiency of the system at other sites and to turn off when not in use.

CHOICE OF SUCTION APPARATUS

When selecting a suction apparatus for a particular purpose, the following points should be considered:

- Must it be portable? If so, should it be manually operated (Fig. 24.11) or powered by a gas cylinder using an injector? If not, should it be powered (by electric motor) at the site where it is used, or connected to a pipeline system?
- Is a high displacement needed?
- Is a high vacuum needed?
- What size should the collection vessel be?

It is also important to ascertain, for an electrically driven suction machine, whether it is rated for continuous or intermittent use, as some are intended for intermittent use only and prolonged periods of operation could lead to the motor overheating and failing. Such units are labelled appropriately.

High-volume aspirators, as used in dental surgery, that use a pump similar to a vacuum cleaner usually have three suction tubes of different diameters or with different nozzles (Fig. 24.3). Under no circumstances should those nozzles that are not in use be obstructed, since the

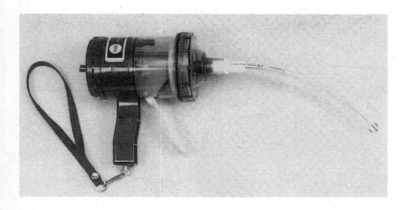

Figure 24.11 Vitalograph hand-operated suction apparatus with applicator.

free air passing through them is used to cool the motor, which may otherwise overheat. These suction machines are needed especially where a jet or spray of water is used for cooling the operation of the high-speed turbine drill.

STANDARDS AND TESTING

As with all other medical equipment there are published Standards for design and manufacture. These Standards include descriptions of tests for the safety and efficacy of suction apparatus. The relevant Standards are listed in (Appendix III). Some of these tests are too complex to be performed routinely in the hospital setting.

A simple test to prove the efficiency of a high-vacuum suction apparatus may be performed as follows.

A litre or so of water (at a temperature of 45–50°C) is placed in the collection vessel, which is then placed in its operating position. The vacuum source is then applied and the patient end of the delivery tube is occluded. By the time the vacuum has built up to its maximum, the water should be boiling.

FURTHER READING

HTM 2022 (1994) (Suppl.) Permit to Work Systems. London: HMSO.

Rosen M, Hillard EK (1960) The use of suction in clinical medicine. *British Journal of Anaesthesia* **32**: 486–503.

CLEANING AND STERILIZATION

Contents

INTRODUCTION

When patients present for either a local or general anaesthetic, they would expect that:

- the equipment used on them would be in a state of cleanliness that would do them no harm;
- items supplied from a manufacturer would be free of risk from noxious particles used in the manufacturing process which might be injected or inhaled, as well as free from the possibility of acquiring an infection from organic contaminants;
- reusable equipment be free from risk of passing on an infection from a previous use.

It is agreed that the degree of risk increases with the proximity of the equipment to the patient and methods employed to minimize this should be tailored accordingly. The stages in the process are therefore:

1. general cleaning and decontamination, and then, if required:
2. sterilization;
3. disinfection.

DECONTAMINATION

This consists of the physical removal of infected matter (micro-organisms and the organic material on which

they survive) and can be achieved by a thorough soaking, scrubbing and washing using a detergent. Modern devices include the following.

Automatic washing machines (washer/disinfectors). These often combine decontamination with subsequent disinfection (see below). An example of this is the 'Scotts' washer (Fig. 25.1), which resembles a dishwasher with special racks for holding anaesthetic breathing hose, endotracheal tubes and facemasks. It cleans by pumping treated water with detergent through holes in the racks so that it passes through the internal parts of the equipment, and then disinfects it by circulating hot water at 80°C and holding it at that level for 10 min (pasteurization).

The ultrasonic washer This is another example of a decontaminator that is particularly useful for small pieces of equipment, and for equipment of intricate shape. It consists of a bath of water in which the objects are immersed and in which they are subjected to ultrasonic vibration. The water contains detergent, and for specialized purposes, as in the dental operatory, other chemicals such as ammonia may be used to break up the resins and alginates that are common contaminants.

It should be noted that decontamination is very important. If foreign material remains on or in the equipment, then further processing using some of the methods described below may not be totally successful as the surfaces of the items may not be fully exposed to the

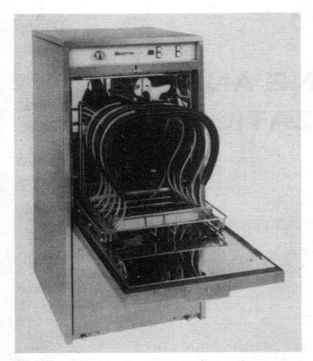

Figure 25.1 The Scotts SL40 anaesthetic apparatus decontaminator. Note that different trays may be used in the same machine to wash and disinfect other equipment, including surgical instruments.

process. For example, cases of cross-infection have been documented from equipment that was insufficiently cleaned and which was subsequently sterilized using ethylene oxide.

This process is sufficient for *low-risk* items, particularly those that are not introduced into the patient.

DISINFECTION

This implies the removal or killing of most or all infective organisms, with the exception of the most resistant ones such as bacterial spores. Those that are not killed are reduced to a level that is not harmful to health. This is regarded as adequate for many purposes and may be applied to *intermediate-risk items*. These include items that come into contact with intact skin or mucous membranes. They may be treated by the following methods.

Cold Chemical Methods

Several organic agents possess the ability to kill bacteria and viruses. The efficacy of these compounds depends

on their concentration, the length of time in contact with the article to be treated and their individual potency. Most are in the form of liquids, into which the various objects to be treated are immersed. The liquid may also be impregnated onto a cloth, which is then used for wiping down smooth surfaces. The agent (if suitable) may be employed as a nebulized mist or fog (see below). Some agents may exist as a gas or vapour at room temperature, and can be blown through equipment or even whole rooms (fumigation).

Liquids Alcohol, in the form of 70% ethyl or isopropyl alcohol in water, is a fairly efficient disinfectant. (Pure alcohol is not as effective as the aqueous mixture.) It is used mainly to wipe down hard surfaces such as anaesthetic machines.

Chlorhexidine may be used in various concentrations. It is a non-detergent chemical disinfectant. Facemasks may be soaked for 30 min in a 0.05% solution in water. Quicker disinfection (2 min) may be attained by using a 0.5% solution in 70% alcohol. This solution is also useful for swabbing down equipment such as anaesthetic machines. Detergent chemicals should be avoided because they may cause damage to the rubber parts of anaesthetic apparatus.

Chloroxylenol has frequently been used, particularly for facemasks. A dilute solution should be used and the facemasks rinsed in clear water for 2 h after immersion. However, there is a danger that the patient may develop facial skin rashes as a result of sensitivity to chloroxylenol, which is absorbed into the rubber of the facemask, so this agent is best avoided.

Hypochlorite solutions (bleach) have recently been shown to be highly effective in decontaminating and disinfecting material infected with the human immunodeficiency virus.

Several agents have been used to disinfect ventilators. These include 70% alcohol in water, hydrogen peroxide, various aldehyde preparations and a proprietary mixture of dimethyl phenols in an alcoholic/detergent base. Alcohol should not be used to disinfect a ventilator that is electrically powered, where a risk of explosion exists. The ventilators should then be run for several hours in fresh air to clear the disinfectant from the tubing and the internal parts of the breathing systems.

Pasteurization

This is particularly suitable for materials that do not withstand well the higher temperatures of autoclaving, and is especially appropriate for anaesthetic equipment. The process consists of heating the article to a temperature of 70°C for 20 min or 80°C for 10 min. It is most conveniently done in a water bath or as part of the cycle in a Scotts washer after the decontamination process. It may also be done in the low-pressure autoclave. It is not as efficient as boiling, but does kill most infective agents and is usually considered adequate for perishable articles and where absolute sterility is not necessarily required. Whereas plastic and rubber articles may soon lose their shape and antistatic properties as a result of repeated boiling, they are less damaged by pasteurization. The antistatic properties may be restored, where this is still required, by the weekly application of a suitable spray.

One of the problems arising in the use of the water bath is that rigid discipline is required to ensure that it continues for the necessary length of time. Not only must the temperature be maintained but one must also prevent the addition of extra items while the process is continuing, thus recontaminating those already being treated.

Boiling

Relatively small articles, including facemasks, may be boiled in water for 5 min. This is a fairly efficient method of disinfection, provided that one maintains the discipline mentioned above for pasteurization. Boiling is satisfactory for any article made entirely of metal and also for those made of rubber or neoprene. The process should be timed from the point when the water returns to boiling after the introduction of the last item to be treated. Large, cold articles may lower the temperature significantly!

STERILIZATION

This is a process designed to destroy all organic material such as viruses, bacteria and their spores. It is the best process for minimizing the risk of passing on an infection to a patient. It should be used on all items that constitute a *high risk to the patient*, i.e. items that come into contact with a break in the skin or mucous membranes or are introduced into a sterile body area. The principal methods of sterilization are discussed below.

Autoclaving

In autoclaving, the most effective method of sterilization, the articles to be treated are prepacked in envelopes or boxes of suitable material and the pack sealed with a special adhesive tape that shows, by colour changes, that the heat process has been adequate. They are then placed in a chamber with a gas-tight door. Steam is admitted not only to the chamber, but also to the jacket surrounding it, in order to raise the temperature within. The vari-

ous stages of the process are usually controlled automatically, and finish with a vacuum stage in which the remaining moisture is removed. The steam is at a temperature considerably above the boiling point of water and therefore at a high pressure. The time required depends on both the pressure and temperature developed, as shown in Table 25.1.

Autoclaving is the most efficient, quickest, simplest and probably the most cost-efficient means of sterilization for use in the hospital. Other methods of sterilization mentioned below are appropriate only when autoclaving is contraindicated for items that would be irreparably damaged by this process.

Table 25.1 Sterilization times for autoclaves at different temperatures and pressures

Time (min)	Pressure (psi/kPa)	Temperature (°C)
30	15/101.3	122
10	20/135.0	126
3	30/202.6	134

Low Pressure, Low Temperature Steam (LTS)

This is performed in a chamber somewhat similar to the high-temperature autoclave. However, the pressure within is about 37 kPa (5.5 psi) absolute (in other words subatmospheric) in order to maintain the steam as a vapour at approximately 74°C. This is efficient at disinfection in that it kills most vegetative organisms, but not spores.

The addition of formaldehyde vapour to this, called low pressure steam and formaldehyde (LTSF), renders this process very much more efficient and kills many, if not all, spores. It does, however, require very careful programming, including vacuum extraction, and 'pulsing' of the steam and formaldehyde. This is a process in which the latter are pumped in and out of the chamber, so that the changes in pressure assure that the vapours penetrate completely all the articles being treated.

Relatively small LTSF chambers of about 4 cubic feet may be used to sterilize fibrescopes, whereas others, with doors at both ends, may be so large that articles such as anaesthetic machines or even bedsteads may be wheeled in. The development of LTSF would seem to be at a stage when there are still difficulties in assuring its reliability, but some authorities consider that they may well replace ethylene oxide for many purposes.

Formaldehyde Cabinets

The Dräger Aseptor is an entire system in which a 'dirty' and a 'clean' room may be separated by the cabinet, into which large items of equipment may be wheeled, or in which small items may be attached to the nozzles through which formaldehyde vapour is introduced. In earlier models the formaldehyde was then neutralized with ammonia, but in later models this is no longer necessary, because the formaldehyde does not adhere to surfaces. This is because the temperature and humidity are controlled at suitable levels: approximately 45°C and 90% relative humidity.

It would seem that with the use of formaldehyde alone, the incidence of damage to even domestic electronic equipment, such as television sets, is very rare.

Dry Heating

Some articles are suitable for sterilization by dry heat. They may be wrapped in special craft paper and then placed in a thermostatically controlled hot air oven at 150–170°C for 20–30 min. This method is not suitable for plastics or rubber. All-glass syringes may be sterilized by dry heat, provided that the temperature is raised and lowered slowly to prevent breakage by uneven expansion. Most lubricants deteriorate and should not be used on syringes. Metal plungers should be removed from the barrel of the syringe before heating, or the barrel will be fractured. Dry heat is the method of choice for some ophthalmic instruments.

Gas Sterilization (Ethylene Oxide or Propylene Oxide)

Ethylene oxide or propylene oxide gas may be used for sterilizing equipment and in particular those articles that are damaged by other methods. The difficulty is that a special sterilizer is required. This consists of a chamber resembling an autoclave, in which both humidity and temperature are controlled. The process is expensive and takes several hours. Ethylene oxide is very flammable, and is used in a 5–10% mixture with a gas such as carbon dioxide or 'Arcton 12' (dichlorodifluromethane) to prevent explosion risk. Heat and water vapour are also required. The expense and mechanical difficulties of this method usually limit it to use in specialist departments and for perishable items.

Provided that it is properly used, ethylene oxide is an efficient sterilizing agent, but makeshift arrangements, such as enclosing large items of equipment in plastic bags, may prove unsatisfactory.

After sterilization in ethylene oxide, a period of 5–7 days must elapse before the gas is entirely eliminated from rubber and plastic. This period of 'elution' may be speeded by the use of an aeration chamber.

Ethylene oxide cannot be used to sterilize polystyrene, because it has an adverse effect on this material.

Gamma Irradiation

The use of gamma rays requires a large, expensive and sophisticated plant, which is appropriate to the sterilization of large quantities of disposable goods, rather than the resterilization of individual pieces of equipment in repeated use. This method is quite inappropriate for any but the largest of hospital groups and will not therefore be described here.

Chemical Compounds

Several compounds in liquid solutions of suitable concentrations exhibit sterilizing properties against organic pathogens. The concentrations of agent and the exposure times required to sterilize equipment may vary with the agent and can be found on the product labelling.

Stabilized gluteraldehyde (Cidex) is popular as it is non-corrosive to equipment. However, users may suffer from skin and mucous membrane irritation as a result of contact with the liquid or inhalation of the fumes. Developed allergy to these agents is well known. Such reactions mentioned above would be drastically reduced if these agents were regularly handled in a fume-extraction cabinet as recommended.

Stabilized buffered peracetic acid solution (Nu-Cidex) is a more recently introduced agent that acts as an oxidizing agent on both the cell walls and the nuclei of microorganisms so disrupting and destroying enzyme systems. It is supplied in a container that keeps the concentrate and the diluent/stabilizing solution separate (Fig. 25.2). When required for use, the design of the

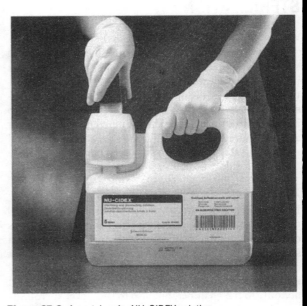

Figure 25.2 A container for NU-CIDEX solution.

container allows the two solutions to mix safely without risk to the operator or contaminating the local environment. The 'in-use' concentration of 0.35% is claimed to be a mild and transient irritant on the skin and produces a much lower vapour concentration of the agent and other volatile components (such as hydrogen peroxide and acetic acid).

TREATMENT OF ANAESTHETIC EQUIPMENT

The last few years have seen a major increase in the availability of single-use items of anaesthetic equipment such as facemasks, airways, endotracheal tubes, laryngoscopes, breathing systems, reservoir bags, self-inflating bags, soda-lime canisters and one-way, non-rebreathing and even APL valves. Together with the advent of low-resistance bacterial and viral (breathing system) filters (see later) to protect ventilators and non-disposable breathing systems, a major reappraisal of the policies recommended for cleaning and sterilization procedures may well be required in many hospitals. Although all these items are available, only the wealthiest of healthcare systems can afford to use all of these items on routine cases, and many of the more expensive items are still manufactured to be reusable. However, items such as airways, endotracheal tubes and breathing hoses can now be produced at competitive cost for single use.

In the UK it is difficult to find any nationally agreed policy on the definitive treatment of reusable items. Locally agreed hospital policies are the norm except where there is a specific recommendation by a manufacturer. In countries where the professional bodies have issued guidelines (e.g. Australian and New Zealand College of Anaesthetists, Policy on infection control in anaesthesia P28 (1995)), there is sometimes a discrepancy between what is considered adequate and the manufacturer's recommendation for an item of equipment. For example, items such as laryngoscopes need only be disinfected but laryngeal masks, which are placed in the same area, are required to be sterile!

The Anaesthetist

Practitioners should wear gloves when handling items of equipment that have been, or may come, into contact with a patient's blood or saliva (airways, endotracheal tubes, etc.). These should be removed before handling other items such as the components of the anaesthetic machine or ventilator so that contamination is minimized.

Endotracheal Tubes and Airways

Preferably, these should be single-use items supplied by the manufacturer as clean, sterile and in packets. Where items are intended for reuse such as laryngeal masks or some types of endotracheal tubes, they should be dropped into a bucket of soap solution immediately after use to prevent drying and crusting of blood or saliva as this will make the decontamination process more difficult. They should later be cleaned out with a long narrow brush specially made for the purpose (Fig. 25.3), thoroughly rinsed and then autoclaved as this is undoubtedly the most efficient method of sterilization, even though this reduces the lifespan of the items.

Endotracheal tubes often have a self-sealing attachment on the cuff inflation tube. In this case it should be confirmed that no water or air remains in the cuff, or the self-sealing end should be maintained open by a dummy syringe without a plunger, otherwise during autoclaving the cuff may become overdistended and rupture. The cuff should be tested at some time during the process to ensure that there are no leaks.

Laryngoscopes

The blades should be washed and scrubbed in between cases, using a disinfectant solution. Particular attention

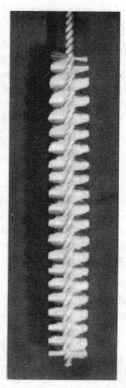

Figure 25.3 A brush for cleaning endotracheal tubes, etc.

should be paid to recesses through which the light carrier passes. The handle should also be decontaminated between uses.

Facemasks

Reusable facemasks may be made solely from rubber or silicone rubber or from combinations of materials. Some rubber ones may have a wire gauze stiffener; others may have a polycarbonate body which is rigid and surrounded by an inflatable seal made from rubber or silicone rubber. Rubber deteriorates rapidly when autoclaved in high-pressure steam to become stiff and brittle after two to three cycles. Silicone rubber is more resilient, but will have its lifespan reduced by as much as 50% if so treated. Fortunately, most authorities agree that these items can be treated satisfactorily by decontamination and disinfection.

Immediately after use, facemasks may be immersed in soap solution. At the end of every session the facemasks should be taken out and put through an automatic washer–disinfector. They should not be cleaned with detergents or with substances such as trichloroethylene, because these tend to damage the surface and make them sticky. (This damage is particularly likely in the case of facemasks made of rubber with a silicone rubber finish.)

Breathing Systems

Historically, it has been difficult to substantiate significant evidence of cross-infection between healthy patients when the same breathing system was used, and as the cost of disposable and individually clean reusable systems was substantial, the latter were only used following a known infected case or following a set number of cases. However, as it is impossible to identify every potentially infectious patient, and as the cost of providing either a single use breathing system or a disposable breathing filter is now reasonable, there is no justification in failing to provide every patient with either, or where expedient, a reusable system that has been disinfected. Where the latter has been used, the components should be separated and the corrugated hose, reservoir bags, APL valves, elbows and catheter mounts placed in a washer–disinfector that has a drying cycle.

Monitoring Equipment

Some Wright's-type respirometers are autoclavable, especially those that transfer the data electronically to a separate display. (The older, mechanical type is not autoclavable and requires ethylene oxide sterilization.) They may also be protected by a bacterial filter. This may be preferable as it prevents condensation on the vanes of those types that are not heated electrically.

Gas monitoring devices may be mainstream or sidestream samplers:

- Mainstream samplers are sited within the breathing system and therefore should be autoclavable.
- Sidestream samplers are sited away from the breathing system and are supplied by a gas sampling line. These do not need to be sterilized. If the gas is returned to the breathing system it must pass through a viral filter.

Bacterial Filters

These should be placed as close to the patient as possible (Fig. 25.4) so as to maximize the protection conferred to the breathing system and ventilator. They are discussed in more detail in Chapter 13.

Anaesthetic Machines

At the end of every day's work, the external surfaces of the anaesthetic machine should be thoroughly cleaned with a solution containing soap or 70% alcohol or with a suitable disinfectant solution, such as 0.5% chlorhexidine (Hibitane) in 70% alcohol. Special attention should be paid to the flowmeter knobs as these are most frequently handled by the hands of the anaesthetist, which may have been contaminated inadvertently by a patient's saliva or blood.

Circle Absorbers

Some circle absorbers are constructed of materials that would be damaged by heat sterilization, in which case the following is advised. The reservoir bag and corru-

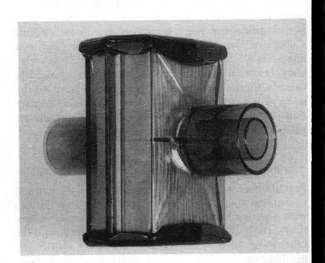

Figure 25.4 A bacterial filter.

gated hose should be treated as above. The domes on the unidirectional valves may be unscrewed and the valve discs carefully removed and cleaned, and the dome wiped out with a spirituous solution, such as 70% alcohol, or a 0.5% chlorhexidine solution. When refitting the dome one should make sure that the sealing washer is in place. When the soda lime canister is emptied, it should be thoroughly cleaned. This is partly to disinfect it, and partly to remove small particles of soda lime from the thread of the canister, which otherwise would cause

corrosion and wear and might prevent an airtight fit.

The contamination of circle absorbers may be reduced if, during use, the hoses are allowed to fall in a deep U-loop. This tends to cause droplets of moisture that may contain infection to 'fall out' before they reach the absorber. Bacterial filters, as described in Chapter 13, should be used in the breathing system to protect the absorber from infection.

Many modern circle absorbers may be autoclaved, and this is obviously more satisfactory.

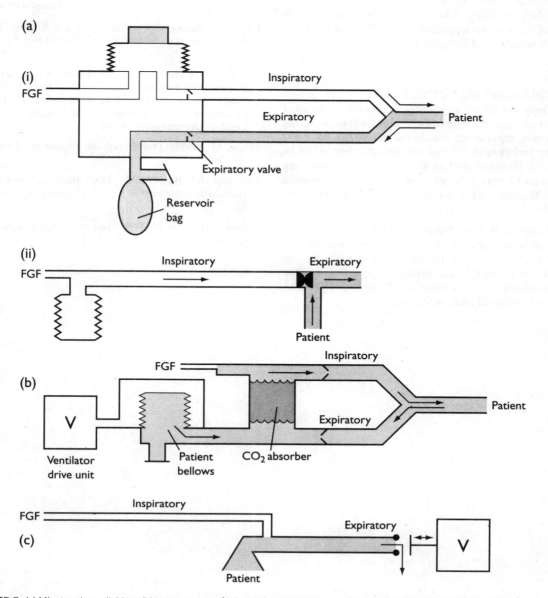

Figure 25.5 (a) Minute volume dividers; (b) bag squeezers; (c) T-piece occluders. The shading shows the extent of contamination of a ventilator system according to its application.

Ventilators

Part or all of the gas pathway through the ventilator may become contaminated depending on its design and application.

- *Minute volume dividers*. The inspiratory pathway should not become contaminated (Fig. 25.5) but the expiratory pathway can be and so should be detachable for autoclaving.
- *Bag squeezers*. The whole gas pathway can become contaminated including the bellows and should therefore be detachable and autoclavable.
- *'T'-piece occluders*. The reservoir limb and patient valve can become contaminated and should therefore be detachable and autoclavable.

Special Precautions for Infected Cases

As it may not always be possible to identify an infected case in advance, the best hygiene standards for selecting and using equipment should be employed on every patient and as such 'special precautions' should not be required. However, the handling of equipment following its use on a known infected patient merits consideration if only to comply with various hospital policies on its disposal:

- All disposable items should be placed in a plastic bag, which is then labelled a biohazard and incinerated.
- All reusable items should be placed in a labelled bag and sent to the relevant sterilizing department rather than mixed in with similar items from other patients, in order to avoid cross-infection.

- The work surfaces of the anaesthetic machine (including flowmeter knobs) should be wiped down after the case rather than at the end of the day.

FURTHER READING

Australian and New Zealand College of Anaesthetists (1995) *Policy on Infection Control in Anaesthesia*, P28. Melbourne: Australian and New Zealand College of Anaesthetists.

Central Sterilising Club (1986) *Report of a Working Party on Sterilization and Disinfection of Heat-Labile Equipment*. CSC.

Department of Health (1991) *Decontamination of Equipment, Linen or Other Surfaces Contaminated with Hepatitis B and/or Human Immunodeficiency Viruses*, Microbiology Advisory Committee to the Department of Health, July 1991. London: Department of Health.

Fraise AP (1995) Disinfection in endoscopy. *Lancet* **34**: 787–788.

Luttropp HH, Berntman L (1993) Bacterial filters protect anaesthetic equipment in a low flow system. *Anaesthesia* **48**: 520–523.

Snowdon SL (1994) Hygiene standards for breathing systems? *British Journal of Anaesthesia* **72**: 143–144.

—26—

ELECTRICAL HAZARDS AND THEIR PREVENTION

THE MAINS ELECTRICITY SUPPLY

Since many items of anaesthetic apparatus and monitors are powered by electricity, it is important to understand some of the principles involved. The 'mains' electricity supply is not direct current, flowing uninterruptedly in the same direction, as is produced by a battery; for good engineering reasons it provides an alternating current, in which the flow is constantly changing from one direction to the other in a rapid and regular manner. The number of complete cycles of this change of direction, or its *frequency*, is 50 per second in the UK and 60 per second in some other countries, for example the USA. The two conductors in a cable therefore cannot be said to be positive and negative, as would be the case with direct current, but because one conductor is at, or at about, the same potential as earth (because it is connected to earth at the source), this is said to be 'neutral' or 'return', and the other conductor to be 'live'. Because of this earthing of the neutral conductor, any person (or object) who is also connected to earth would complete an electric circuit by touching the live conductor, even if no contact were made with the neutral one. Figure 26.1 shows how under certain conditions the circuit may be completed by, say, an earthed diathermy plate, resulting in fatal electrocution. (In most modern diathermy machines the plate is 'earth-free'.) Stringent precautions should be taken to ensure that the polarities are correctly identified and connected for all mains electrical apparatus. Furthermore, the interruption of the neutral conductor alone could result in apparatus being at a live potential and yet not operating. Any contact with apparatus in this condition could, if it has not been disconnected from the

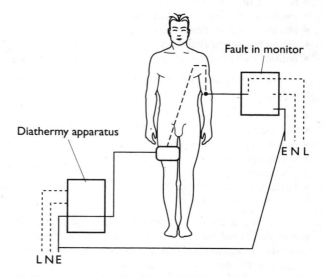

Figure 26.1 A fault in a monitor may cause the patient to come into contact with a live wire, the current being returned to earth via a metal object such as a diathermy plate (in those types of diathermy machine in which the plate is earthed). L, live; N, neutral; E, earth conductors.

mains supply, lead to electrocution. It cannot be over-emphasized that if a fault exists, the services of a competent technician should be sought.

The inclusion in an electric supply cable of a third conductor that connects the metal chassis, frame and enclosure of the apparatus to the earthed point of the supply ensures that under faulty conditions, such as an internal short in the equipment, the chassis and enclosure would not be rendered live. This wire is said to be the earth conductor.

Fuses interrupt the electric supply in the event that the current passing through them exceeds a predetermined level that might cause overheating or damage. They may be installed in the mains supply circuit, in the plug-top at the end of the lead to the apparatus, or in the apparatus itself. They usually consist of a fine-gauge wire, which melts if the current passing through them exceeds that against which they are intended to offer protection.

PATHOPHYSIOLOGICAL EFFECTS OF ELECTRICITY

Electric current passing through the human body may have several pathophysiological effects, the magnitude of which is dependent upon the current, the time and the frequency:

- resistive heating of the tissue;
- electrical stimulation of excitable tissues;
- electrochemical effects;
- arcing leading to charring;
- ignition of flammable material in contact with the body.

The factors that determine the severity of electrical injury are:

- resistance of the tissues;
- current (amperes);
- potential difference (volts);
- current pathway;
- duration;
- environmental factors;
- pre-existing health.

Heating of the tissues depends upon the energy or power dissipated by the tissues; this, in turn, depends upon the voltage applied and the resistance of the tissues. In general the body may be considered as an electrolyte solution (a good conductor) contained in a leathery bag (a poor conductor). However, the resistance of the integument is very variable (Table 26.1). This may be compared with the resistance of the internal tissues (Table 26.2).

However, there is a strange non-linear effect in that although the total body impedance (a.c. resistance)

Table 26.1 Skin resistance

	Skin resistance (ohms/cm²)
Mucous membranes	100
Vascular areas (volar arm, inner thigh)	300–10 000
Wet skin	
in the bath	1200–1500
sweat	2500
Other dry skin	10 000–40 000
Sole of foot	100 000–200 000
Heavily calloused palm	1 000 000–2 000 000

Table 26.2 Resistance of body tissues

Lowest	*Intermediate*
Nerves	Dry skin
Blood	
Mucous membranes	*Highest*
Muscle	Tendon
	Fat
	Bone

varies with the state of the skin and the area of the skin contact at low voltages (25–100 V), at 250 V and higher the total body resistance falls to around 2000–5000 ohms irrespective of the contact area and the current pathway (Beiglemeier 1987).

The effects of electric current upon excitable tissues such as muscle and nerve depend not only upon the current and time but also upon the frequency (IEC 1984, 1987). It is one of those ironies of life that the commonly used mains frequencies of 50 Hz or 60 Hz are the frequencies at which the excitable tissues are at greatest risk of excitation and damage (Fig. 26.2).

At greatest danger is the heart, as it is susceptible to induced arrhythmias as well as permanent damage. The current pathway is also important when considering the heart. Clinical studies suggest that sudden death from ventricular fibrillation is more likely with current passing 'horizontally' from hand to hand whereas heart muscle damage is more often associated with a 'vertical' current pathway (Fontanarosa 1993).

In general, the effects of hand-to-hand 50 Hz alternating current on the body are shown in Table 26.3 (Sykes et al 1991).

Direct current electric shock tends to produce:

- single muscle spasm;
- victim thrown from source;
- blunt mechanical trauma;
- disturbance of heart rhythm.

Even very low, imperceptible, direct current may produce chemical burns if the currents is allowed to pass for long enough.

Alternating current shock:

- is about three times more dangerous ampere-for-ampere;
- produces continuous muscle contraction (tetany) with 40–110 Hz;
- induces grip and pull as flexor muscles are much stronger than extensor muscles – this prolongs the duration of the current;
- induces local diaphoresis, which reduces skin resistance.

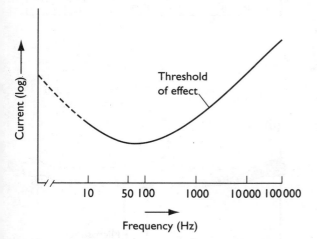

Figure 26.2 Variation of the threshold of pathophysiological effects of electric current with frequency.

Table 26.3 The effects of hand-to-hand 50 Hz alternating current

50 Hz current (mA)	Effect
1	Tingling sensation
5	Pain
15	Severe pain with local muscle spasm
50	Respiratory muscle spasm
80–100	Dysrhythmias with pump failure

ACCIDENTS ASSOCIATED WITH THE MAINS ELECTRIC SUPPLY

There are four ways in which the mains electric current, or equipment powered by it, may endanger the patient in the operating theatre:

- electrocution
- burns
- electrochemical
- ingnition of flammable materials, leading to fire or explosion.

Electrocution

Electrocution may cause death relatively slowly by the tonic contraction of the respiratory muscles, leading to asphyxia, or more rapidly by ventricular fibrillation. The onset of ventricular fibrillation may be somewhat delayed, being preceded by ventricular tachycardia, which causes circulatory failure, but which may revert to normal rhythm if stopped in time.

It will be remembered that the neutral pole of the mains electric supply is connected to earth at a point remote from the patient. Since all conductors have some resistance, however low, a loss known as *volts drop* occurs along these conductors, so that the neutral conductor is not exactly at earth potential at the patient end of the circuit. This difference in potential can cause 'stray voltage' and may lead to a 'stray current'.

Since earthed electrodes may be attached to more than one part of the patient, and from more than one piece of apparatus supplied by different mains sockets, it is recommended that the earth connections on all the socket outlets in a single clinical area be interconnected by a conductor of low resistance to minimize voltage differences between them. Similarly, all exposed metal objects such as radiators, water pipes, etc. are interconnected to a good earth.

Microshock

So far, only *macroshock* has been discussed. Figure 26.3 a–c shows the effect of a current passing between the extremities. When it passes across the patient's trunk only a small part of it passes through the heart. However, recent advances in medicine and surgery have led to the placement of electrodes on, within or close to the heart. Under these circumstances a very much smaller current, possibly as low as 100 μA, can result in ventricular fibrillation (Fig. 26.3d) because all the current passes through the heart. A very small potential, such as the stray voltage in the mains neutral lead, could be sufficient to produce electrocution in this way. This phenomenon is known as *microshock*.

Shock Protection

There are two ways of preventing accidents caused by unwanted currents returning to earth:

- install an isolating transformer, the output of which is carefully isolated from earth;
- Detect unwanted currents passing earth by a device that may then either sound a warning or automatically switch off the supply.

Both have advantages and disadvantages. An isolating transformer may supply all the outlets for a whole

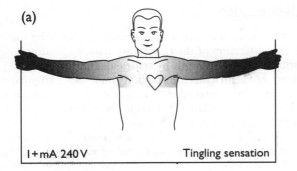

(a)

1+mA 240V   Tingling sensation

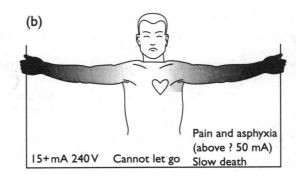

(b)

15+mA 240V   Cannot let go

Pain and asphyxia
(above ? 50 mA)
Slow death

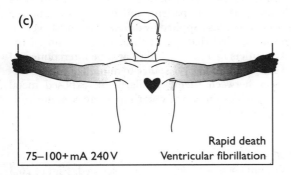

(c)

75–100+mA 240V   Rapid death
Ventricular fibrillation

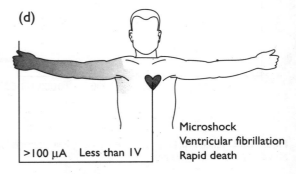

(d)

>100 μA   Less than 1V

Microshock
Ventricular fibrillation
Rapid death

Figure 26.3 (a) A current in excess of 1 mA passing through the body may produce a tingling sensation. (b) If the current exceeds about 15 mA, muscles are held in tonic spasm; the victim cannot let go and will eventually die of asphyxia. (c) When the current exceeds 100 mA, ventricular fibrillation and rapid death will occur. (d) If one electrode is applied to the right ventricle of the heart itself, a very small current can result in ventricular fibrillation.

operating room or theatre suite. This is referred to as safe patient power (Fig. 26.4). Apart from the expense, the problems are that if there are several appliances in use, and each of these has a small earth leakage current that is harmless in itself, the sum of all these currents may be sufficient to trip the relay and cut off the power to some piece of vital life-support equipment. Similarly, a fault in one piece of equipment may cause the cessation of power to another. If the relay operates a warning device rather than a circuit breaker, it may be observed too late or be unheeded by staff who do not appreciate its importance. Isolating transformers may be used in another more satisfactory manner. A small one may be included in the circuitry of each individual item of mains-operated electromedical equipment that can be connected to a patient. The patient circuit is earth-free and said to be *fully floating*. The enclosure of the equipment may be earthed or completely insulated.

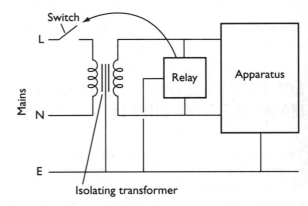

Figure 26.4 Safe patient power. The output of the isolating transformer is free from earth. Should earth leakage occur above a prearranged level, the relay will either disconnect the supply to the input of the transformer or sound a warning device. L, live; N, neutral; E, earth connectors.

The second method of improving safety is to install a current-operated earth-leakage circuit breaker (COELCB, also known as an 'earth trip' or residual current circuit breaker or RCCB) (Figs. 26.5 and 26.6). This may be installed in the electric supply to a whole operating room or theatre suite; or may be installed in each item of equipment. The live and neutral conductors each take a couple of turns or so (both exactly the same) around the core of a toroidal transformer. A third winding is connected directly to the coil of the relay that operates the circuit breaker. If the current in the live and neutral conductors is the same, the magnetic fluxes cancel themselves out. If they differ, there is a resultant field which induces a current in the third winding and this causes the relay to operate and break the circuit. A difference of as little as 30 mA can trip the COELCB in as short a time as 0.03 s. It may be manually reset, and may also have a test button to check its operation.

A similar device may be used instead merely to give a warning of excess earth leakage, or it may perform both functions.

COELCBs may present problems similar to those of isolating transformers, except that they are less expensive. They operate so quickly, and as a result of such a low earth leakage current, that they very greatly reduce the possibility of serious electric shock.

In the UK electrical safety in clinical areas is achieved by a high standard of earthing of the fixed wiring, by good earthing of enclosures and by fully floating patient circuits where appropriate. Safety may be further improved by using battery-operated equipment. In some cases the battery may be recharged between periods of use by 'plugging in' to the mains supply.

Burns

Where an electric current passes through the skin, whether intentionally or not, electrical resistance leads to the generation of heat. Depending on the amount of heat produced, the area over which it is applied and the rate of cooling by the blood circulation, burns may result. This matter is discussed further in Chapter 27, in connection with diathermy.

Fire

Sparks occurring at switches or from the interruption of the supply by the removal of a plug could ignite flammable vapours. They may be prevented in the operating theatre by the installation of sparkproof switches (Fig. 26.7), and electrical socket outlets that 'capture' the plug, preventing its withdrawal while the switch is turned on. All electrical apparatus in the operating theatre that does not comply with these precautions is kept outside the 'zone of risk', as described later in this chapter. Note that this 'zone of risk' no longer includes the whole operating theatre.

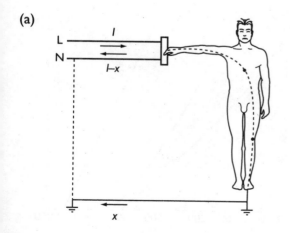
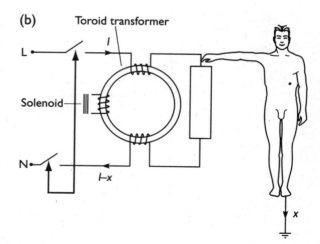

Figure 26.5 (a) If a load is taking a current of I amps from the live conductor L and x amps is returning via the patient and earth, then the current in the neutral conductor N will be $(I-x)$ amps. (b) A current-operated earth-leakage circuit breaker (COELCB). The imbalance between the currents in the live L and neutral N conductors is sufficient to set up a field in the toroidal transformer sufficient to induce in the third winding a current that will trip the solenoid and therefore disconnect both the live and neutral supply.

(a)

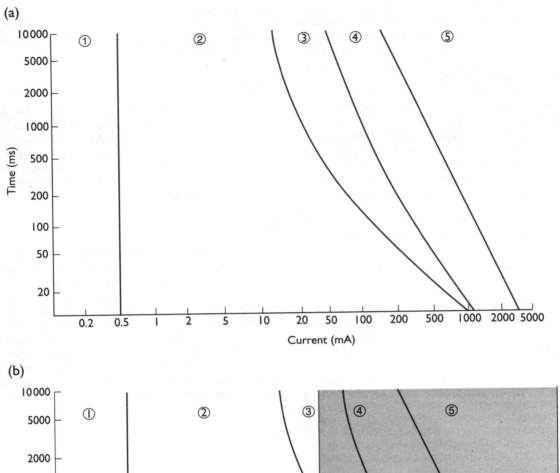

(b)

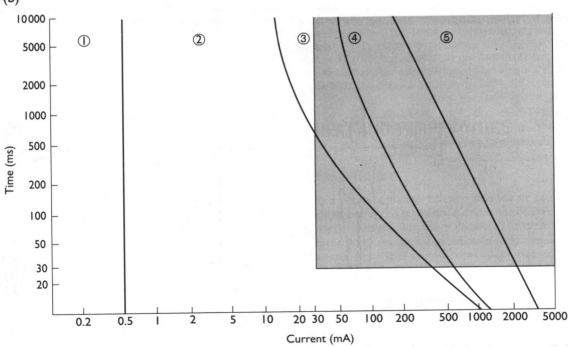

Figure 26.6 (a) The effects of a current passing through the human body (hand to hand or hand to foot). Zone 1, usually no effect; zone 2, usually no dangerous effect; zone 3, usually no danger of ventricular fibrillation; zone 4, ventricular fibrillation possible; zone 5, ventricular fibrillation probable. (b) The shaded area denotes the protection given by a COELCB.

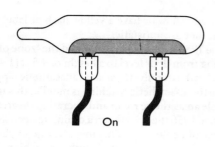

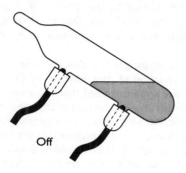

Figure 26.7 The contact of a sparkless mercury tip switch.

Fire and Explosion

For these to occur there are three prerequisites: combustible material, oxygen to support combustion, and a source of ignition. The risks arise from three sources:

- the use of high-pressure oxygen and high concentrations of oxygen at atmospheric pressure;
- the use of flammable solvents for cleaning and skin preparation;
- the use of flammable anaesthetic agents.

Burning consists of the chemical combination of a 'combustible' material with oxygen. Energy is liberated in the form of heat, and if it takes place in a confined space the pressure may be increased greatly. Rapid liberation of heat and the rise of pressure result in an explosion.

High-pressure Oxygen

When there is a rise in the pressure of a gas, heat is generated. If a flammable material such as oil or grease, in a confined area, is suddenly subjected to oxygen at the pressure of a full cylinder (approximately 2000 psi (140 000 kPa)), the heat generated is sufficient to ignite it and cause an explosion. This, incidentally, is the principle of the compression–ignition (diesel) engine.

Therefore, oil, grease or other flammable materials should be kept away from apparatus in which high-pressure oxygen is used.

Under some conditions nitrous oxide may dissociate, producing nitrogen and oxygen, and the latter gives rise to the risk of an explosion. Therefore nitrous oxide cylinders should be treated with similar care.

Anaesthetic Agents

Cyclopropane, most ethers and ethyl chloride are explosive in anaesthetic concentrations. They are no longer in common use in the developed world.

Carbon dioxide, halothane (Fluothane) and enflurane (Ethrane) are not flammable, nor is nitrous oxide at atmospheric pressure. However, nitrous oxide does support combustion even more fiercely than oxygen. Trichloroethylene also is non-flammable under the conditions in which it is used by the anaesthetist. (It should be noted that halothane is flammable in oxygen but at much higher concentrations than are used clinically.)

Fire or explosion may be caused by the ignition of gases or vapours within the anaesthetic equipment, or escaping from it, or of the vapour of a flammable substance that has been accidentally spilled or used for purposes such as the cleansing of the patient's skin.

Ignition of flammable mixtures may be caused by sparks from static electricity, from faulty electrical apparatus, from the cautery and diathermy apparatus, from electric motors, or from an electric plug-top being pulled out of the socket when the switch is turned on and current is flowing. Naked flames are seldom employed in operating theatres now, but they may be encountered in ophthalmic or dental surgery.

Static Electricity

Static electrical discharges have probably been responsible for most of the explosions that have occurred.

Today, when nylon and other manmade fibre clothes are so popular, the 'clicking' from sparks as static electricity is discharged is commonplace. Similar static charges are developed on dressing trolleys, operating tables and anaesthetic machines.

Although the quantity of static electricity generated in the operating theatre is relatively small, there is sufficient energy in the spark, when it is rapidly discharged, to ignite flammable vapours such as cyclopropane and ether. Arrangements should therefore be made not only to prevent the generation of static electricity but also to discharge slowly to earth any that does occur.

There is therefore an upper and a lower limit to the permissible electrical resistance between any part of the antistatic floor and earth. The resistance between two electrodes set 2 ft (60 cm) apart should nowhere be less than 20 000 ohms or more than 5 000 000 ohms. All mobile equipment in the operating theatre and anaesthetic rooms should make electrical contact with the floor. Trolleys, anaesthetic machines, etc. have wheels, the tyres of which are constructed of antistatic (conducting) rubber. In the absence of such precautions a metal chain, one end of which is attached to the frame of the trolley, is allowed to dangle onto the floor in such a way that at least three links are in contact with the floor. Such chains may become damaged or detached, and are sometimes wound round the frame so that they do not reach the floor. They are therefore a poor substitute for conducting rubber wheels and should be used only where it is necessary to update old equipment.

All footwear worn by the staff should contain conducting material. Tests should be made periodically with an instrument such as a Megger resistance meter to confirm that the electrical conductivity of the above items remains within the prescribed limits.

If flammable agents are being used, the most important precaution, however, is the use of antistatic (conducting) rubber or neoprene in the construction of the components of breathing attachments and other flexible parts of anaesthetic machines. As recently as 1982 an explosion occurred with cyclopropane, where a co-axial breathing attachment, the outer tube of which was of a non-conducting material, was damaged. Fortunately it was not in use with a patient at the time.

Sparks may also be caused by the striking of metal against stone, as occurs when the metal end adaptor of a corrugated hose is dropped on a terrazzo floor.

Zone of Risk

In 1956 a working party set up in the UK by the Ministry of Health reported on the risk and prevention of anaesthetic explosions. This followed a period of 7 years during which 36 explosions had been reported, some of them fatal.

The term *zone of risk* was used to denote the area in which explosive mixtures were deemed to be liable to exist during routine anaesthetic practice.

Within the 'zone of risk' the following precautions were advised:

- There should be no naked flames.
- All electric switches should be sparkproof and electric plugs should be 'captive' while the switch is turned on.
- All parts, especially rubber tubing, etc., of anaesthetic apparatus should be constructed of conductive (antistatic) rubber or other material, and the operating theatre floor should be antistatic. Antistatic rubber, containing carbon, has sufficient conductivity to leach away static electricity, and yet has sufficient resistance to prevent so fast a discharge that a spark occurs.

All trolleys, stools and other mobile equipment should have tyres or feet of a conducting material. These are painted yellow or have a yellow flash or label to indicate that they are antistatic.

The 1956 working party defined the 'zone of risk' as extending from floor level to a height of 4.5 ft (1.4 m) and 4 ft (1.2 m) laterally from any anaesthetic apparatus. Because the anaesthetic machine is mobile, this included the whole anaesthetic room and operating theatre.

Since 1956 there has been a dramatic decrease in the incidence of explosions. This must be due in part to the advent, 2 years later, of halothane, which quickly replaced cyclopropane and ether to a very great extent.

In 1968 Professor Vickers (1970, 1973) of Cardiff enquired into the possibility that the expensive precautions taken were more stringent than was really necessary.

Following investigations described in a paper in 1970, the Association of Anaesthetists of Great Britain and Ireland has recommended that the zone of risk be reduced to 25 cm around any part of the gas pathways of the anaesthetic machine or its breathing attachment.

In the UK and other countries this smaller zone of risk has been accepted. It is considered safe to install switches and socket outlets that are not sparkproof in the operating theatre provided that they are permanently attached to the wall. It is also recommended that they be at a height of approximately 15 inches (40 cm) above the floor. This reduces the risk of damage to flexible cables. All mobile electrical apparatus, and socket outlets on the operating table or floor, should comply with the criteria for sparkproof precautions, since they may be placed within the zone of risk.

The above regulations do not seem to take account of the fact that an anaesthetic machine may be pushed up against a wall at a place where an electric fitting is positioned.

It would seem that the most important precaution for the prevention of explosions where inflammable agents are employed is the use of antistatic materials in the breathing attachments. Certainly, explosions are more likely on a cold, winter Monday morning when the air is dry, the water vapour having been precipitated as frost, and the operating list has not been running long enough to generate sufficient steam or water vapour to humidify the air within the operating theatre suite.

Other Causes of Fires

There are two other modern causes of burns and fire in the operating theatre: (a) fibreoptic light sources, and (b) surgical lasers.

Powerful visible light sources are now commonplace in the operating theatre to provide illumination for endoscopic procedures. These sources, even at the patient end of a fibreoptic light cable, produce a concentrated amount of heat as well as light. The carelessly placed end of the cable may cause a burn directly or set fire to surgical drapes or other flammable material. This situation becomes more dangerous if the drapes have a high concentration of oxygen or flammable vapour beneath them.

FURTHER READING

Beiglemeier G (1987) *Effects of Current Passing Through the Human Body and the Electrical Impedance of the Human Body. A Guide to IEC Report 479*. Berlin: vde-Verlag gmbh.

British Standard (1989) *Medical Electrical Equipment Part 1. General Requirements for Safety*, BS 5724: Part 1 1989 (IEC 601–1: 1988). Milton Keynes, UK: BSI.

Fontanarosa PB (1993) Electric shock and lightning strike. *Annals of Emergency Medicine* **22**: 378–387.

IEC (1984) *Effects of Current Passing Through the Human Body, IEC 479–1, General Aspects*. Geneva: Bureau Central de la Commission Electrotechnique Internationale.

IEC (1987) *Effects of Current Passing Through the Human Body, IEC 479–2, Special Aspects*. Geneva: Bureau Central de la Commission Electrotechnique Internationale.

Sykes MK, Vickers MD, Hull CJ (1991) *Principles of Measurement and Monitoring in Anaesthesia and Intensive Care*. Oxford: Blackwell Scientific.

Vickers MD (1970) Explosion hazards. *Anaesthesia* **25**: 130–131; 482–492.

Vickers MD (1973) Hazards in the operating theatre. Fires and explosions. *Annals of the Royal College of Surgeons of England* **52**: 354–357.

— 27 —

SURGICAL DIATHERMY

Contents

INTRODUCTION

The anaesthetist and his or her assistants are often responsible for the correct connection of the diathermy machine. Therefore they should know something of those aspects of the use of diathermy that will concern them.

Radiofrequency (RF) surgical diathermy or electrosurgery uses the heat generated by an electric current to cut, destroy or vaporize living tissue and to maintain haemostasis by causing coagulation and sealing small blood vessels. Passing an electric current through the body causes all the tissue through which the current passes to heat up. To make use of this effect requires an understanding of the concept of current density.

Current Density

Current density refers to the current per unit cross-sectional area. With a large conductive area there is a very low current density and although the amount of heat generated is the same as at the active electrode, the heat is rapidly conducted away. At the contact point of the active electrode, the current density is very high and the same amount of heat is generated over a very small area, thereby creating a surgical effect (Fig. 27.1)

It is necessary to pass considerable currents through the human body to produce enough heat to have these effects. Under normal circumstances the acciden-tal passage of an electric current through the body has several deleterious effects, including sudden death. However, it was found experimentally, many years ago, that although living tissues, especially conducting and contractile tissues, are very sensitive to direct current and low-frequency alternating current, this sensitivity markedly decreases as the frequency is increased beyond 10 kHz (Fig. 27.2).

The frequencies used in surgery, although not standardized, are in the region of 0.4–1.5 MHz. RF diathermy machines are in fact powerful radio transmitters and would cause severe interference to radio receivers even at some distance. For this reason, by international agreement only certain spot frequencies are used.

A sine-waveform is used for cutting and a damped waveform for coagulation (Fig. 27.3). A combined waveform is also available usually referred to as 'blended', which is commonly used during cystoscopic resection of tumour or prostate.

A block diagram of an RF diathermy machine is shown in Fig. 27.4. A high-power, high-frequency oscillator or generator is controlled by a modulator to produce the necessary waveforms. The output of the generator is led through coupling circuits to the 'indifferent' electrode and the 'active' electrode. The indifferent lead (i.e. the plate) is at earth potential in many diathermy sets and it is therefore important that it is connected to the correct terminal of the diathermy apparatus. If the plate were accidentally connected to the active terminal, the patient might be burned where

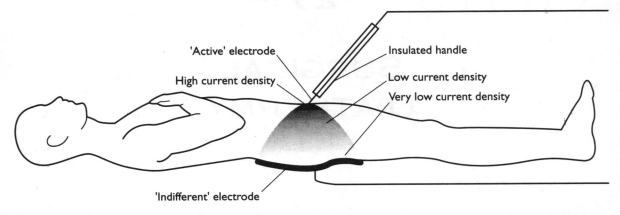

Figure 27.1 The concept of 'current density' or the current per unit cross-sectional area. In areas of low current density the heat generated is quickly dissipated whereas in the area of high current density the heating effect is very high.

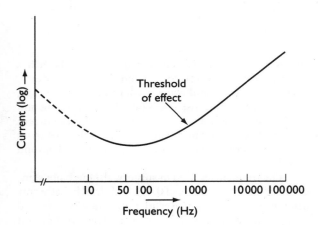

Figure 27.2 Variation of the pathophysiological effects of electric current with frequency. As the frequency increases, a higher current can be passed before there is stimulation of nerve or muscle tissue; as the current is increased the heating effect is increased.

his/her body was in contact with those parts of the operating table at earth potential, when the foot switch was depressed.

The above description is of a unipolar arrangement. However, some diathermy sets are capable of being used with a bipolar system in which the current passes from one blade of a pair of forceps to the other. The circuit is earth-free and the current does not pass through any part of the patient's body other than that grasped by the forceps (Fig. 27.5). The power required is small and it is electrically safer, but it is suitable only for the coagulation of small pieces of tissue or blood vessels. It is particularly suitable for ophthalmic and neurosurgical procedures; however, from a safety point of view it should be used whenever possible.

ACCIDENTS DUE TO THE USE OR MISUSE OF RF DIATHERMY

These may be divided into two groups: first, where the patient receives electrical burns, and second, where fires or explosions are caused by the use of diathermy in the presence of flammable vapours.

The second group of accidents may also be caused by hot wire cautery.

Electrical Burns

Electrical burns may be the result of:

1. Accidental depression of the foot switch when the forceps or cutting electrode is in contact with some part of the patient that it was not intended to burn. This may be prevented by keeping the forceps in an insulated 'quiver' when not in use, and it is also minimized by the installation of a buzzer within the diathermy machine that sounds when the foot switch is depressed. The indicator light on the machine is useful as a confirmation that the apparatus is working, but is not usually heeded as a warning when it is accidentally operated.
2. They may also result from poor contact between the plate and the patient, a burn occurring where it actually does touch because of the high current density caused by the small area of contact. Some diathermy machines give an audible warning if the plate lead is

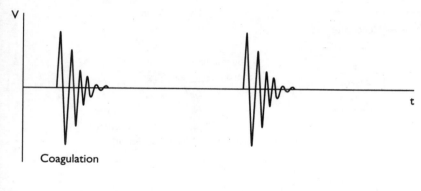

Coagulation

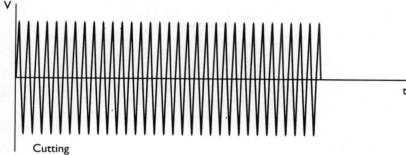

Cutting

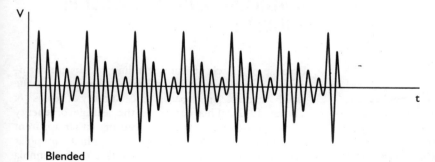

Blended

Figure 27.3 The waveforms commonly used for surgical diathermy.

not plugged in, or if the electrical continuity of the lead is broken. However, the fact that the warning is not given is not proof that the plate has been applied to the patient. Some transistorized sets have a fully floating output and the patient is unharmed if the indifferent electrode is neglected. Where the old–fashioned saline pad is used, it may have dried out, or too dilute a solution of saline may have been used. The plate may have been applied too loosely. The pad must completely envelop the plate and its terminal, otherwise metal parts might touch the patient's skin and cause burning or mechanical injury.

3. Burns can also be caused by the electrical circuit being completed via the operating table and the floor, or other points through which the patient may be earthed, which may occur if the plate is not applied. It

has been known for the tracheal mucous membranes to be severely damaged when the patient was earthed through the damp endotracheal tube and the anaesthetic machine.

4. Another danger seldom appreciated is the risk of infarction when unipolar diathermy is used on an organ that has been temporarily raised on its vascular pedicle. The classical injury is that caused to the testis when raised from the scrotum on its vas. Figure 27.6 shows how the current density is greatly increased in the vas thus causing its destruction. If unipolar diathermy must be used, then the exposed testis must remain in contact with the rest of the body and its electrical conduction improved by the interspersion of a saline-soaked swab.

5. Burns caused by capacitive coupling through intact

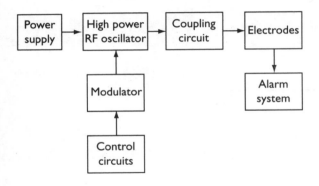

Figure 27.4 Block diagram of a surgical diathermy unit.

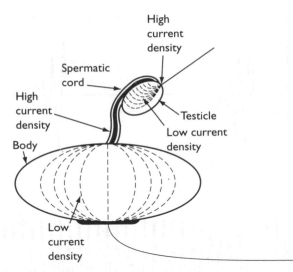

Figure 27.6 The danger of high current density at areas other than that intended, during surgical diathermy.

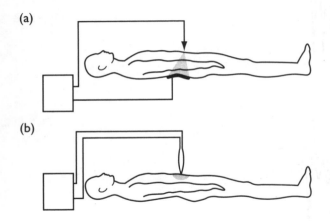

Figure 27.5 (a) Unipolar and (b) bipolar diathermy. Note that the current passes through a much smaller volume of tissue with bipolar diathermy.

DIATHERMY AND LAPAROSCOPIC SURGERY

Because of a lack of understanding of physical principles, a new danger has become apparent with the rapid increase in laparoscopic surgery (Voyles & Tucker 1992). This danger is the leakage of energy from laparoscopic instruments causing either apparent malfunction of laparoscopically applied unipolar diathermy and/or actual tissue damage at the cannula site or at other sites out of the field of vision of the laparoscope.

This 'stray' current pathway may be due to:

- insulation breaks in the diathermy applicator;
- capacitive coupling through intact insulation;
- direct coupling between the active electrode and other organs or metal instruments outside the field of vision.

The problem of insulation breakdown is obvious except that small cracks in insulation may be invisible to the naked eye and their effect may be amplified by conductive fluids such as saline and Hartmann's solution. The combination of a diathermy electrode, the insulation of the cannula and the body tissues form a capacitor (Fig. 27.7). This problem is not improved by using all-plastic cannulas. To make matters worse, there is a tendency to use smaller-diameter cannulas, thus producing smaller scars. The smaller the diameter of the cannula the higher the value of capacitance and the greater the

insulation. Capacitive coupling is not so easy to visualize without some theoretical background. Any two conductors separated by an insulator form a capacitor; one property of a capacitor is to have an infinitely high resistance to direct current but a progressively lower resistance as the frequency of the current is increased (Fig. 27.7). Burns caused by capacitive coupling may occur to the surgeon's fingers if he or she is in contact with any other conductive surface, to the vaginal wall during cervical cautery, and during laparoscopic surgery (see below).

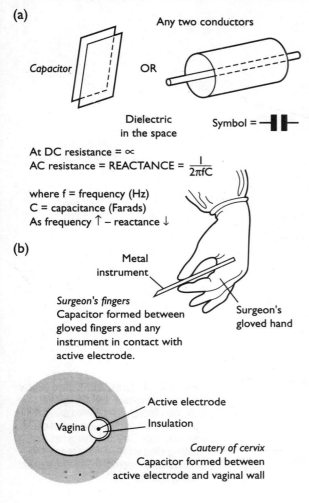

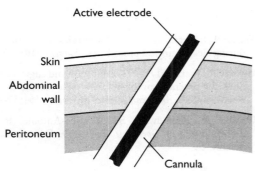

Figure 27.7 The concept of capacitive coupling. (a) A capacitor is formed between any conductive surfaces separated by an insulator (dielectric). At d.c. a capacitor is a pure insulator; as the frequency increases, its resistance (reactance, impedance) decreases. (b) Inadvertant capacitors may be formed between an instrument and the surgeon's fingers, the active electrode and other tissue (e.g. the vaginal wall) or between the (insulated) active electrode and the abdominal wall during laparoscopic surgery.

current passed at any particular frequency. Figure 27.8 shows the difference in the amount of power lost between commonly used 5 mm and 11 mm diameter cannulas.

Inadvertant direct coupling to tissues other than the intended site of diathermy is more common during laparoscopic surgery owing to the small field of vision; this may be protected against by using instruments that are insulated their entire length except at the very tip.

All of these dangers may be avoided by the use of bipolar diathermy; instruments for laparoscopic bipolar diathermy are now becoming available.

DIATHERMY AND PACEMAKERS

The use of RF diathermy should be avoided in patients with internal or temporary external cardiac pacemakers as there is a risk of inhibition or even permanent damage. There is also the risk of causing intracardiac burns at the conductive sites of the pacing wire by alteration of current density patterns. If diathermy must be used, the bipolar variety should be used and then only away from the anatomical site of the pacemaker and its wiring. This is further discussed in Chapter 28.

FIRES AND EXPLOSIONS

Fires and explosions may be caused in the presence of any flammable vapour or liquid (see also Chapter 26). It should be remembered that not only are some anaesthetic agents flammable, but so are ethyl and isopropyl alcohol, which are often used for cleaning the skin prior to an operation. They may be soaked up by, and remain in, the drapes. This is particularly dangerous, because alcohol flames are barely visible under the strong illumination of a theatre lamp.

The cause of fire may be a spark at the active electrode itself, or a faulty mains lead, plug or foot switch.

Real safety lies in the abandoning of flammable vapours and liquids.

The external cases (enclosures) of most diathermy machines are made airtight, i.e. gas-proof, but this state is difficult to maintain when the machine is to be wheeled about into rooms of varying temperature, so that pressures are developed across the gas-proof seal. Also if, owing to overuse or electrical fault, the interior is heated and fumes are generated, a dangerous increase of pressure may occur, leading to rupture.

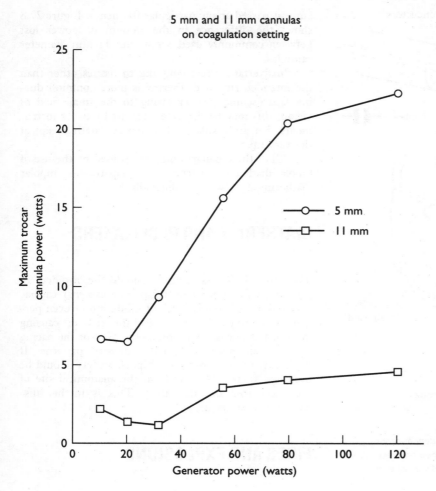

5 mm and 11 mm cannulas on coagulation setting

Figure 27.8 During laparoscopic surgery the maximum power 'lost' through the cannula (through capacitive coupling from a 5 mm electrode) with a 5 mm versus an 11 mm electrode. This 'lost' energy has a heating effect at the cannula site and may cause a burn. (Reproduced from Voyles and Tucker (1992).)

FURTHER READING

Department of Health (1994) *Safety Action Bulletin – Diathermy Injury During Laparoscopic Surgery*, SAB(94)38 September 1994. London: Department of Health.

Haag R, Cuschieri A (1993) Recent advances in high frequency electrosurgery: development of automated systems. *Journal of the Royal College of Surgeons of Edinburgh* **38**: 354–364.

Tucker RD, Ferguson S (1991) Do surgical gloves protect staff during electrosurgical procedures? *Surgery* **110**: 892–895.

Voyles CR, Tucker TD (1992) Education and engineering solutions for potential problems with laparoscopic monopolar electrosurgery. *American Journal of Surgery* **164**: 57–62.

Wattiez A, Khandwala S, Maurice-Antoine B (1995) *Electrosurgery in Operative Endoscopy*. Oxford: Blackwell Scientific.

—28—

DEFIBRILLATORS AND PACEMAKERS

Contents

INTRODUCTION

Although not strictly anaesthetic equipment, it is vital that the anaesthetist understands the principles of pacemakers and defibrillators. Simple devices of a decade ago are now more complex and versatile. Defibrillators apply single large electric shocks to counteract abnormal cardiac rhythms by producing synchronous depolarization of all heart muscle cells, which hopefully leads to a normal heart rhythm. Defibrillators are conventionally 'external' but, recently, *implantable* defibrillators have become available for patients at risk of sudden death due to recurrent unstable tachyarrythmias or ventricular fibrillation. Pacemakers produce a small electrical stimulus in the form of a low voltage pulse at the required heart rate, when the heart's own pacemaker has failed. Temporary pacemakers may be used when there is a high likelihood of the natural pacemaker recovering or until a permanent implanted system has been surgically inserted. Temporary pacemakers were only available for use invasively via a transvenous electrode wire. A recent advance is the external pacemaker.

DEFIBRILLATORS

The earliest forms of defibrillator were simple devices that basically consisted of a transformer and a switch. Several cycles of 100–300 V root-mean-square (rms) alternating current were applied either directly across the heart or twice that amount across the chest externally. However, it was soon realized that a single pulse of direct current (d.c.) had fewer deleterious effects.

The basic d.c. defibrillator consists of a large capacitor which after charging to a predetermined voltage, is discharged across the cardiac axis, usually externally via large area electrodes. A schematic diagram of the basic d.c. defibrillator is shown in Fig. 28.1. As most defibrillators are designed to be immediately usable away from a mains power source, a rechargeable low-voltage battery powers a high-current oscillator which drives a variable-voltage step-up transformer. The very high voltage from the transformer charges a high-voltage capacitor of between 10 and 50 μF. The patient is defibrillated by discharging this capacitor across the chest. The output of a d.c. defibrillator is commonly variable between 20 J (watt-seconds) for children and internal use in adults, and 400 J maximum. The energy stored in the capacitor is given by the equation:

$$E = \frac{CV^2}{2}$$

where E = energy in joules, C = capacity in farads and V = potential difference across the capacitor in volts. Thus for the maximum 400 J the voltage required to charge the capacitor will vary between 2000 and 9000 V depending upon the value of the capacitor. Owing to losses in the circuit and electrode paddles, the actual charge applied to the patient is often much lower than selected.

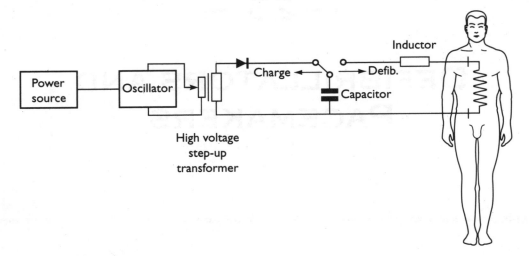

Figure 28.1 Schematic diagram of a basic d.c. defibrillator.

Refinements to the basic circuit include:

- inductance to improve the waveform of the applied charge;
- monitoring of the actual discharge applied to the patient;
- optional ECG synchronization of the discharge.

The synchronized defibrillator or cardioverter applies the electric shock shortly after the occurrence of an R wave and is used for the correction of tachyarrhythmias. It is more complex than the basic defibrillator (Fig. 28.2) in that it must include an ECG monitor. The ECG is detected via conventional ECG electrodes or through the defibrillator 'paddle' electrodes.

The paddle electrodes of defibrillators must have a large enough surface area to pass the required current without causing skin burns, but not too large otherwise the current density between them through the body will be too low. The paddles must also have a highly insulated handle, which must remain dry and free of conductive electrode jelly, to protect the user from inadvertant electrocution. To improve the conduction between the hard surface of the paddle electrode and the patient, some form of flexible paste or gel conductive medium is placed between the paddle and the skin. It is important that this medium is restricted to the area under the paddle as it may reduce the effect of the shock if some of the energy is 'leaked away' by the medium. There is a risk of serious skin damage if such a medium is not used at all, as the area of contact will be much smaller with a higher concentration of electric current.

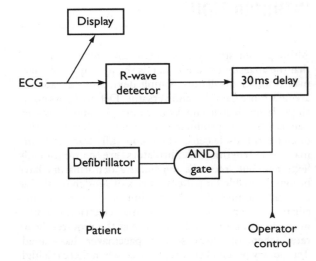

	Operator	
R-wave	control	Defib.
0	0	0
0	1	0
1	0	0
1	1	1

Figure 28.2 Basic principle of a cardioverter. The ECG is monitored, the R wave is fed to one input of an AND-gate, and operator control is to the other input of the gate. Defibrillation occurs 30 ms after the first R wave, when the operator depresses the control button.

The Automatic Implantable Cardioverter-Defibrillator

For patients with recurrent ventricular tachycardia that is refractory to drug treatment and for those with recurrent ventricular fibrillation, sudden death is a constant fear. This fear has been alleviated to a certain extent by the development of the automatic implantable cardioverter-defibrillator (AICD) This is a miniature synchronized defibrillator of approximately 11 cm × 2 cm × 8 cm, which contains its own power source and is implanted in a similar way to the conventional implantable pacemaker (see below). The output of the AICD may be set to between 0.1 and 30 J. The electrical activity of the heart is sensed via a lead placed transvenously but the shocking electrodes are in the form of a metallic mesh and are stitched to the outside of the ventricular walls. The latest versions shock via a lead placed transvenously, which avoids major thoracic surgery necessary with earlier versions. The sensing electronics not only sense the heart rate but also analyse the morphology of the complexes. The batteries last approximately 2–3 years or 100 shocks, which ever is the least. It is possible to control the AICD externally with a magnet, and most provide some form of telemetry so that their history of use can be analysed.

PACEMAKERS

Electronic pacemakers are used in conditions where otherwise the heart rate would be too slow to maintain active normal life. The indications for electronic pacemakers are (Kusumoto & Goldschlager 1996):

- sinus-node dysfunction
- atrioventricular block
- bifascicular or trifascicular block
- neurogenic syncope
- cardiomyopathy.

Pacemakers may be either temporary or permanent; it is usual to use a temporary pacemaker in the first instance, until the necessity of a permanent implanted system is assessed. In the majority of cases a temporary pacemaker is all that is required in the acute situation until the heart's pacemaker or conduction system has recovered from some insult such as myocardial infarction. Tempory pacemakers are also sometimes necessary as prophylaxis during general anaesthesia in patients with early heart block.

The most common type of pacemaker (Fig. 28.3) is basically an electronic pulse generator with variable rate and output, 'connected' to the heart with a co-axial lead and inserted via a central vein to the right ventricle.

The pacing wire is inserted aseptically, under fluoroscopic control, so that the tip is placed in the apex of the right ventricle. In an emergency it is possible to place the wire without X-ray control, by connecting an ECG monitor to the pacemaker wire and observing the trace of the existing activity on the monitor (Fig. 28.4).

All pacemakers have two main modes of operation: (a) asynchronous or free running at a fixed rate, and (b) synchronous or 'demand'.

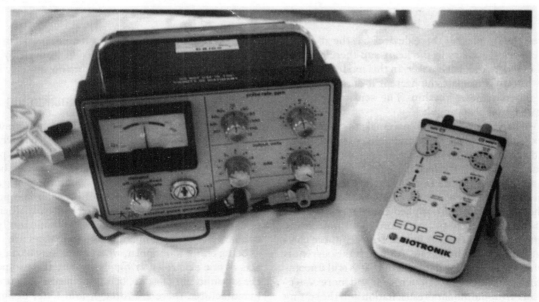

Figure 28.3 Typical external pacemakers.

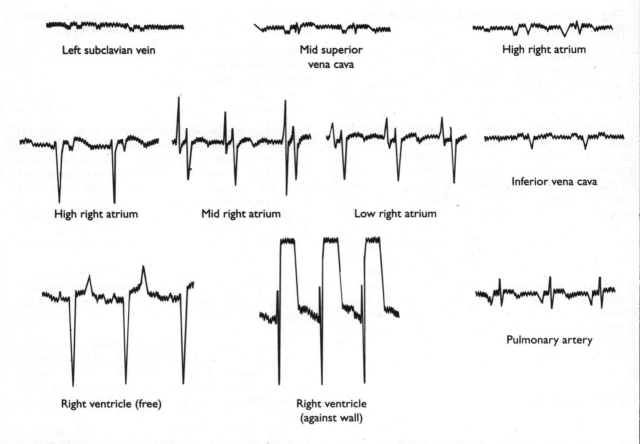

Figure 28.4 Pacemaker electrode locations as recorded by intracardiac ECG. (Reproduced with permission from Bing *et al.* (1972).)

Even the simplest of these devices has the ability to 'sense' electrical activity in the heart and therefore may be used as a 'demand' pacemaker. In this mode, the pacemaker will only stimulate the heart if it does not detect regular inherent heart rhythm. The sensitivity of the sensing system is also variable.

More advanced external pacemakers with more complex wires are able to sense and deliver stimuli to the atria and ventricles separately in sequence, thus producing a more physiological effect.

In an emergency, the transcutaneous pacer is now the quickest and easiest option (Fig. 28.5). Two large, self-adhesive electrodes are applied either across the axis of the heart or, better still, anteriorily and posteriorly across the heart; a current is pulsed between these electrodes at the required heart rate. Although the current is very much lower than for defibrillation, it is still uncomfortable for the patient but is much safer and more convenient than cardiopulmonary resuscitation and the setting up of an isoprenaline infusion whilst preparations are being made for the insertion of a temporary pacing wire. This type of pacemaker may even be applied by emergency medical technicians away from hospital facilities.

Implantable Permanent Cardiac Pacing

If the heart's own pacemaker or conduction system do not recover from whatever acute pathology has occurred, it becomes necessary to install an implantable permanent pacing system (Fig. 28.6). These system are becoming ever more complex and are beyond the scope of this book. They all basically consist of the same components as external systems, in miniature, and with their own power source all contained in a sealed biologically inert container. Modern implantable pacemakers are classed as being either monopolar, where the casing of the device acts as one electrode, or bipolar, where the two poles of the stimulus are close to, or in, the heart. Whatever the manufacturer, there is a three or four letter designation for the pacing mode (Table 28.1).

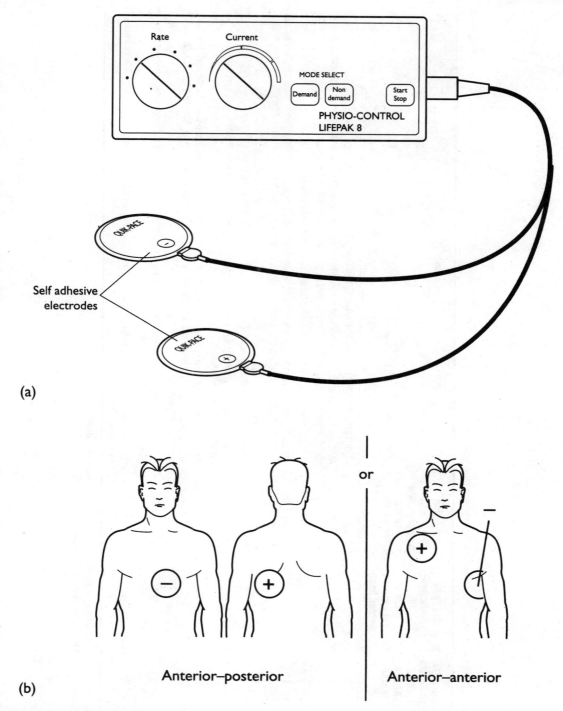

Figure 28.5 The transcutaneous temporary pacemaker.

Table 28.1 Explanation of the three- and four-letter designations for commonly used pacing modes.*

1st Letter (Indicates the chamber paced)	2nd Letter (Indicates the chamber sensed)	3rd Letter (Indicates the mode of response to sensed beat)	4th Letter (Indicates programmable features present)	Description
A	A	—	—	Atrial pacing on demand; output inhibited by sensed atrial signals.
A	A	—	R	Atrial pacing on demand; output inhibited by sensed atrial signals. Atrial pacing rates can decrease and increase in response to sensor input, up to the programmed sensor-based upper limit of the rate.
V	V	—	—	Ventricular pacing on demand; output inhibited by sensed ventricular signals.
V	V	—	R	Ventricular pacing on demand; output inhibited by sensed ventricular signals. Ventricular pacing rates can decrease and increase in response to sensor input, up to the programmed sensor-based upper limit of the rate.
V	D	D	—	Paces the ventricle; senses in both the atrium and the ventricle; synchronizes with atrial activity and paces the ventricle after a preset atrioventricular interval up to the programmed upper limit of the rate.
D	D	—	—	Paces and senses in both the atrium and the ventricle; the only response to a sensed P or R wave is inhibition. No tracking of intrinsic atrial activity.
D	D	—	R	Paces and senses in both the atrium and the ventricle; the only response to a sensed P or R wave is inhibition. Atrial and ventricular pacing rates increase and decrease independently in response to sensor input. Atrioventricular synchrony may not be achieved.
D	D	D	—	Paces and senses in both the atrium and the ventricle; paces the ventricle in response to sensed atrial activity up to the programmed upper limit of the rate.
D	D	D	R	Atrial and ventricular pacing rates can increase and decrease in response to sensor input up to the programmed sensor-based upper limit of the rate.

* In the designations, A denotes atrial, I inhibited, R rate-adaptive, V ventricular, and D dual.
Reproduced with permission from Kusumoto and Goldschlager (1996).

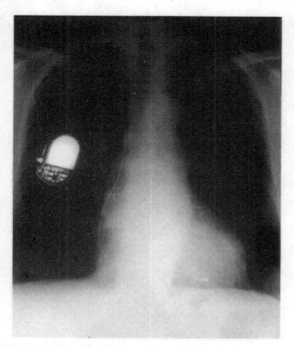

Figure 28.6 Chest X-ray of an implanted cardiac pacemaker system.

Pacemakers and Anaesthesia

As already mentioned, it may be necessary to have a temporary pacemaker inserted in patients with incipient heart block as a prophylactic measure before the administration of anaesthesia. Patients with temporary or permanent pacemakers undergoing surgery and anaesthesia have remarkably stable heart rhythms for obvious reasons!

The biggest danger during anaesthesia and surgery is interference and even permanent damage to pacemaker systems with surgical RF diathermy. Diathermy must be avoided if at all possible in patients with pacemakers, either internal or external. The risks involved are:

- permanent damage to the device;
- upsetting the rhythm by inhibiting the device;
- electrical burns around the implanted device or at the contacts within the heart.

Pacemakers are also very susceptible to high electrical or magnetic fields. One reason for this is that localized magnetic fields are used for preprogramming and also setting pacemakers into asynchronous mode.

Magnets should not be used to set the asynchronous mode during surgery as any preprogramming may be upset by the use of diathermy.

Patients with implanted systems must keep away from magnetic resonance imaging scanners, heavy-current power systems such as electrical substations and also from radio transmitters.

If diathermy is unavoidable:

- bipolar diathermy must be used;
- the generator should be kept well away from the site of the pacemaker as radiated EMI from the generator itself may affect the pacemaker;
- only a short burst of diathermy should be used;
- cutting mode should be avoided.

There is not enough evidence about the safety of implanted systems and the use of cellular telephones.

FURTHER READING

Bing OHL, McDowell JW, Hantman J (1972) Pacemaker placement by electrocardiographic monitoring. *New England Journal of Medicine* 278: 651.

Fitzpatric A, Sutton R (1992) A guide to temporary pacing. *British Medical Journal* 304: 365–369.

Kusumoto FM, Goldschlager N (1996) Cardiac pacing. *New England Journal of Medicine* 334: 89–98.

Munter DW, DeLacey WA (1994) Automatic implantable cardioverter–defibrillators. *Emergency Medicine Clinics of North America* 12: 379–395.

Vukmir RB (1993) Emergency cardiac pacing. *American Journal of Emergency Medicine* 11: 167–176.

Wattiez A, Khandwala S, Maurice-Antoine B (1995) Electromagnetic interference with pacemakers. In *Electrosurgery in Operative Endoscopy*. Oxford: Blackwell Scientific.

—29—

LASERS

PRINCIPLES

Anaesthetists should be aware of the principles of lasers as they are finding increasing application in medicine and surgery and their employment gives rise to several dangers.

The term 'laser' is an acronym derived from Light Amplification by Stimulated Emission of Radiation. The laser produces an intense beam of pure monochromatic light, that is light of a single wavelength or colour. The output beam may be of very small cross-sectional area and is virtually non-divergent. These properties mean that large amounts of energy may be delivered to very small areas of tissue with great accuracy. The wavelength of a laser is determined by the lasing medium used.

Although there are many more complex laser systems, the basic components of a laser are shown in Fig. 29.1. The lasing medium, which may be a gas, liquid or solid, is chosen from a study of the atomic electron energy levels upon which the laser depends. The atoms of the lasing medium are excited to high energy levels by a 'pumping' source, which may be a high-voltage discharge in the case of a gas, or an intense flash of light from a flashtube. Figure 29.2 shows the excitation and emission processes possible in a gaseous lasing medium. A photon of energy from the pumping source may be absorbed by a stable atom in its so-called 'ground state', which then becomes an excited atom with an electron in a higher energy level. Spontaneous emission of a photon

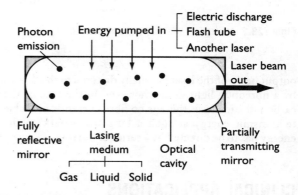

Figure 29.1 Basic components of a laser.

of energy occurs as the excited atom falls back to the ground energy level. If a further photon of pumping energy at the correct wavelength is applied to an atom in its excited state, then as it falls to the ground state two photons of energy will be emitted instead of one. This is known as stimulated emission. The emitted photons thus produced are in phase with, have the same polarization as, and travel in the same direction as the stimulating radiation. This mechanism is amplified by many of the escaping photons being reflected back into the lasing medium by the mirrors. Thus a chain reaction occurs, producing an intense source of light energy, some of which is allowed to escape through the partially reflecting mirror at the output end of the lasing medium. The

Absorption

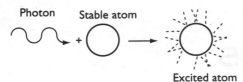

Spontaneous emission

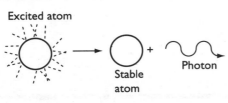

Stimulated emissions

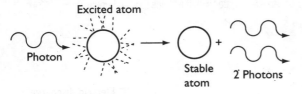

Figure 29.2 Absorption, excitation and emission processes.

output beam of the laser is usually directed to the tissues by a fibreoptic light guide; however, in the case of the carbon dioxide laser there is no fibre currently available to transmit energy at such a long wavelength so the energy has to be directed by a series of mirrors.

CLINICAL APPLICATIONS

The clinical use of lasers depends upon a compromise between:

- laser–tissue interaction;
- absorption and penetration depth;
- availability of a laser of the correct wavelength and power;
- availability of a suitable method of transmission.

Table 29.1 shows the currently available lasers in medical use.

Table 29.1 Currently available medical lasers

	Wavelength (nm)	Colour	Transmission
Excimer	193–355	UV	Mirrors
Tunable dye laser	360–670	Blue to red	Optical fibre
Krypton	476, 521, 568, 647	Blue to red	Optical fibre
Argon	488–515	Blue/green	Optical fibre
Nd-YAG-KTP	532	Green	Optical fibre
Helium–neon	633	Red	Optical fibre
Ruby	694	Red	Optical fibre
Nd-YAG	1064	Near IR	Optical fibre
Holmium	2100	IR	Mirrors
Er-YAG	2940	IR	Mirrors
CO_2	100 600	Far IR	Mirrors

The graph in Fig. 29.3 shows the spectrum of absorption by haemoglobin, melanin and water. Monochromatic energy is absorbed by tissue of *complementary* colour.

The carbon dioxide laser energy at 10.6 μm is absorbed by water and thus the intracellular water is rapidly vaporized. The main use of the carbon dioxide laser is as a 'bloodless scalpel'. The blue–green argon laser beam is maximally absorbed by substances with the complementary colour, i.e. red. Thus the argon laser is used to coagulate blood in small vessels with very little effect on other more transparent tissues, for example the retina. The Nd: YAG (neodymium:yittrium–aluminium garnet) laser has a solid lasing medium and produces energy in the near-infrared region of the spectrum, which is absorbed deeply in the tissues. When invisible infrared lasers are used, it is common practice to make use of a low-powered, visible-light laser such as a helium:neon laser at the same time, in order to aid in aiming the therapeutic laser accurately.

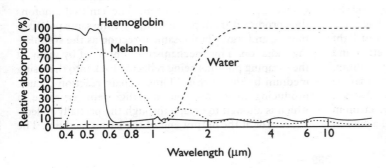

Figure 29.3 Absorption characteristics of tissue constituents.

SAFETY ASPECTS

Apart from the danger to the patient from the beam of laser energy if it is misused, there is a risk to the operator and other persons in the operating environment. This is because of the long range of laser light due to the virtual non-divergence of the beam; thus increased distance from the source has little safety benefit. Even reflected laser light may be very dangerous to the eyes. Visible laser light transmitted to the retina of the eye may burn it irreparably, leaving a blind spot in the field of vision. A similar lesion over the optic nerve may result in total blindness of that eye. The cornea, lens and aqueous and vitreous humours partially or totally absorb far-infrared laser radiation and therefore these tissues are more susceptible to damage than the retina.

Laser radiation on the skin may be felt as a burning sensation, which is therefore self-protective provided that the victim is conscious and has not received an analgesic.

There is an international classification for lasers, which is shown in Table 29.2.

Table 29.2 International Classification of continuously working lasers

Class I	Powers not to excede MPE for the eye
Class II	Visible laser beams only
	Powers up to 1 mW
	Eye protected by blink-reflex time of 0.25 s
Class IIIa	Relaxation of Class II to 5 mW for radiation provided beam is expanded so that the eye is still protected by the blink-reflex
Class IIIb	Powers up to 0.5 W
	Direct viewing hazardous
Class IV	Powers over 0.5 W. Extremely hazardous

MPE, maximum permissible exposure.

Protective Eyeware

Protective eyeware may be in the form of goggles or spectacles. Spectacles generally do not give as complete peripheral protection as goggles. It should be noted that different eyeware is required for different wavelengths of laser.

Anaesthetic-Related Risks

A further risk that is of special importance to the anaesthetist is the danger of fire caused by oxygen enrichment of the local environment in which the laser is being used. This problem occurs not only during ENT surgery but also when the laser is inadvertently directed towards drapes under which high concentrations of oxygen and nitrous oxide may be present. The following precautions should be taken:

- No flammable anaesthetic agents or nitrous oxide should be used. (Nitrous oxide supports combustion *better than* oxygen.)
- Non-reflective (matt black) instruments should be used, as the reflected laser beam is almost as powerful as the main beam.
- Inspired oxygen concentration should be no greater than 25% if possible.
- Non-flammable endotracheal tubes, either using special materials or by covering a conventional tube with aluminium tape, should be used. Other tissues should be protected with wet swabs.
- Protective goggles *appropriate to the wavelength of the laser* in use should be worn be *everybody* in the operating theatre, including the patient.
- Doors to the operating area should be locked and all windows should be covered to protect those outside the operating area.

SAFETY CODES

In the UK the Department of Health has published guidance (1984) on laser safety. This should form the basis of a set of local rules, a Safety Code, and the appointment of a Laser Protection Supervisor in every area in which a laser is in use. The Laser Protection Supervisor must not be the operator of the laser but should be observing the safety aspects during its use. The most important duty of the Laser Protection Supervisor is to make sure that all staff are wearing the correct eye protection throughout the laser session.

FURTHER READING

Department of Health & Social Security (1984) *Guidance on the Safe Use of Lasers in Medical Practice*. London: DHSS.

Jacques SL (1992) Laser – tissue interactions. *Surgical Clinics of North America* 72: 531–558.

Sliney DH (1995) Laser safety. *Lasers in Surgery and Medicine* 16: 215–225.

van der Speck AFL, Spargo PM, Norton ML (1988) The physics of lasers and implications for their use during airway surgery. *British Journal of Anaesthesia* 60: 709–729.

PROVISION OF ANAESTHESIA IN DIFFICULT SITUATIONS AND IN THE DEVELOPING WORLD

Contents

INTRODUCTION

There are certain situations in which it would be difficult or impractical to provide sophisticated, heavy and bulky anaesthetic equipment on the scale to which we are accustomed in hospital operating theatres. Examples are:

- sites in hospital but away from the operation theatres;
- anaesthesia in underdeveloped countries;
- anaesthesia on the battlefield;
- resuscitation and anaesthesia at the site of an accident or disaster;
- domiciliary anaesthesia.

In all of these situations the following problems may occur:

- poor control of environmental factors;
- lack of supply of cylinder oxygen and nitrous oxide;
- lack of electricity supply;
- difficulty with transport of equipment;
- lack of adequate maintenance facilities;
- lack of skilled assistance;
- in the case of underdeveloped countries, lack of finance for equipment and drugs.

Other principles involved in these situations are:

- transfer patients to hospitals with better facilities if this is possible and the patient's condition allows;
- use local or regional anaesthetic techniques if at all possible;
- consideration should be given to modern total intravenous anaesthesia (TIVA) with provision for respiratory support if necessary.

SITES IN HOSPITALS BUT AWAY FROM THE OPERATING THEATRES

In these areas the equipment may be up-to-date. There are certain key points:

- Apart from basic anaesthetic and monitoring equipment, it is necessary to have the full range of resuscitation equipment and drugs.
- There is a risk of tampering and 'knob twiddling' in all unattended equipment.
- Checking and maintenance are less likely to be adhered to.

- These environments will not have antispark/static precautions and therefore flammable agents must never be used.
- Due regard must be paid to the level of experience of the anaesthetist and his or her assistant.
- There must be easy communication between the anaesthetist at the remote site and other anaesthetic staff in case of emergency.

Each area has its own special problems:

Accident & Emergency Department
- Usually standard anaesthetic and monitoring equipment but anaesthetic machines may have recently been used as a source of oxygen or suction.

Imaging Department
- ionizing radiation risk;
- usually restricted access to the patient or patient's head;
- facility to arrest respiration for some seconds to stop image blurring;
- high risk of sparks;
- lack of piped oxygen/suction.

Magnetic Resonance Imaging (MRI)
- The risks associated with occupational exposure to intense magnetic radiation are not entirely elucidated.
- No metallic or otherwise electrically conductive materials should come into the magnetic zone of risk.
- There is a special risk associated with pacemakers, implanted or external.
- Special fibreoptic monitoring equipment should be used for pulse plethysmography and oximetry.
- There is an especially high electromagnetic interference (EMI) risk in the vicinity of MRI equipment, which may interfere with monitoring, infusion and other electronic equipment at some distance from the supposed area of risk.

Electroconvulsive Therapy (ECT)
- Usually somewhere a considerable distance from conventional forms of medicine and surgery.
- Staff involved usually have a singular lack of knowledge about *anything* technical!

Radiotherapy
- intense ionizing radiation;
- impossible to remain in the same room as the patient during treatment;
- vision via glass–liquid–glass window or closed circuit television (colour distortion);
- multiple treatments over short period (week(s));
- with head and neck treatment: 'applicator' obstructs head;
- 'sedation' by infusion;
- laryngeal mask if general anaesthesia necessary.

THE MAJOR ACCIDENT

In this situation there may be many casualties and the incident always occurs unexpectedly. The territory is often unfamiliar to those working, and this can often pose problems to all concerned. Exposure to high temperatures and dehydration in the tropics can be matched in its importance by extremes of cold climate, which may be found even in so-called temperate zones such as the UK. Low temperatures may not only incapacitate those working and harm the injured, but may also preclude the use of some anaesthetic agents, such as Entonox. Altitude may also pose problems with the administration of nitrous oxide and the volatile agents.

The lines of communication between the rescue workers and their patients, and the removal of the patients to safety, may be rendered very difficult by local conditions, as, for example, in an underground railway disaster or a mining accident. Darkness, dust and cramped conditions may preclude the carrying or employment of sophisticated equipment. If emergency amputation or disentanglement of patients from wreckage is required, this may well be achieved under intravenous or intramuscular anaesthesia with ketamine, but even so oxygen (bearing in mind flammability) and Entonox may be required. The greatest need may be for resuscitation, including endotracheal intubation, and this should be borne in mind when selecting equipment.

ANAESTHESIA IN UNDERDEVELOPED COUNTRIES

In some underdeveloped countries, problems may arise not only on account of apparatus but also because of the experience and training of the anaesthetist. It is not within the scope of this book to discuss the desirability of employing nurse-anaesthetists, but it seems certain that in many countries anaesthetics will have to be given by these 'medical assistants' for many years to come. Furthermore, it may well be argued that a medical assistant who has been well trained may be more efficient at anaesthetizing patients than a doctor who has received little or no training in anaesthesia.

Let us consider the personnel first. In many hospitals there may be one doctor who is helped by several medical assistants. In these cases he or she may well induce anaesthesia and intubate the patient and then hand over to the assistant while he or she performs the operation, returning to the role of anaesthetist at the end. It is quite obvious that the maintenance of a clear airway is one of the paramount duties of the assistant and this will be greatly facilitated if the patient has been intubated.

Therefore, under these conditions, endotracheal intubation may be more common than elsewhere, and this should be borne in mind when considering the provision for endotracheal equipment. The anaesthetic apparatus used should be as simple as possible so that there are few controls to operate and the least possible chance of malfunction or maladjustment.

Because of the unreliability of pressurized oxygen and gas supplies, the use of air and draw-over type vaporizers is usually the best choice. A combination of the Epstein–Macintosh–Oxford (EMO) vaporizer (Fig 30.1), the Oxford Miniature vaporizer (OMV) (equipped and calibrated for both halothane and trichloroethylene), together with a means of inflation such as a manual resuscitator or Oxford bellows, a Ruben or similar valve, and a facepiece or endotracheal connector may well be the most practical equipment available under these circumstances. The facility for the addition of a supply of oxygen would be desirable. Other draw-over arrangements are shown diagramatically in Fig. 30.2. The working prin-

ciples of the commonly available draw-over vaporizers are shown in Fig. 30.3. Although medical oxygen in cylinders would be the ideal, cylinders of oxygen for industrial use are sometimes available but it must be remembered that there may well be an increased level of impurities in such supplies. An inexhaustible supply of high quality oxygen of up to 95% concentration may be obtained by the use of an oxygen concentrator. The principles of oxygen concentration are described in Chapter 2. The power source for the concentration of oxygen may, in theory, be electrical (high or low voltage) or mechanical. The maintenance of the oxygen concentrator may be carried out by anyone with the competence to repair refrigerators as the technology is similar.

Oxygen at high concentration may also be generated by a chemical reaction as in the Genox apparatus (Bhimsan et al 1994). This is a small portable apparatus that generates oxygen by the combination of manganese dioxide and sodium percarbonate with water. Each sachet of chemicals produces approximately 36 litres of pure oxygen when water is added.

The other vital piece of anaesthetic equipment that is essential is some form of efficient medical suction.

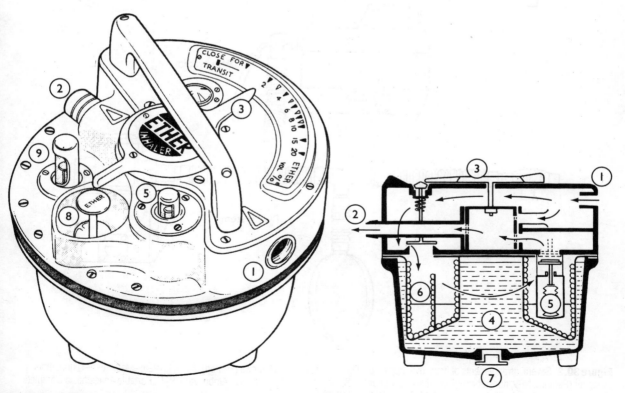

Figure 30.1 EMO ether vaporizer. (1) Inlet port, (2) outlet port, (3) concentration control, (4) water jacket, (5) thermocompensator valve, (6) vaporizing chamber, (7) filling port for water, (8) filling port for anaesthetic, (9) anaesthetic-level indicator. (Reproduced with permission of WHO from Dobson (1988).)

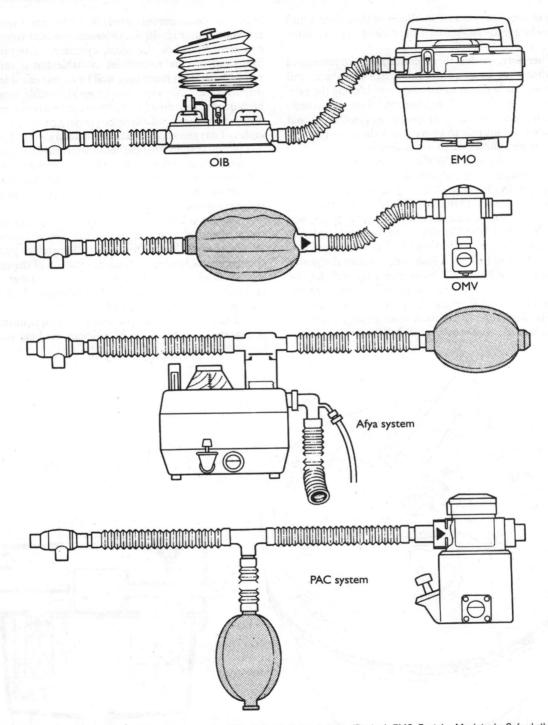

Figure 30.2 Several arrangements of draw-over apparatus: OIB, Oxford inflating bellows (Penlon); EMO, Epstein–Macintosh–Oxford ether vaporizer (Penlon); NRV, non-rebreathing valve (e.g. Ruben); SIB, self-inflating bag (Laerdal, Ambu, etc.); PAC, Portable Anaesthesia Complete (Ohmeda). (Reproduced with permission of WHO from Dobson (1988).)

(a)

(b)

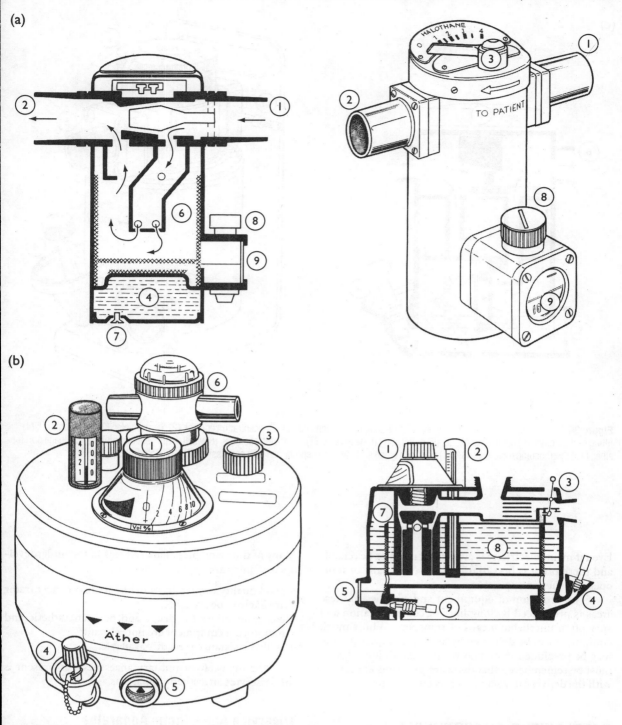

Figure 30.3 Draw-over vaporizers (a) OMV. (1) Inlet port, (2) outlet port, (3) concentration control, (4) heat sink, (6) vaporizing chamber, (7) filling port for water, (8) filling port for anaesthetic, (9) anaesthetic-level indicator. (b) Afya vaporizer (Dräger). (1) Concentration control, (2) thermometer, (3) on/off control, (4) filling port for ether, (5) ether-level gauge, (6) outlet and one-way valve, (7) vaporizing chamber, (8) water-filled heat reservoir, (9) drainage port for ether. (Reproduced with permission of WHO from Dobson (1988).)

(c)

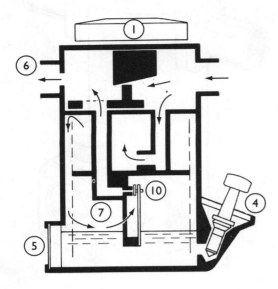

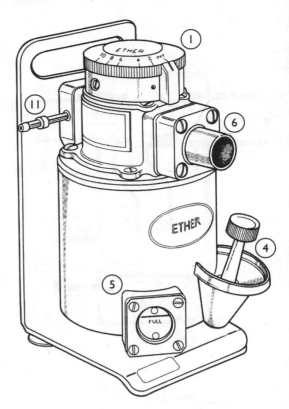

Figure 30.3 (continued) Draw-over vaporizers (c) PAC vaporizer (Ohmeda). (1) Concentration control, (2) thermometer, (3) on/off control, (4) filling port for ether, (5) ether-level gauge, (6) outlet and one-way valve, (7) vaporizing chamber, (8) water-filled heat reservoir, (9) drainage port for ether, (10) thermocompensator valve, (11) port for oxygen enrichment. (Reproduced with permission of WHO from Dobson (1988).)

Even if mains electricity is available it may not be reliable and therefore it is best to use either a manually or foot-operated suction apparatus.

The provision of equipment and supplies to these areas is prejudiced by long lines of communication and very often unreliable means of transport. Whilst much equipment can be delivered by air, this is expensive and may be precluded in certain weather conditions. Also it must be remembered that there are problems concerned with the delivery of agents such as ether by air.

BATTLEFIELD ANAESTHESIA

Anaesthesia close to the front line of any conflict should be limited to resuscitation and for life-saving surgery.

Many of the principles of anaesthesia in the underdeveloped country are applicable but:

- good quality oxygen from cylinders or a concentrator are likely to be available;
- cost constraints for drugs and both anaesthetic and monitoring equipment are not relevant;
- skilled assistance is readily available.

The mainstay of military anaesthesia at present is the Triservice anaesthetic apparatus.

Triservice Anaesthetic Apparatus

This compendium of anaesthetic and resuscitation equipment (Fig. 30.4) has been designed by the three British armed forces in order to provide a versatile but standardized system which, with the exception of the

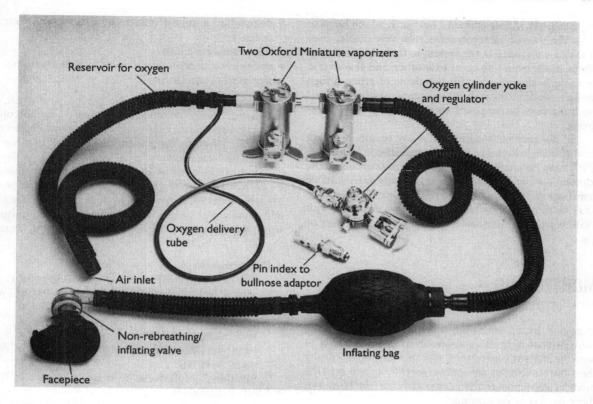

Figure 30.4 The Triservice apparatus. The patient may breathe spontaneously, drawing air through the two Oxford Miniature vaporizers and the inflating bag. There is a valve mounted on the facepiece that prevents rebreathing. The air drawn in through the inlet may be enriched with oxygen from a cylinder which is attached to the cylinder yoke, with the pin index to bullnose adaptor if required. During expiration, the oxygen is stored in the reservoir tubing. The two Oxford Miniature vaporizers may be used for a variety of anaesthetic agents, there being interchangeable calibration labels for each. In the case of induction with ether, with spontaneous ventilation, both vaporizers will be required so as to produce an adequate vapour concentration. However, with spontaneous ventilation, if halothane is employed in the first vaporizer, it may be found convenient to use trichloroethylene in the second in order to make good the deficiency of analgesia caused by the exclusion of nitrous oxide. These vaporizers may be easily cleaned to remove traces of previous anaesthetic agents. For controlled or assisted ventilation, the inflating bag may be squeezed manually or it may be replaced by a mechanical ventilator of the bag-squeezing type. The choice is dictated to some extent by the type of power source available. As an alternative to the inflating bag shown, the Laerdal folding silicone rubber bag may be used.

oxygen cylinder, is all housed in a box of rugged construction that can be dropped by parachute and weighs no more than 25 kg.

The basis of the compendium is a breathing system, which includes a Laerdal folding manual resuscitator and two OMVs. During spontaneous ventilation the patient draws in air through the OMVs, and if it is desired to enrich it with oxygen the reservoir tubing is added to conserve the oxygen during the expiratory phase. During expiration the exhaled gases are voided to air through a valve mounted adjacent to the facepiece.

The OMVs are a modified version: they have three folding feet that enable them to be stood on a flat surface, and their capacity has been increased to 50 ml. The calibration scale for one agent may be detached and replaced

by that for another – halothane or trichloroethylene (Trilene) may be used. Since the wicks in the vaporizing chamber are of metal, and therefore non-absorbent, one agent may be drained out, and after 'rinsing out' the vaporization chamber with a little of the new agent and then discarding it, it may then be filled with the new agent. When the control is turned to '0' (off) the contents will not spill if the vaporizer is accidentally inverted, although during transport it is preferable to empty out the agent. If the control is not turned to '0', the vaporizer should be maintained stationary and upright, in the vertical position, for a few minutes before use, so that any liquid agent that has entered the bypass or the vapour control mechanism may drain back into the sump. Although the OMV is not temperature compensated, it does contain a heat sink, which helps to keep the output concentration relatively stable. Two OMVs are included in the system so that a quick change can be made from one agent to another, and also so that by using both, in series, for halothane or ether, a high enough concentration of those agents may be obtained for induction (as opposed to maintenance) of anaesthesia.

If the patient is apnoeic for any reason, whether arising from collapse or from the anaesthetic technique, IPPV may be instituted by manual compression of the resuscitator bag or by a ventilator, if available. A suitable ventilator is shown in Fig. 30.5; the compPAC (pneuPAC Ltd) is a time-cycled, volume preset, flow generator with a safety pressure limit and may be powered by battery or gas.

MONITORING

In any of the situations discussed that are away from a conventional hospital, consideration must be given to how the patient's condition will be monitored. Ideally the same monitoring equipment should be used as in the modern western anaesthetic operating theatre. However, there are several constraints:

- capital cost;
- power source (mains? battery availability?);
- disposable supplies (electrodes, catheters, transducers);
- maintenance facilities;
- ability of the user to interpret sophisticated results;
- transport of equipment.

Safe emergency anaesthesia can be performed, if necessary, using minimal equipment: stethoscope, sphygmomanometer, eyes on the patient and finger on the pulse. However the patient's safety will increase if more sophisticated equipment is available.

Individual items of monitoring equipment should be chosen bearing in mind how much information is available from each item and whether that information adds to safety or quality of anaesthesia; in remote situations, safety is more important than quality of anaesthesia:

- Pulse oximeter
  heart rate and rhythm (changes in cardiac output)
  arterial blood pressure in conjunction with a sphygmomanometer
- Capnograph
  end-tidal carbon dioxide
  respiratory depression
  respiratory rate
  breathing circuit disconnection
- Electrocardiogram
  heart rate
  heart rhythm
  cardiac ischaemia

ANAESTHESIA AT ABNORMAL AMBIENT PRESSURES

Emergency anaesthesia may have to be administered at low ambient pressure at high altitude or at high ambient pressure in a barochamber. There are considerable changes in physiology and pathophysiology at abnormal ambient pressure; this is not the subject of this section. This section considers only the effects of the change in ambient pressure upon the anaesthetic equipment.

Anaesthetic Equipment at High Altitude

- Low oxygen content of air.
- Anaesthetic and analgesic efficiency of nitrous oxide decreases as altitude increases because of the reduced partial pressure.
- Saturated vapour pressure (SVP) of volatile anaesthetic agents depends upon temperature, not ambient pressure, therefore although the partial pressure of the

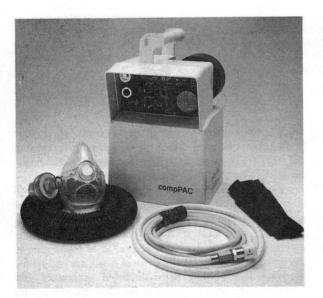

Figure 30.5 compPAC battery/gas-powered emergency rescue, transport and anaesthesia ventilator for military and civilian use. The compPAC is a time-cycled, volume preset flow generator.

agent remains constant for a given vaporizer setting, the *percentage concentration of the agent rises with increase in altitude*. Because all vaporizers are calibrated in per cent, this scale becomes progressively more inaccurate as altitude increases, with a higher percentage emitted than indicated.

- Most gas analysers actually measure the *partial pressure* (the number of molecules) of the gas under test *but are calibrated in per cent* (the proportion of the gas or vapour in the carrier gas) at sea level. Most analysers therefore *under-read* at high altitude if they have been calibrated at sea level.
- The density of any gas decreases with increase in altitude (viscosity changes little with pressure although it is affected by temperature). Variable orifice, constant differential pressure flowmeters are calibrated at 760 mmHg at 20°C. With increase in altitude this type of flowmeter progressively *under-reads* as altitude increases.

Anaesthetic Equipment in the Hyperbaric Environment

- Claustrophobic working environment.
- Usually a *variable pressure* environment.
- Increased risk of fire and explosion.
- The pharmokinetics of *intravenously* administered drugs and local anaesthetics are altered.
- The effect on vaporizers calibrated in volume-percentage is that *less* volatile agent is emitted than is indicated.
- Variable orifice, constant differential pressure flowmeters *over-read*.
- Gas analysers measure partial pressure of gases and are usually calibrated at sea level to indicate volume-percentage and are therefore very unreliable in the hyperbaric environment.
- Blood samples for gas-analysis must be analysed with a machine inside the hyperbaric chamber. If samples are passed through an air-lock to be analysed at normal atmospheric pressure, most of the gases to be measured will bubble out of the sample in the air-lock.
- As rapid changes of ambient pressure may occur, the cuffs of endotracheal tubes should be inflated with water rather than air.

RESTRICTED ARTICLES REGULATIONS

The International Air Transport Association publishes regulations concerning the precautions to be taken when transporting by air the following: flammable gas, oxidizers, corrosives, explosives, poisons, non-flammable compressed gas, flammable liquids and radioactive material. These regulations are accepted throughout most of the world, and are concerned with the labelling, the general packing requirements and the handling and loading of restricted articles. The labels are all diamond shaped, of different colours, and bear both a word and a symbol to denote the danger.

Agents such as trichloroethylene and chloroform may be carried in both passenger and cargo aircraft, but subject to a restriction in quantity; in both cases 40 litres. Halothane, unfortunately, is not as yet mentioned. Ether is not accepted at all in passenger aircraft and a maximum of 40 litres may be carried in cargo aircraft. One litre of ethyl alcohol may be carried in a suitable container in passenger aircraft and up to 40 litres in cargo aircraft. Up to 70 kg of both nitrous oxide and gaseous oxygen may be carried in passenger aircraft and up to 140 kg in cargo aircraft. Liquid oxygen is not acceptable as cargo in any aircraft, in either a non-pressurized or pressurized package. Up to 70 kg of gaseous or liquefied carbon dioxide may be carried in passenger aircraft and up to 140 kg in cargo aircraft; there is no restriction for solid carbon dioxide.

MAINTENANCE OF EQUIPMENT

In some countries there are good standards of equipment and work, but maintenance may be a problem. One of the authors' experiences in an island in the Indian Ocean with a population of less than one million was that the personnel in all categories were well trained. However, problems arose owing to the distance that had to be travelled by service engineers, and so even relatively small matters of maintenance became a problem. It would be difficult to justify the full-time employment of an engineer for just an occasional task, and yet the cost of transporting an engineer by air to perform the work is very expensive. For this reason it is better to avoid complicated and sophisticated equipment such as the larger ventilators, which may need frequent attention and adjustment. Supplies of oxygen and nitrous oxide may be available but very expensive, and consideration should be given to the use of closed, low-flow breathing systems and oxygen concentrators.

When ordering equipment for these areas, consideration should be given to the provision of adequate spares and it may well be deemed advisable to have one of the anaesthetists trained in some of the less-complicated mechanical manipulations required in servicing.

FURTHER READING

Bhimsan NR, Rout CC, Murray WB (1994) Laboratory assessment of a user-assembled oxygen generation kit. *Anaesthesia* 49: 419–421.

Boulton TB (1966) Anaesthesia in difficult situations III. *Anaesthesia* 21: 513–545.

Boulton TB, Cole P (1966) Anaesthesia in difficult situations I, II. *Anaesthesia* 21: 268–276; 379–399.

Dobson M (1988) *Anaesthesia in the District Hospital*. Geneva: World Health Organization.

Dobson M, Peel D, Khallaf N (1996) Field trial of oxygen concentrators in upper Egypt. *Lancet* 347: 1597–1599.

Farman JV (1973) *Anaesthesia and the EMO System*. London: English Universities Press.

Friesen RM (1992) Oxygen concentrators and the practice of anaesthesia. *Canadian Journal of Anaesthesia* 39: R80–R84.

Jowett MD (1984) Anaesthesia ashore in the Falklands. *Annals of the Royal College of Surgeons of England* 66: 197–200.

King MH (ed.) (1986) *Primary Anaesthesia*. Oxford: Oxford University Press.

Pedersen J, Nyrop M (1991) Anaesthetic equipment for a developing country. *British Journal of Anaesthesia* 66: 264–270.

— 31 —

RISK
MANAGEMENT

Contents ━━━━━━━━━━━━━━━━━━━━━━━━━━━━━━━━━━━━━━

INTRODUCTION

Risk is defined in the Oxford English Dictionary as the 'chance of danger, injury, loss etc.' or the 'person or thing causing risk'. *Risk management* in anaesthesia has been defined by Runciman (1993) as: the cost effective reduction of risk to levels perceived to be acceptable to society.

PRINCIPLES OF RISK MANAGEMENT

Risks may be catagorized into three main groups (Secker–Walker 1994):

- those that have a direct impact upon the patient;
- those that have a impact upon the efficiency of patient care;
- health and safety risks related to the carers.

There are five stages in the management of risk (DoH 1994) and these are shown in Fig. 31.1. There needs to be continual awareness that adverse events may occur so that they may be *identified*. This is done by asking:

- what could go wrong?
- how could it happen?
- what would be the effect?

One must also be aware that there may be a combination of causes leading to a risk. The risk having been identified needs to be *analysed and evaluated*:

- how often could it happen?
- what is it likely to cost?
- how severe would the effects be?

The next step is to control the risk if at all possible:

- how can it be eliminated?
- how can it be avoided?
- how can it be made less likely?
- how can it be made less costly?

There are many ways of controlling risk, many of which are cheaply applied, such as:

- *checklists* to make sure that everything is available and functioning properly;
- *interlocks* on equipment so that it must be operated correctly (e.g. hypoxia prevention, one vaporizer at a time in use);
- *protocols* for handling specific situations;
- *training* and, if necessary, certification in the use of equipment or procedures.

Difficult decisions may have to be made when considering the cost of risk management when it is cheaper to pay for damage done to a patient that may be a very rare occurrence, when it is known that this risk could be eliminated entirely if enormous amounts of money were

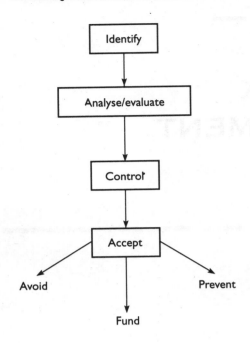

Figure 31.1 Stages in risk management. (Reproduced with permission from the Department of Health (1994).)

poured into the problem. Which is more important: money or patient well-being?

In controlling a risk it is possible to:

- avoid the risk;
- accept the risk and its consequences;
- prevent the risk.

Obviously, if at all possible the risk should be avoided or prevented but if it is impossible or extremely expensive to do this then the risk has to be accepted and funds made available to cover any claims. These funds may be built into the cost of the overall procedure or may be transfered to some form of insurance. The insurers are likely to want to be involved in the risk management procedure.

RISK REDUCTION RELATED TO EQUIPMENT

Risks arising from equipment are related to the following areas:

- equipment must be used only for the purpose for which it was designed;
- it must be designed and built to comply with the relevant International Standards;
- it must be installed by engineers trained by the manufacturers;
- it must be operated only by clinicians who have been trained in its use;
- it must be maintained by trained service engineers at the specified intervals;
- it must be taken out of service when faults occur;
- periodical preventative maintenance is more appropriate than repair of breakdowns.

It should be borne in mind that manufacturers of medical equipment bear a *product liability*, which means that the manufacturer is liable for injury to operator or patient if the injury is due to malfunction of the equipment. However, the manufacturer is liable only if:

- the equipment is being used as in the operating manual;
- the equipment has not been modified in any way;
- installation and maintenance have been carried out as per their instructions by engineers trained by them to do so.

FURTHER READING

DoH (1994) *Risk Management in the NHS*. London: Department of Health.

Runciman WB (1993) Risk assessment in the formulation of anaesthesia safety standards. *European Journal of Anaesthesiology* **10** (suppl 7): 26–32.

Secker-Walker J (1994) Quality and management of risk. In: *Quality and Safety in Anaesthesia*. London: BMJ Publishing Group.

Appendix I
Directory of Manufacturers

Abbott Laboratories Ltd, Hospital Products Division, Abbott House, Norden Road, Maidenhead, Berkshire SL6 4XE, UK. Tel: 01628–773355; Fax 01628–644305.

Actamed Ltd, Trinity House, Borough Road, Wakefield WF1 3AZ, UK. Tel: 01924–200550; Fax 01924–200518.

Advanced Medical Devices, Mantra House, Keighley, West Yorkshire BD21 1SX, UK. Tel: 01535–610078; Fax 01535–608028.

Ambu International (UK) Ltd, Charlton Road, Midsomer Norton, Bath BA3 4DR, UK. Tel: 01761–416868; Fax 01761–419429.

or **Ambu International A/S,** Sondre Ringvej 49, PO Box 215, DK 2600, Denmark. Tel: +45 43 63 01 11.

AVL Medical Instruments UK Ltd, Unit 24, Whitebridge Industrial Estate, Whitebridge Lane, Stone, Staffordshire ST15 8LQ, UK. Tel: 01785–815987; Fax 01785–816863.

B Braun Medical Ltd, Braun House, Aylesbury Vale Industrial Park, Stocklake, Aylesbury, Buckinghamshire HP20 1DQ, UK. Tel: 01296–393900; Fax 01296–435714.

Baxter Healthcare Ltd, Wallingford Road, Compton, Newbury, Berkshire RG16 0QW, UK. Tel: 01635–200020; Fax 01635–578800.

Becton Dickinson, Between Towns Road, Cowley, Oxford OX4 3LY, UK. Tel: 01865–748844; Fax 01865–781503.

Biomedical Sensors Ltd, PO Box 88, 5 Manor Court Yard, Hughendon Avenue, High Wycombe, Buckinghamshire HP13 5RE, UK. Tel: 01494–446651; Fax 01494–534489.

Bird Products, 8 Lansdown Place, Lansdown Road, Cheltenham, Gloucestershire GL50 2HU, UK. Tel: 01242 250818.

or **Bird Products Corporation,** 3101 East Alejo Road, Palm Springs, CA 92262, USA. Tel: +1 619 778 7200.

Blease, Deansway, Chesham, Buckinghamshire HP5 2NX, UK. Tel: 01494–784422; Fax 01494–791497.

Brüel & Kjaer, Harrow Weald Lodge, 92 Uxbridge Road, Harrow, Middlesex HA3 6BZ, UK. Tel: 0181–954 2366; Fax 0181–954 9504

Cardiac Recorders International Plc, Unit 2, Watermill Business Centre, Edison Road, Millmarsh Lane, Enfield, London EN3 7XF, UK. Tel: 0181–364 7000; Fax 0181–364 7716.

Cardiokinetics Ltd, 2 Kansas Avenue, Salford M5 2GL, UK. Tel: 0161–872 8287; Fax 0161–848 7916.

Central Medical Supplies Ltd, CMS House, Town Yard Ind. Estate, Station Street, Leek, Staffordshire ST13 8BP, UK. Tel: 01538–399541; Fax 01538–399572.

Childerhouse Medical (Division CDL), 310A Upper Richmond Road West, East Sheen, London SW14 7JN, UK. Tel: 0181–876 6040; Fax 0181–876 4078.

CIBA Corning Diagnostics Ltd, Colchester Road, Halstead, Essex CO9 2DX, UK. Tel: 01787–472461; Fax 01787–475088.

Cory Brothers Ltd, 6 Bittacy Business Centre, Bittay Hill, London NW7 1BA, UK. Tel: 0181–349 1081; Fax 0181–349 1962.

Critikon, The Braccans, London Road, Bracknell, Berkshire RG12 2AT, UK. Tel: 01344–871000; Fax 01344–872599.

Datascope Medical Co Ltd, Lakeview Court, Ermine Business Park, Huntingdon, Cambs PE18 6XR, UK. Tel: 01480–433477; Fax 01480–434051.

or **Datascope Corporation,** 580 Winters Avenue, PO Box 5, Paramus, New Jersey, 07653–005, USA. Tel: +1 201 265 8800.

Dräger Medical Ltd, The Willows, Mark Road, Hemel Hempstead, Hertfordshire HP2 7BW, UK. Tel: 01442–213542; Fax 01442–240327.

or **Drägerwerk,** Aktiengesellschaft, Postfach 1339,

Moislinger Allee 53–55, D-2400 Lübeck 1, Germany. Tel: +49 451 8820.

or **North American Dräger**, 148B Quarry Road, Telford, PA 18969, USA. Tel: +1 215 723 9824.

East Healthcare Ltd, Sandy Lane West, Littlemore, Oxford OX4 5JT, UK. Tel: 01865–714242; Fax 01865–747249.

EME Tricomed Ltd, 17 Bristol Gardens, Brighton, Sussex BN2 5JR, UK. Tel: 01273–609101; Fax 01273–694254.

Engström, Gambro Ltd, Lundia House, 124 Station Road, Sidcup, Kent DA15 7AS, UK Tel: 0181–309 7800.

or **Gambro Engström**, AB, Box 20109, S-161 20 Bromma, Sweden. Tel: +46 8 98 82 80.

Eschmann, Peter Road, Lancing, West Sussex BN15 8TJ, UK. Tel: 01903–761122.

Ferraris Medical Ltd, 26 Lea Valley Trading Estate, Angel Road, Edmonton, London N18 3JD, UK. Tel: 0181–807 3636; Fax 0181–807 4886.

Graseby Medical Ltd, Colonial Way, Watford WD2 4LG, UK. Tel: 01923–246434; Fax 01923–231595.

Hawksley and Sons Ltd, Marlborough Road, Lancing, West Sussex BN15 8TN, UK. Tel 01903–752815; Fax 01903–766050.

Hellige (UK) Ltd, 8 Weller Drive, Hogwood Lane Industrial Estate, Finchampstead, Berkshire RG11 4QW, UK. Tel: 01734–733844; Fax 01734–730254.

Henleys Medical Supplies Ltd, Brownfields, Welwyn Garden City, Hertfordshire AL7 1AN, UK. Tel: 01707–333164; Fax 01707–334795.

Hewlett-Packard Ltd, Amen Corner, Cain Road, Bracknell, Berkshire RG12 1HN, UK. Tel: 01344–363344.

or **Hewlett-Packard Company**, 3000 Hanover Street, Palo Alto, CA 94304, USA. Tel: +1 415 857 1501.

HG Wallace Ltd, Commerce Way, Colchester, Essex CO2 8HH, UK. Tel: 01206–792800; Fax 01206–798434.

Huntleigh Nesbit Evans Healthcare, 310–312 Dallow Road, Luton, Bedfordshire LU1 1SS, UK. Tel: 01582–413104; Fax 01582–459100.

Instrumentation Laboratory (UK) Ltd, Kelvin Close, Birchwood, Warrington, Cheshire WA3 7PB, UK. Tel: 01925–810141 (ext. 224); Fax 01925–826708.

Ivac, Intec 2 Building, Wade Road, Basingstoke, Hampshire RG24 0NE, UK. Tel: 01256–474455; Fax 01256–463770.

KeyMed, KeyMed House, Stock Road, Southend-on-Sea, Essex SS2 5QH, UK. Tel: 01702–616333; Fax 01702–465677.

Kontron Instruments Ltd, Blackmoor Lane, Croxley Centre, Watford, Hertfordshire WD1 8XQ, UK. Tel: 01923–245991; Fax 01923–220666.

Laerdal, Laerdal House, Goodmead Road, Orpington, Kent BR6 0XH, UK. Tel: 01689–876634; Fax 01689–873800.

or **Asmund S. Laerdal**, PO Box 377, N-4001 Stavanger, Norway. Tel: +47 4 511 700.

McKesson Equipment Company (of Great Britain), Tradent House, Park Road, Chesterfield, S40 2JX, UK. Tel: 01246–276111; Fax: 01246–230825.

Mallinckrodt Medical (UK) Ltd, 11 North Portway Close, Round Spinney, Northampton NN3 4RQ, UK. Tel: 01604–646132; Fax 01604–646884.

or **Mallinckrodt Medical Incorporated**, 675 McDonnell Boulevard, PO Box 5840, St Louis, MO 63134, USA. Tel: +1 314 895 2000.

Marquette Electronics (GB) Ltd, Unit 7, Priestley Road, Worsley, Manchester M28 5NJ, UK. Tel: 0161–794 8114; Fax 0161–794 6295.

Medex Medical Inc, St Crispin Way, Haslingden, Rossendale, Lancashire BB4 4PW, UK. Tel: 01706–212236; Fax 01706–218834.

Ohmeda, Ohmeda House, 71 Great North Road, Hatfield, Hertfordshire AL9 5EN, UK. Tel: 01707–263570; Fax 01707–260065.

Olympus Optical Company Ltd, 1–22–2 San-ei, Building, Nishi Shinjuka, Shinjuka, Tokyo, Japan. Tel: +81 340 2111.

Pall Biomedical, A division of Pall Europe Limited, Europa House, Havant Street, Portsmouth PO1 9PD, UK. Tel: 01705–303303; Fax 01705–302505.

Penlon Ltd, Radley Road, Abingdon, Oxon OX14 3PH, UK. Tel: 01235–554222; Fax 01235–555252.

Physio-Control UK, Intec 2, Units 10–20, Wade Road, Basingstoke, Hampshire RG24 0NE, UK. Tel: 01256–474455; Fax 01256–463770.

or **Physio Control Corporate Headquarters**, 11811 Willow Road North East, PO Box 97006, Washington 98073–9706, USA. Tel: +1 206 867 4000.

Pneupac Ltd, Crescent Road, Luton, Bedfordshire LU2 0AH, UK. Tel: 01582–453303; Fax 01582–453103.

Portex Ltd, Hythe, Kent CT21 6JL, UK. Tel: 01303–260551; Fax 01303–266761.

or **Concord/Portex**, 15 Kit Streett, Keene, New Hampshire 03431, USA. Tel: +1 603 352 3812.

Puritan-Bennett, Unit 1, Heathrow Causeway Estate, 152–176 Great South West Road, Hounslow, Middlesex TW4 6JS, UK. Tel: 0181–577 1870; Fax 0181–577 7762.

or **Puritan-Bennett International Corporation**, 9401 Indian-Creek Parkway, PO Box 25905 Overland Park, Kansas 66225, USA. Tel: +1 913 661 0444.

Radiometer Ltd, Manor Court, Manor Royal, Crawley, West Sussex RH10 2PY, UK. Tel: 01293–517599; Fax 01293–531597.

Rimer-Alco Ltd, Dumballs Road, Cardiff CF1 6JE, UK. Tel: 01222–378421.

or **Rimer-Alco North America Ltd**, 15 Jefferson Street, Box 749 Morden, Manitoba, Canada, R0G 1J0. Tel: +1 204 822 6595.

Rocket of London Ltd, Imperial Way, Watford, Hertfordshire WD2 4XX, UK. Tel: 01923–239791; Fax 01923–230212.

Rotameter Ltd, KDG-Mobray Ltd, Crompton Way, Crawley, West Sussex RH10 2YZ, UK. Tel: 01293–525151.

Rusch UK Ltd, PO Box 138, Halifax Road, Cressex Industrial Estate, High Wycombe, Buckinghamshire HP12 3NB, UK. Tel: 01494–532761; Fax 01494–524650.

or **Willy Rusch AG**, Strasse 4–10, Postfach 1633, D-7050 Waiblingen, Germany. Tel: +49 71514060.

or **Rusch Inc.**, 2450 Meadowbrook Parkway, Duluth, GA 30136, USA. Tel: +1 404 623 0816.

S&W Vickers Ltd, Ruxley Corner, Sidcup, Kent DA14 5BL, UK. Tel: 0181–309 0433; Fax 0181–309 0919.

Servomex Plc, Crowborough, Sussex TN6 3DU, UK. Tel. 01892–652181; Fax 01892–662253.

Siemens Plc Medical Engineering, Siemens House, Oldbury, Bracknell, Berkshire RG12 8FZ, UK. Tel: 01344–396421; Fax 01344–396496.

or **Siemens Aktiengesellschaft**, Bereich Medizinische Technik, Henkestrasse 127, Postfach 3260, D-8520 Erlangen, Germany. Tel: +49 91 31 840.

3M Health Care Ltd, 3M House, Morley Street, Loughborough, Leicestershire LE11 1EP, UK. Tel: 01509–611611.

or **3M Inc**, 3M Center, St Paul, MN 55144–1000, USA. Tel: +1 612 733 1110.

Tricomed Ltd, Unit 2, Chiltonian Industrial Estate, Manor Lane, London SE12 0TX, UK. Tel: 0181–463 0933.

VA Howe & Co Ltd, Beaumont Close, Banbury, Oxon OX16 7RG, UK. Tel: 01295–252600/252666 (customer support); Fax 01295–268096.

Viggo-Spectramed, Faraday Road, Dorcan, Swindon, Wiltshire SN3 5HZ, UK. Tel: 01793–430388; Fax 01793–430031.

Vitalograph Ltd, Maids Moreton House, Buckingham MK18 1SW, UK. Tel: 01280–822811; Fax 01280–823302.

Vygon (UK) Ltd, Bridge Road, Cirencester, Gloucestershire GL7 1PT, UK. Tel: 01285–657051; Fax 01285–650293.

Weatherall Equipment & Instruments Ltd, PO Box 69, Tring, Hertfordshire HP23 6PL, UK. Tel: 01494–758110; Fax 01494–758014.

or **Riken Keiki Fine Instrument Co. Ltd**, 2–7–6 Azusawa, Itabashi-ku, Tokyo, Japan. Tel: +03 966 1111.

Appendix II
SI Units and Table of Conversions

Although SI units (Système International d'Unités) have been adopted for scientific purposes, they are not yet universally used in anaesthetic practice. As many pieces of anaesthetic and oxygen therapy apparatus will survive for many years, the older units in which they are calibrated have been retained throughout this book.

SI UNITS

The SI units applicable to anaesthesia are as follows:

Function	SI Unit
Mass	kilogram (kg)
Length	metre (m)
Force	newton (N) – accelerates a mass of 1 kg by 1 m/s² (1 N = 10⁵ dynes)
Pressure	pascal (Pa) = 1 N/m² (NB 1 bar = 10⁵ Pa)
Energy	joule (J) – force of 1 newton acting through 1 metre (1 J = 10⁷ ergs)
Power	watt (W) = 1 J/s
Temperature	kelvin (K) = °C (0 K = −273°C)
Frequency	hertz (Hz) = 1 cycle/s
Capacity	litre (l)

TABLE OF CONVERSIONS

1 metre	=	1.0936 yards = 3.2808 feet = 39.3696 inches
1 kilogram	=	2.2046 pounds = 35.2736 ounces
1 litre	=	0.22 (imperial) gallons = 1.76 pints
	=	35.2 fluid ounces
	=	0.27 US gallons
1 kilopascal	=	0.146 psi
[1 mmHg	=	1.36 cmH₂O = 133.3 N/m² = 0.0194 psi]
1 joule	=	10⁷ ergs = 0.239 calories
0 kelvin (K)	=	−273° Celsius ('absolute zero')
273.15K	=	0°C = 32°F
373.16K	=	100°C = 212°F
°C	=	(°F −32) × 5/9
°F	=	(°C × 9/5) + 32

APPENDIX III
STANDARDS

BS 1319: 1976≡ISO/R32, ISO 407
Specification for medical gas cylinders, valves and yoke connections

BS 1319C: 1976
Colours for the identification of the contents of medical gas cylinders

BS 3353: 1987≡ISO 5262: 1986
Specification for anaesthetic reservoir bags

BS 3487: Part 1: 1989≡ISO 5361–1
Tracheal tubes. Specification for all types of tubes

BS 3487: Part 2: 1993≡ISO 5361–2: 1993
Tracheal tubes. Oro-tracheal and naso-tracheal tubes of the Magill type (plain and cuffed)

BS 3487: Part 3: 1986 (1992)≡ISO 5361–3: 1984
Tracheal tubes. Specification for tubes of the Murphy type

BS 3487: Part 4: 1988 (1993)≡ISO 5361–4
Tracheal tubes. Specification for tubes of the Cole type

BS 3487: Part 5: 1986 (1991)≡ISO 5361–5: 1984
Tracheal tubes. Specification and methods of test for tube collapse and cuff herniation

BS 3849: Part 1: 1988 (1993)≡ISO 5356–1
Conical connectors for anaesthetic and respiratory equipment. Specification for cones and sockets (excluding 8.5 mm size)

BS 3849: Part 2: 1988 (1993)≡ISO 5356–2
Conical connectors for anaesthetic and respiratory equipment. Specification for screw-threaded weight-bearing connectors

BS 3849: Part 4: 1990 (1993)
Conical connectors for anaesthetic and respiratory equipment. Specification for 8.5 mm cones and sockets

BS 4272: Part 1: 1968
Specification for anaesthetic and analgesic machines. Anaesthetic machines of the on-demand type supplied with nitrous oxide and oxygen from separate containers

BS 4272: Part 2: 1996
Anaesthetic and analgesic machines. Specification for intermittent (demand) flow analgesic machines for use with 50/50% (V/V) nitrous oxide and oxygen

BS 4272: Part 3: 1989 Similar to ISO 5358
Anaesthetic and analgesic machines. Specification for continuous flow anaesthetic machines

BS 5682: 1984 (1992) Similar to ISO 5359
Specification for terminal units, hose assemblies and their connectors for use with medical gas pipeline systems

BS 5724: Part 2: Section 2.4: 1985 (1994)≡IEC 601–2–4: 1993
Medical electrical equipment. Particular requirements for safety. Specification for cardiac defibrillators and cardiac defibrillator-monitors

BS 5724: Part 2: Section 2.10: 1988≡IEC 601–2–10: 1987
Medical electrical equipment. Particular requirements for safety. Specification for nerve and muscle stimulators

BS 5724: Part 2: Section 2.12: 1990≡IEC 601–2–12: 1988
Medical electrical equipment. Particular requirements for safety. Specification for lung ventilators

BS 5724: Part 2: Section 2.13: 1990≡IEC 601–2–13: 1989
Medical electrical equipment. Particular requirements for safety. Specification for anaesthetic machines

BS 5724: Part 2: Section 2.23: 1989≡ISO 8359: 1988
Medical electrical equipment. Particular requirements for safety. Specification for oxygen concentrators

BS 5724: Part 2: Section 2.24: 1989≡ISO 8185
Medical electrical equipment. Particular requirements for safety. Specification for humidifiers

BS 5724: Part 2: Section 2.27: 1989≡ISO 7767: 1988
Medical electrical equipment. Particular requirements for safety. Specification for oxygen analysers for monitoring patient breathing mixtures

BS 5724: Part 3: Section 3.12: 1991
Medical electrical equipment. Particular requirements for performance. Method of declaring parameters for lung ventilators

BS 6149: Part 1: 1987 (1992)≡ISO 5366/1: 1986
Tracheostomy tubes. Specification for connectors

BS 6149: Part 2: 1993≡ISO 5366/2: 1993
Tracheostomy tubes. Basic requirements for tubes for adults

BS 6151: 1992≡ISO 5367: 1991
Specification for breathing tubes for use with anaesthetic apparatus and ventilators

BS 6546: 1994≡ISO 7228: 1993
Specification for tracheal tube connectors

BS 6834: 1987 (1992)
Specification for active anaesthetic gas scavenging systems

BS 6850: 1987 (1992) Similar to ISO 8382
Specification for ventilatory resuscitators

BS 7143: 1989
Specification for catheter mounds (flexible adaptors) for use with medical breathing systems

BS 7634: 1993≡ISO 10083: 1992
Specification for oxygen concentrators for use with medical gas pipeline systems

BS 7711: Part 1: 1994
Respiratory therapy equipment. Specification for tubing and connectors

BS 7711: Part 2: 1994
Respiratory therapy equipment. Specification for air entrainment devices

BS 7711: Part 3: 1994
Respiratory therapy equipment. Specification for gas-powered nebulizers for the delivery of drugs

BS 7734: 1994≡ISO 8835–2: 1993
Specification for anaesthetic circle breathing systems

BS ISO 11195: 1995
Gas mixers for medical use. Stand-alone gas mixers

BS EN 475: 1995≡EN 475: 1995 and Similar to ISO 9703–1: 1992 and ISO 9703–2: 1994
Medical devices. Electrically-generated alarm signals

BS EN 540: 1993 EN 540: 1993
Clinical investigation of medical devices for human subjects

BS EN 1281–2: 1996
Anaesthetic and respiratory equipment. Conical connectors. Screw-threaded, weight-bearing connectors

BS EN 60601–2–2: 1993≡EN 60601–2–2: 1993 and IEC 601–2–2: 1991
Medical electrical equipment. Particular requirements for safety. Specification for high frequency surgical equipment

APPENDIX IV
CHECKLIST FOR ANAESTHETIC APPARATUS

Reproduced from *Checklist for Anaesthetic Machines: A Recommended Procedure Based on the Use of an Oxygen Analyser* (1997) with permission of the Association of Anaesthetists of Great Britain and Ireland, London.

The following checks should be made prior to each operating session.

1. **Check that the anaesthetic machine is connected to the electricity supply (if appropriate) and switched on.**

- Take note of any information or labelling on the anaesthetic machine referring to the current status of the machine. Particular attention should be paid to recent servicing. Servicing labels should be fixed in the service logbook.

2. **Check that an oxygen analyser is present on the anaesthetic machine.**

- Ensure that the analyser is switched on, checked and calibrated.
- The oxygen sensor should be placed where it can monitor the composition of the gases leaving the common gas outlet.

3. **Identify and take note of the gases which are being supplied by pipeline, confirming with a 'tug-test' that each pipeline is correctly inserted into the appropriate gas supply terminal.**
   Note: Carbon dioxide cylinders should not be present on the anaesthetic machine unless requested by the anaesthetist. A blanking plug should be fitted to any empty cylinder yoke.

- Check that the anaesthetic machine is connected to a supply of oxygen and that an adequate supply of oxygen is available from a reserve oxygen cylinder.
- Check that adequate supplies of other gases (nitrous oxide, air) are available and connected as appropriate.

- Check that all pipeline pressure gauges in use on the anaesthetic machine indicate 400 kPa.

4. **Check the operation of flowmeters.**

- Ensure that each flow control valve operates smoothly and that the bobbin moves freely throughout its range.
- Check the operation of the emergency oxygen bypass control.

5. **Check the vaporizer(s):**

- Ensure that each vaporizer is adequately but not over filled.
- Ensure that each vaporizer is correctly seated on the back bar and not tilted.

  Check the vaporizer for leaks (*with vaporizer on and off*) by temporarily occluding the common gas outlet. When checks have been completed turn the vaporizer(s) off.
  A leak test should be performed immediately after changing any vaporizer.

6. **Check the breathing system to be employed.**

- The system should be visually inspected for correct configuration. All connections should be secured by 'push and twist'.
- A pressure leak test should be performed on the breathing system by occluding the patient port and compressing the reservoir bag.

- The correct operation of unidirectional valves should be carefully checked.

7. **Check that the ventilator is configured appropriately for its intended use.**

- Ensure that the ventilator tubing is correctly configured and securely attached.
- Set the controls for use and ensure that an adequate pressure is generated during the inspiratory phase.
- Check that the pressure relief valve functions.
- Check that the disconnect alarm functions correctly.
- Ensure that an alternative means to ventilate the patient's lungs is available.

8. **Check that the anaesthetic gas scavenging system is switched on and is functioning correctly.**

- Ensure that the tubing is attached to the appropriate expiratory port(s) of the breathing system or ventilator.

9. **Check that all ancillary equipment which may be needed is present and working.**

- This includes laryngoscopes, intubation aids, intubation forceps, bougies etc. and appropriately sized facemasks, airways, tracheal tubes and connectors.
- Check that the suction apparatus is functioning and that all connections are secure.
- Check that the patient can be tilted head-down on the trolley, operating table or bed.

10. **Ensure that the appropriate monitoring equipment is present, switched on and calibrated ready for use.**

- Set all default alarm limits as appropriate. (It may be necessary to place the monitors in the stand-by mode to avoid unnecessary alarms before being connected to the patient.)

INDEX

Page numbers in **bold** indicate tables; numbers in *italics* indicate illustrations